Reduce Your Healthcare Costs
through
Natural Medicine

ISBN-13: 978-0-9819478-6-0

To buy more copies of this book,
or to contact Guy go to **myoptimalhealthcare.com**

This book is printed on recycled paper

Printed in the United States of America

Reduce Your Healthcare Costs through Natural Medicine

By

Guy Daniels, M.S., M.H.

Dedication

This book is dedicated to my two wonderful boys
whom I cherish with all my heart.

Acknowledgements

Recognition must clearly been given to the many ethical, passionate, and competent researchers and practitioners in the fields of nutrition, biochemistry, and medicine who have over the years, sometimes under adversity, advanced our knowledge and understanding of the human body to this point in time where we are on the verge of amazing things, despite the head-winds of corruption.

Table of Contents

Introduction

Americans are moving to natural medicine in record numbers, and the goal of this book is to help you in that endeavor. Patients are tired of being sick. They are tired of being told that their symptoms are in their head when a doctor can't come up with a unifying diagnosis in the few minutes allotted to them. Many patients have seen multiple doctors in an attempt to get well, and after years of frustration and expense, are no better off, and perhaps worse. Patients are finally questioning their doctor's word, and are slowly becoming advocates for their own care. In this time of fiscal irresponsibility, deception, internet access, and greed, patients are beginning to take matters into their own hands, as well they should.

Although mostly corrupt, our federal government grasps the financial aspects of our ill-health. In an op-ed article written by Senator Tom Harkin during the healthcare debate (as if it has ended) he wrote, "…we currently do not have a healthcare system in the United States, we have a sick care system. We spend twice as much per capita on healthcare as European countries, but we are twice as sick with chronic disease. The problem is that we have systemically neglected wellness and disease prevention." He went on to cite from Dean Ornish's testimony before the Senate health committee: "Studies have shown that changing [one's] lifestyle could prevent at least 90% of all heart disease."

The question is: "Whose advice do you heed?" There are many large companies with money at stake. Some authorities tell you one thing, while others say the opposite. You, the average consumer, with all of the other aspects of life in balance, require an honest broker in the most important aspect of life itself, your health. There are facets of natural medicine unknown to you, which may help diminish the negative effects of stress, toxins, adulterated foods, genetic flaws, and other issues that impact our health.

I wrote this to empower you as the biggest advocate and practitioner in your family's healthcare. I provide extensive clinical data to support the use of natural medicine, and to help guide you in your endeavors to save

1

money, time, and frustration. So let's take a step back and take some bearings.

The type of medicine we are accustomed to here in America is modern/western/conventional/allopathic medicine, which will simply be referred to as modern or conventional medicine. You know it well. Natural medicine is a bit more complex to define. Natural medicine will use conventional and non-conventional diagnostics, nutrition, exercise, and supplements based on the biochemistry of the human genome to better your health. Natural medicine has many uses, but in fairness, modern medicine does as well, and using the best of both worlds together is what's referred to as integrative medicine. We will not look into yoga, spirituality, biofeedback, hypnosis, bodywork, homeopathy, and chiropractic medicine, all of which fall under the umbrella of alternative medicine. The focus of this book is on hard science known to us in nutrition, biochemistry, and supplements.

Unlike many other books on the shelf that try to sell you some miracle at the expense of your money, I will provide honest and well researched data, and supply both sides of an argument when applicable. I will mention no products or companies by name. I find that adults can't be told to do something like a child can, but value must be shown, and only then can an independent decision be made. I will try to show you value through data and reason. As you probably already know, researchers often don't agree, which is why you are so confused about what to eat, what to take, and what to do. I will do my best to clarify this confusion for you. There are enormous sums of money at stake here in the "healthcare game". Companies pushing foods, drugs, insurance, healthcare, supplements, and more have both mutual and conflicting interests. You, the consumer, are left to fend for yourself, trying to distill fact from fiction, doing the best you can for your own health.

I am excited to bring you some amazing information, some of which may be familiar, but most you've likely never seen before. Many of the topics are highly debatable, but I bring you cutting edge research and opinions, not from someone with questionable motives, but from someone with a vested interest in doing the right thing. I am passionate about natural medicine, because it has helped to save me, and it can

2

potentially do the same for you or a loved one. I have compiled some of the most interesting topics from 25 years of research. Within each chapter I'll support controversial statements with data, turning upside-down much of what you've heard about health.

There are several central aspects to this book, one of which is to inspire you to become the primary caregiver in your own healthcare. The days of the "doctor knows all" are rapidly disappearing. The way medicine is conducted these days leaves you to fulfill your own needs. Patients cannot walk into the practitioner's office expecting a crystal ball diagnosis and some Rx "magic in a bottle". Nor should we expect to buy a bottle of supplements expecting a miracle either. You are an active participant in this process, and the process may be longer and more challenging than you'd like. Those can be the facts, and I won't mislead you.

Natural medicine is very tricky business. There is still so much we do not know about the human body. Amazingly, we do know a good bit, but it's buried in research that doesn't often see the light of day, and thus practitioners are not working with all the information. Historical perceptions, money, power, and marketing can sway many a mind. This is why many patients, conventional doctors, and even practitioners in natural medicine are looking for answers. Consider the data presented, and with independence of thought, make up your own mind. Don't be a lemming.

This book will not provide all answers to all conditions, but will show you the power of natural medicine, nutrition, and non-conventional diagnostics through multiple common examples that may pertain to you. As a proponent and critic of natural medicine, I'll help highlight some of the pitfalls within the profession as well. On the one hand, there are some talented practitioners out there doing wonderful things with natural medicine in autism, gastrointestinal disorders, and much more. However, there are many highly questionable ones as well. How do you get to the right provider, and avoid quackery and greed, so you don't waste time and money? Have you been given guarantees when it comes to your health? If so, do they back it up with their wallet? I doubt it. They usually back it up with yours. So, whether you're considering a first visit to a natural practitioner, or a frustrating one-more-last-chance visit, this book may help. Although practitioners may hang a shingle that says "natural medicine", it doesn't mean they know what they're doing. In your life, you've interacted with many people who have a given title or degree, but you've found that it doesn't mean they are any good at what they profess. Healthcare providers are human like the rest of us. Some are better at what they do, and some take their job more seriously than others.

On a different level, there is a love-hate battle going on between conventional and natural medicine. We all read the articles bashing supplements and/or natural medicine, and yet people know there's "something to it", and display that with their wallets. Conventional doctors will often dismiss natural medicine, although they know next to nothing about it. What they also don't know is that big-pharma and big business are very much in bed with natural medicine. For example, have you heard of Lovaza, formerly Omacor? It's a fish oil. It may be prescription, but it's still a fish oil. The company that owns Lovaza, Reliant Pharmaceuticals Inc, had the "ability" to get it passed as a prescription item, which is thus conveniently covered by Medicare. Do you want another example? Perhaps you've heard of Resveratrol. A Harvard researcher was able to increase the life span of mice using this interesting polyphenol from the skin of red grapes. He co-founded a company named Sirtris, based on a resveratrol proprietary formulation and sold it to GlaxoSmithKline for $720 million. It's currently in phase 2 trials for diabetes. How about another? Have you heard of Folate? Of course you have. It's a B vitamin. There is more than one form of folate available in the market. You can buy folic acid, which is less expensive and widely utilized, or you can also buy a product known as 5-MTHF, or "active" folate. There is only one source for 5-MTHF, and it's pricey. Guess who owns it? Merck of Germany. "Big Pharma" sees the potential healing in natural medicine, and all the money the public spends on supplements doesn't go unnoticed. If big-pharma is on board, maybe it's time for those of you who view big pharma as the solution to get on board too.

Chapter 1   Our Current Healthcare Model

The current healthcare system in this country is mostly broken, and it's almost everyone's fault. Patients want instant solutions in their busy lives. Providers have less time to be practitioners, and can't be an expert in everything. HMO's struggle to balance the needs of their subscribers, the needs of the providers, and the survivability of the organization. Hospitals take all-comers, and if the percent of uninsured is too high they may not survive. Employers work to provide medical benefits at an affordable cost that doesn't compromise the bottom line. Pharmaceutical companies spend exorbitant sums of money to try to bring a product to market, but when they do they make out like bandits. The success of big-pharma and the state of ill-health of our nation can be measured by the fact that many street intersections in America have one or more pharmacies open for business. Let me try to give you an example of our modern paradigm of medicine. It should sound familiar to you.

Mrs. Jones eats the standard American diet, which consists mostly of highly processed denatured foods such as white flour, simple sugars, fried foods, lots of dairy, high saturated fat, with one of many other bonuses heaped on top. She essentially never exercises, especially intensely, has a busy and fairly stressful life, doesn't get enough sleep, nor enough sunlight. She likely has some type of nutritional deficiency like many others. She has put on some extra weight as a result, may smoke or drink, and lacks energy. Like many other Americans she gets medical coverage through her employer, which goes up every year in cost. It may be the deduction from the paycheck that goes up, it may be the annual deductable that must first be met, it may be copays, it may be all of the above.

She isn't feeling well, and goes to the doctor complaining of symptoms that have been nagging for some time. She was hoping they'd go away, but they haven't quite done so. As a part of the current healthcare model the provider has on average about 7-9 minutes to spend with her. If the doctor is in a group practice, this time is likely mandated to keep up with productivity. She reveals the symptoms in a few minutes while the doctor takes notes. The routine check-up is done and the doctor is left with making a quick educated guess. He writes a prescription to treat the symptoms and informs Mrs. Jones that if the drug doesn't work she should come back in a month for a different one.

After departing the doctor's office, the physician is racing around like a crazy person as well. The individual wants, needs, and concerns of Mrs. Jones are gone and replaced by those of others. He has ceased to give thought to her, as he has others waiting for his attention. Like the patient, the life of the provider is no less stressful. He went to school for many years, and is now wondering *why* on occasion. Four years of pre-med, four years of med-school, and as a PCP he probably had 1-3 years of residency. Ten years of school and the doctor is practicing assembly-line medicine and not getting paid as well as he probably should. If the doctor is on staff, then he's likely salaried, which is enough to survive to pay the bills, which include extensive college loans. If the doctor owns the practice (group or individual) he may be older, in which case he may have made some money before things really got bad, but now has to work hard to stay above water. In either event, the HMOs are killing the practice. The reimbursements from the HMOs go down every year, while the cost of insurance goes up from mostly ridiculous litigation. The doctor has to hire a series of staff members just to chase down the HMOs to get paid. This extra staff comes at a cost, of course. Reimbursements from the state Medicaid is not any better, and could be worse.

Mrs. Jones takes the medication for a week and begins to notice an improvement in symptoms, which will likely be temporary. Likely, neither the patient nor the provider has addressed the underlying cause for the disease; they have simply alleviated the symptoms. The symptoms are the way the body tells the brain that something isn't quite right. It's the brain's job to give it some thought and propose some solutions. But we have relegated that role to the doctor, whom we trust to know all. Of course the doctor is human too. The doctor can't know all. There are too many drugs, too many conditions, and too many symptoms that could be attributed to more than one condition. The doctors do the best they can in the time allotted to make you happy. Why? Because you're the customer.

That's right, you're the customer. If the practice loses you, they'll lose that little bit of income. They need to keep you, because the model of business is volume, given the low reimbursement rates. Volume is king, since cash is king, and without you, there's no volume. This makes you the king. As Mel Brooks said, "It's good to be the king." So the doctor does the best quick thing they can unless the cause is obvious. You are given a drug to alleviate your symptoms. You feel better, and you think the doctor is a miracle worker.

You know how the rest of the story unfolds. There are multiple doctor visits for other opinions. You get lab-work done, maybe take more drugs, endure possible side effects, and hear different diagnoses. In the end, you may settle on one diagnosis with its applicable drug regimen. It is human nature to want to have our illnesses labeled. Without a "diagnosis" you might be considered weak or a complainer. You probably need a diagnosis for legal reasons as well. Although your symptoms are very real to you, you might even be told, "It's all in your head," and get some catch-all diagnosis like chronic fatigue/fibromyalgia, or none at all. Your symptoms are real, regardless of your condition, and so we all have to have a diagnosis to validate them.

In any event, you now have a name to your complaint, so now you can share your misery with others, because now it's legitimate. Unfortunately, these diagnoses can become a crutch for many. Instead of working or doing something fun, you tell the world, "I can't do it because I have condition X." I'm sure you've heard someone say that, or you've said it yourself. This is at the root of the problem. You must find the underlying cause, and at the very least attempt to resolve it; otherwise, your option is to let it take over your life. Do not let your disease state rule your life, as I have so often seen. If your provider has failed you, seek another more competent one. It's not in your head. There is a biochemical explanation for what's happening inside your body. It's no coincidence that so many people are sick with chronic degenerative diseases at this moment in time.

With all this in mind, more people are turning to natural medicine as a solution. Americans don't know much about natural medicine, because that is not how most of us were raised, and our parents before us. The old philosophy of "the doctor is always right" is slowly disappearing and turning into "the doctor isn't helping." My hope is that you'll be empowered to be the biggest advocate and most energetic provider of your own health care. I frequently see and hear of patients who have not been helped by many providers in modern medicine, and seek out natural medicine as a last hope. They may have heard of others who got better, come across an article, or simply stumbled upon it.

With this new move to natural medicine, what happens next? Some patients may venture into a health food store and purchase for the least amount of money possible, supplements that may be questionable in quality and dose. The customer most often cannot rely on the store employees for professional advice, and so, often the remedy will not work to the satisfaction of the customer. You may be using a poorly made product, you may be using the wrong product for that disease, you may have the wrong diagnosis, you may not be taking the correct dose, you likely need more than just one bottle of something, or a variety of other possible factors may doom your venture into natural medicine. As your venture into natural medicine has failed you, you return to the same old doctor-drug cycle, because you know that at least the drug will likely result in relief in the near term. Curiously, in the big economic downturn of 2008-2010, while most industries were shrinking, natural medicine grew significantly.

The patient may also venture out to see a provider in natural/integrative medicine, but that can get pricey. Why pay cash when you're already paying money each month for medical benefits? Consider that deductibles have risen so high now, you may be paying cash for most or all of your healthcare anyhow. More often than not the patient will give natural medicine a try in desperation since none of their previous nine doctors covered by their plan have been of much help. Here is when you roll the dice. You may be one of the lucky ones and get a good natural medicine doctor who can help you, or you may get someone less than competent or with questionable integrity. To have success in natural medicine, it helps if you become a very active component, the most active component of your new health care model. If you either get a provider who can't help you, or you do not take the plunge into your new healthcare model seriously and with conviction, then you may find yourself back at your PCP looking for another drug.

Natural medicine is more than just supplements. Natural medicine is a holistic way of treating you. Since your inner workings are connected in various ways, your program must take much into consideration. Natural medicine is not the solution to everything. I don't want to mislead you. There are conditions where it may not help at all. There are other conditions where it may help some, and then there are conditions where it is the total, or near total solution. It must be done properly and thoroughly to stand a chance of success. This is its big challenge, but then again that's also true for "modern medicine".

Prevention of any illness or disability should be, without a doubt, at the forefront of each person's health considerations. However, here in America, the general philosophy is something quite different. Overall, in my interactions, it is the buy-now-pay-later, instant gratification philosophy that drives most Americans. When and if they do become ill, there exists an all-knowing doctor with "magic in a bottle" waiting at the end of their HMO rainbow. Imagine avoiding the above disease cycle altogether. Wouldn't that be great? It requires hours of researching your symptoms/condition in the hopes of getting to the root of your problem. If you value your health, and if you find you can't afford your current healthcare model, there are possibilities in natural medicine, which may augment or replace what you're doing now.

Diving into this lifestyle is a big change for most. It requires a paradigm shift from how you've been raised and marketed to. It's so easy to grab some pre-made food and reheat, or pick up some take-out and watch a movie. It's easy to take a drug for your symptoms. It's sad to say, but this is why there will continue to be plenty of business for many years to come in the field of natural medicine. Consider the vast amount of data within this book to shift your healthcare paradigm. My goal is merely to provide you with information. It is up to you to use it or not. Data can be a powerful driving force in your decisions. Data can give you hope, and it can give you fear.

What do most reasonable people fear most? Death, pain, disease, and loss of a loved one, right? These are the reasons we seek medical care, and they are damn good ones at that. The only problem is the quality of the medical care itself. Is it really helping? In some cases "yes", in other cases "no". Let's just consider overall mortality. We will take a look at several studies and try to tally up the tragic results. These researchers were looking into inadvertent deaths caused by those in our health care system, which are referred to as "iatrogenic" deaths, caused by a physician, procedure, or drug. Yes, we actually have an official name for this, and it happens more than you may think.

The first study we'll examine estimates an annual 106,000 deaths from hospital adverse drug reactions (ADR's) (1) In this meta-analysis (a review of data) published in the *Journal of the American Medical Association (JAMA),* in April of 1998, the author estimated that in 1994 about 221,600 hospitalized patients had serious adverse drug reactions and about 106,000 had fatal ADRs, making these reactions between the fourth and sixth leading cause of death. As a reference, our National Vital Statistics report informs us that 71,599 people are estimated to have died from Alzheimer's disease in 2005. This 106,000 number only includes adverse reactions to drugs either prompting admission or while in hospital care. *This is a fraction of all drug-induced problems.* By the way, twenty times that number had serious side effects from these ADRs. In other words, over 2 million serious side effects occurred just in hospitals. This study comes from the American Medical Association. They clearly don't have a vested interest in publicizing this study, but you have to hand it to them-- they published it.

Our second reference comes to us from the Institute for Medicine (IOM). They looked at medical error in hospitals. According to their website, the IOM is a private, non-profit organization that provides health policy advice under a congressional charter granted to the National Academy of Sciences (NAS). They referenced two studies, which analyzed data out of hospitals in Utah and Colorado, and extrapolated the data for the nation. These researchers state, "At least 44,000 people, and as many as 98,000 people, die in hospitals each year as <u>a result of medical errors that could have been prevented</u>." There is some overlap with the previous study as some of these deaths were caused by drug adverse events; however, drug ADRs were only 19% of all these adverse events. This leaves plenty of room for surgical error and more. Just as a point of reference, our government tells us that in 2005, 75,119 people died from diabetes complications. This is less than the higher estimate from this paper.

Our third study looks at hospital based infections. This paper estimated that in 1995, nosocomial infections (from hospital pathogens) contributed to more than 88,000 deaths (2). Interestingly, this is a 35% percent jump compared to the previous 20 years, possibly attributed to overuse of antibiotics, antibacterial everything products, and a host of other issues. These are real numbers, these infections occur, and they can be quite nasty. We've all heard stories and seen news reports of someone dying in the hospital from a bacterium that was resistant to antibiotics. The estimate of 88,000 here is more than our government reports for all influenza and pneumonia deaths in 2005 at 63,001.

Let's move out of the hospitals now and into outpatient care. To calculate the cost of drug related morbidity and mortality among outpatients in the United States, these next researchers asked pharmacists to *estimate* the probability of adverse outcomes occurring as a result of drug prescriptions. They calculated that these outpatient ADRs resulted in an extra 116 million physician visits, 76 million additional prescriptions, 17 million emergency department visits, 8 million hospital admissions, and 199,000 additional deaths. The total cost was estimated to be $76.6 billion (3) Although estimates can be a very "squishy" calculation, pharmacists are on the front lines out there, and are in an excellent position to estimate outpatient ADR's. Even if it's a quarter of this number, it's concerning. As a point of reference, strokes are estimated to have killed an approximate 143,579 people in 2005.

Our next study looked into unnecessary procedures. What is unnecessary? I think some surgeons will disagree with those in the world of natural medicine. How many cesarean sections, tonsillectomies, appendectomies, hysterectomies, gastrectomies for obesity, breast implants, other cosmetic surgeries, cholestectomies (gall bladder removal) are unnecessary? This data comes to us from our own governmental agency. The Agency for Healthcare Research and Quality (AHRQ), which falls under the umbrella of the U.S. Department of Health and Human Services, estimated that in 2001, about 7.5 million unnecessary surgical procedures were performed, resulting in 37,136 deaths. In comparison, all suicides in 2005 were only 32,637.

Our last reference pertains to mortality and our current healthcare model, which looked at surgery related deaths. I can only assume these were necessary surgeries, as I could find no distinction. These statistics also come from the AHRQ, published in *JAMA* in 2003. (4) They identified medical injuries within 7.45 million hospital discharge abstracts from 994 acute-care hospitals across 28 states in 2000 from the AHRQ Healthcare Cost and Utilization Project Nationwide Inpatient Sample database. It was found that about 32,000 deaths occurred from post-operative sepsis, foreign objects left in the body, surgical wounds reopening, post-op bleeding, and a number of other parameters. Do you fear dying from homicide? Well, in 2005, our government informs us that 18,124 people died from homicide in America. That is far fewer than the 32,000 from this other government report. Perhaps you should re-evaluate the basis of your fears.

Since we have some overlap in these studies, it's hard to come up with a reasonable estimate. I think we can safely say iatrogenic deaths are <u>at least</u> the third leading cause of death in our country. Even The American Medical Association admitted in 2000 that the medical system was the third leading cause of death in the US, behind heart disease and cancer. They used their own studies and published it in their own journal, the *Journal of the American Medical Association.* THE THIRD LEADING CAUSE OF DEATH. From the AMA. I'll bet you haven't seen this on the nightly news.

The following death rates are taken from this article, and add up to 225,000.

- Unnecessary surgery: 12,000
- Medication errors in hospitals: 7,000
- Other errors in hospitals: 20,000
- Infections in hospitals: 80,000
- Non-error, negative effects of drugs (drugs given correctly, taken correctly, but the unknown side effect was death!): 106,000

An unfortunate fact hidden in all of this is that it is *widely feared and understood that these numbers are under-reported.* Multiple sources quote that as few as 1.5% and up to only about 30% of iatrogenic events are reported.

Varying studies show reporting to range from 1.5% (5), to 25% (6), to 5-30% (7). Why? The answer is simple. It is to protect the staff's reputations, jobs, and money from lawsuits. Do I sound like a conspiracy theorist? Well, the *Psychiatric Times* published an article in April 2000 that states that doctors are afraid they'll be sued if they bring up a medical error. Curiously, they also stated that the AMA strongly opposes mandatory reporting of medical errors. So who's reporting these adverse events? Often times, it's surviving loved ones. The industry will tell you it's hard to separate drug side effects and cause of death from the disease sometimes, and this may be true. Consider information from one of the original Harvard researchers that started all of these analyses back in the 1984. This New York State study reviewed the medical records of 30,121 patients admitted to 51 acute care hospitals. In this, the author cites several autopsy studies that show missed diagnosis as the cause of death for upwards of 35-40% of the patients. (9) Missed diagnosis. How do these numbers fall into our previous estimates?

Let's take a look at something closer to home, NSAID use. NSAID is short for nonsteroidal anti-inflammatory drug, which you may know by their compound name: ibuprofen, aspirin, naproxen, and celecoxib, to name a few. Their trade names include: Aleve, Celebrex, Advil, and Motrin. These NSAIDs are just one of many items from the modern armamentarium of potentially harmful agents not covered previously in our analyses. These aren't surgeries, infections, or drugs. NSAIDs are ubiquitous in our society, popped daily and hourly for pain. Yet another researcher published in the year 2000 estimated that 103,000 individuals are hospitalized annually in the U.S. for NSAID related serious GI complications. (9) He also estimated that 16,500 NSAID related deaths occur each year among patients with rheumatoid and osteoarthritis. How do they die? From internal bleeding. That's just two disease states, by the way. Two other researchers in 2002 estimated 3,443 U.S. deaths caused per year from NSAIDS, due to GI bleeding for all cases. This is much lower than the previous estimate, yet still concerning (10). Respected herbalist James Duke, PhD, the former head of the USDA's botanical division, estimates that while the risk of death from NSAIDs is 1 in 10,000 the risk of death from supplements is a mere 1 in 1,000,000.

Perhaps you don't use NSAIDs for your pain. Perhaps you take acetaminophen instead, which is the active compound in Tylenol. According to estimates from 2006, acetaminophen accounts for about 56,000 emergency room visits, 26,000 hospitalizations, and more than 450 deaths from liver failure. (11) What's our national cost for just this one over-the-counter product? Not only is there a well-known link between Tylenol and alcohol consumption, but there is data to support a link to fasting as well. How many of you don't eat when you're sick? The maximum recommended dose of 4,000 mg per day can be exceeded unknowingly by concomitantly taking other products that contain acetaminophen, such as Vicoden, Percocet, or some cold and flu products.

A 2005 article on Medpage Today, which referenced a 2005 paper in *Hepatology*, stated, "Liver toxicity from acetaminophen poisoning is by far the most common cause of acute liver failure in the United States." It is in response to this that our government considered some action. As experienced in the U.K. and France, restrictions on over-the-counter sales of acetaminophen have significantly reduced hepatotoxic events. An FDA panel proposed in June of 2009 to do the same. Understandably, patients who manage their pain with these compounds are concerned. Imagine if you could get to the root cause of the problem, and eliminate both the pain and the medicines. By the way, did you know that modern medicine uses IV N-acetylcysteine (NAC) as primary treatment for liver toxicity triggered by acetaminophen overdose? NAC is also a routinely used supplement. Who says supplements don't work?

I would also like to add some of my own recent experiences to this risk equation in our health model. I'm sure you could add a few stories as well. In just the past week in the midst of writing this chapter, I have come across more depressing information on our "modern medical establishment". One of my patients told me about her mother's experience, which happened years ago but is relevant to our conversation. Her mother suffered from a hospital surgical error, which then lead to a nosocomial infection, and then another medical error in follow-up, and then her death. If that's not bad enough, the current patient (daughter) suffered from a medical error for a similar operation, and was forced into parental nutrition (tube feeding) and an extended stay to recover. In the same week an acquaintance of mine insisted on having her gallbladder removed. After doing her research online it turns out the surgeon who was to initially perform the procedure had a black mark on his record. What was it? He had performed surgery to remove another patient's gallbladder, but instead he removed a kidney. A KIDNEY!

Armed with all of this information, why in the world would you put your life in the hands of this system? Wouldn't you want to avoid these risks at all costs? We fear murder, plane crashes, drunk drivers, hurricanes, spiders, and so on. Yet, according to reasonable estimates, medical errors in all their forms are at least the third leading killer of Americans. That pharmaceutical magic in a bottle may not be there to save you. The surgeon might do you in. You may pick up a deadly infection from your potentially unnecessary procedure. Wouldn't any reasonable person want to consider natural medicine to overcome an illness, and preventative medicine to avoid others?

Please understand that natural medicine is not a cure-all for all people, all of the time. Modern diagnostics, surgeries, and drugs do have their place. It is up to you to become acquainted with the strengths that each form of medicine has to offer. Of course prevention is the best medicine, which we'll get to in a moment. If you do become ill, and we all will, then natural alternatives may help you live longer and healthier lives based in part on the information previously given. However, if you still want to take your chances, because you can't live with your disease state, and you feel drugs or surgery are your only chances of relief, then think again. The following will summarize a number of clinical trials where use of a natural alternative was compared to the use of a drug.

In one of my favorite clinical trials, researchers studied forty patients with chronic duodenal ulcers of four to twelve years duration, all of whom had been *referred to surgery despite conventional treatment.* (12). Half of the patients were given 3g/d of DGL (a form of licorice root) for eight weeks, and the other half were given 4.5g/d of DGL for 16 weeks. All patients showed substantial improvement, usually within a week, and get this; none required surgery at one-year follow-up. Just for more support, in 1985 another researcher compared DGL, antacids, and cimetidine against each other in confirmed chronic duodenal ulcers (13). Ninety-one

15

percent of all ulcers healed within 12 weeks, with no significant difference in the rate in healing among the groups. Where there were differences was in regards to relapses, where DGL outperformed the other two arms (treatment groups) with half as many.

How about cardiovascular disease, America's number one killer? In 1986, another set of researchers published a fifteen-year evaluation of cholesterol lowering drugs. (14) They found that niacin was the only cholesterol-lowering agent to reduce overall mortality. Now, isn't mortality, and not lab numbers what we're really after here?

Let's now consider rheumatoid arthritis. In just one of several studies, researchers compared 1,200 mg/day curcumin vs 300 mg/day phenylbutazone. (15). Here is a prime example of the side effect benefits of natural medicine. From a symptomological viewpoint, there was no difference in improvement between the curcumin and the drug. However, the curcumin did produce essentially no side effects, compared to multiple ones in the drug arm. Are you treating your arthritis with high dose NSAIDs or acetaminophen? Curcumin is but one option. Of course it's palliative. You still need to get to the root of the matter. In the meantime, it's still nice to reduce the pain.

In pooled data on saw palmetto vs Finasteride for prostate health, urine flow rate was compared, and saw palmetto performed great. In three months, saw palmetto increased flow rate by 38%, while Proscar took twelve months to improve by 16%. (16) In fact, in Germany and Austria, botanical medicines are considered first line therapies for benign prostate hyperplasia (BPH).

In another widely prescribed disease state--depression--St. John's Wort has been researched in at least 25 double-blind trials. In three trials totaling 317 patients, not only did St. John's outperform the drugs on average, but it was better tolerated (17). The average success rate for St. John's Wort was 64% vs 58% for the 3 drugs, as measured by the Hamilton Depression Scale. Dependent on the disease state, protocol chosen, and patient compliance, natural medicine fares an excellent chance as compared to drugs for efficacy, and an even better chance for tolerability. Again, this is disease and patient specific. In some instances the best choice is a drug; in others it is the natural option. However, it is the over-reliance on "life-saving" drugs for every state and every patient, combined with a willingness to disregard healthy habits, that results in our prolific drug taking and unsustainable health care costs.

My goal is not to bash modern medicine; my goal is to supply you with information so that you may make the most informed decision possible. Medicine has done some amazing things for us over the past 100 years or so. Do you know what the top causes of death were in 1900? Number one was pneumonia and influenza combined. Number two was tuberculosis. Number three was diarrhea/enteritis/ulceration of the intestines. You have to get down to the number four cause of death, that of heart disease, to find something that resembles a common disease of today. The average American could expect to live to the age of 49. This is a far cry from today's statistics. The Spanish Flu of 1918-1919 killed an estimated 675,000 Americans. That is ten times more than the number that died in World War One, which ended at the same time. Globally, more people died from the Spanish Flu in a single year than did all people in four years of the infamous black plague in 1347-1351. Today we have the CDC, which is on top of every possible pathogen from New York to the jungles of southeast Asia. We owe a debt of gratitude to many men and women who labored to bring us the benefits of modern medicine. We just have to put its value in perspective.

We simply need a change in how we think about medicine. It's scary how television commercials are filled with drug ads where they spend more time warning you of dangers then trying to sway you with its merits. Yet, T.V. ads work, the numbers don't lie. As Americans we have this knee jerk need to get the drug for a suspected condition as opposed to figuring out the cause. We want pills for everything, and as already discussed, your doctor may likely give them to you to keep you happy since you're the customer. Unfortunately, sometimes it isn't much different in natural/integrative medicine. When trained in natural medicine you are taught to treat the cause of the condition. However I have seen that in some cases the patients have conditioned the providers to treat the symptoms. It all makes perfect sense really. Assume you've started your new integrative medicine practice. In the first year or two you work with patients to address a variety of factors that are likely playing a

17

role in their diagnosis. You're passionate and you want to make a difference. As time passes you find that most patients simply want to walk through your door only to replace their Rx "magic" in a bottle for a supplement "magic" in a bottle. These patients have rightfully learned from somewhere that supplements have fewer, if any side effects, and may even cost less than the drug. Over time, the natural medicine provider too may succumb to just making their patients happy, because they are customers. I know this to be true in many cases because I get questions like the following. "What do you recommend for weight loss"? "What do you recommend for CFS/FM"?

There is no magic product for weight loss. Sorry. Among a number of other factors, one's weight at the most basic level is a balance of energy consumption verses energy expenditure. There are supplements that may aid in weight loss, such as DHEA or L-carnitine, but to rely on them mostly or exclusively is asking for failure. Likewise, I explain that although there may be some supplements that may aid or even resolve one's CFS/FM, such as vitamin D or ribose, you must first uncover the cause of the "disease" instead of shooting blindly in the dark. Providers in natural medicine need to be wary of falling into this trap, where the continuing influx of patients from modern medicine wears you down into their mindset of care.

I'll provide another example of what could be better practice in natural medicine. I was asked if I had any recommendations for erectile dysfunction. I stated that there really aren't any reliable products in the market at this time. I then inquired as to the cause. The patient was suffering from a side effect from his anti-hypertensive drug. Logically, I recommended to the doctor that she address his hypertension, and the ED should then resolve itself. This example highlights two issues. The first is that drugs can have unwanted side effects, which in part explains the influx of patients into natural medicine. The second is that the naturopathic doctor has adopted the symptomological treatment of conditions instead of treating the underlying cause.

The move to integrative medicine is not an entirely easy transition. Medicine is big business, and there are many who stand to lose at the gains of others. It is unfortunate that this more resembles a war, than national healthcare. Although I am a purist of sorts, I am not naive enough to believe that profits can be set aside for the betterment of mankind. It truly is a shame as both natural medicine and modern medicine offer up an array of amazing tools in the treatment of many conditions that have been or still are the scourge of mankind. In its ultimate form, these two fields of medicine overcome the petty grievances and greed to from Integrative Medicine. It is within Integrative Medicine where you seek a well-informed group of grounded visionaries to provide you with your best healthcare. It is the convergence of experts well-versed in all of the data available to us within the many areas of health, to include nutrition, exercise, diagnostics, prescription medicines, natural medicines, and stress reduction. Of course all experts can't agree on all things all the time, but financial interests and unfounded biases aside, given all relevant data, a clearer consensus can be reached.

Human greed has been around as long as the minted coin, and we are for better or worse, no different than our distant ancestors. The pursuit of great things can be fed by recognition, or by want for material things. This greed trait is a double-edged sword. It is hard for an "expert" to give unbiased information when he or she is being paid large sums of money, either directly or for research, while being lavishly treated all the while. Unknown to you the consumer, the financial ties to business interests are not always made known or made clear. You are left to think that their word is gospel, so to speak. This plays into the general level of confusion you have in regards to what is best for your health. You have a busy life, and as such, you can't be an expert in everything. How many of us read through the instruction manual from front to back when we buy some electronics gadget? How many of us read every word of every document at the closing when buying a home? We don't. We rely on people in whom we place our trust. Hopefully the trust is well placed, but as you well know, people don't work for free.

For example, a *Wall Street Journal* article by Winstein and Armstrong attests to healthcare corruption. As they state, "A prominent Massachusetts anesthesiologist allegedly fabricated 21 medical studies that claimed to show benefits from pain killers like Vioxx and Celebrex." This now former chief of acute pain, Dr Scott Reuben, had faked the data. Not surprisingly, we know that at least one pharmaceutical manufacturer,

Pfizer, paid Dr. Reuben to speak and for some of his research. I am not implying Pfizer is complicit. There must be something to this "allegedly" adverb, since the good doctor is on indefinite leave from his hospital post, and no longer holds an appointment as a professor at Tufts University Medical School, a post he held at the time of the article. According to his attorney, "Doctor Reuben deeply regrets that this happened." I'm sure that he regrets getting caught.

Right down the road in good ole Beantown lies Harvard Medical School. In a *New York Times* article published on March 2, 2009, questionable practices at Harvard Medical School litter the paper on which it is printed. Practices listed included: "Pfizer's $1 million annual subsidy for 20 new M.D.s in a two-year program to learn clinical investigation and pursue Harvard Master of Medical Science degrees, including classes taught by Pfizer scientists." Then there's the Merck-built corporate research center across the street, which includes an immunology lab run by a professor who sits on the board for BMS, which paid her nearly $270,000 in 2007. As one doctor stated, "If a school like Harvard can't behave itself, who can?"

In yet another appalling breech of integrity, the topic of ghostwriting has become an issue. In a *New York Times* article by Natasha Singer in August of 2009, she highlights this highly questionable practice among our educational institutions. She states, "A growing body of evidence suggests that doctors at some of the nation's top medical schools have been attaching their names and lending their reputations to scientific papers that were drafted by ghostwriters working for drug companies." So what is this ghostwriting in more detail? There are many medical education companies able to draft research papers at the behest of the drug manufacturers. The publishing of these peer-reviewed research papers is fundamental marketing practice, as you've become accustomed to seeing the results in the news. What you didn't know, was that in some cases, the independent researchers whose names are attached to the paper, did not write them, but just signed off on them.

In fact, recent litigation in a Wyeth case offers a deeper dive into this process. Wyeth had hired a company known as DesignWrite to "prepare an estimated 60 articles favorable to its menopause drugs." In one publication plan, DesignWrite wrote, "The goal of the Wyeth articles was to de-emphasize the risk of breast cancer associated with hormone drugs, promote the (Wyeth) drugs as beneficial, and blunt competing drugs."

Wyeth has since changed its policy, but the practice still continues. She references a professor of cardiology who declined to put his name to a ghostwritten article on a cholesterol-lowering drug. He went on to state that, "This happens all the time." We have to credit Senator Charles Grassley, who has been investigating this issue and is pressuring the NIH, the source of much of the nation's research funding, to crack down on this policy. However, the article goes on to detail how both the NIH and many universities are "reluctant to tackle the issue."

So who's looking out for you? You are outgunned. Between your job, kids, and all the other activities in your life, you don't have the time to do the research. Use this information compiled for your benefit. The marketing of drugs is everywhere, aimed at you and your practitioner. You hear about studies that shoot down natural medicines as an alternative to your medical needs, but yet have heard of others having had success. Who are you to believe in this mess we call medicine?

The irony of the whole thing is that while the modern medical establishment is bashing natural medicine in public, they are trying very hard to get a piece of that pie. They recognize that many Americans do not want the risks and costs associated with drugs and that these natural products do actually work under the right set of conditions. In fact, this previous statement is a bit erroneous. They aren't trying to get a piece of the pie; they are trying to get a bigger piece of it. The intertwining of the two adversaries is especially evident when you consider that many drugs are derived from substances already occurring in nature. I submit to you as evidence some of my examples set forth in the preface. I mentioned how Reliant Pharmaceuticals Inc brought the prescription fish oil to the market, called Lovaza. I covered how GlaxoSmithKline bought a proprietary formulation of resveratrol for $720 million, and that it's currently in phase 2 trials for diabetes. I also mentioned how Merck owns Metfolin, which is the patented form of active folic acid sold to numerous nutraceutical manufacturers. Aspirin is just the trade name for Bayer's acetylsalicylic acid (ASA) preparation, which underwent manufacturing and marketing in the last years of the 1800s. ASA is derived and purified predominantly from the white willow. Its use in medicine goes back to 3,000 B.C. How about another recent "drug" with its roots in nature? Yet another company has brought to the market a "drug" called Limbrel, originating from natural medicine. This has a bit of a twist. Instead of throwing on a molecule to make it synthetic, and thus patentable, they just call it a proprietary formula. They state that it contains flavocoxid, which is their name for a proprietary blend of flavonoids. They went through the FDA hoops and got an indication for osteoarthritis. They even have a clinical trial where they compare their formulation to naproxen (NSAID), and it seems to have the same efficacy. You can get essentially the same product from any number of over the counter supplements already on the market. But this one is special, because it's a "drug".

A company named Medicure Pharma has submitted a "citizen's petition" to the FDA asserting that all dietary supplements containing pyridoxal 5-phosphate, otherwise known as the active form of vitamin B-6, be banned. Why in the world would a pharmaceutical company want to ban the sale of a B vitamin? Surely the health of the public is in danger. I'm quite confident it has nothing to do with the fact that Medicure has developed a vitamin B-6 of their own called MC-1. If they succeed, then Medicure is rich, and you pay more, much more. I'm sure our trusty politicians down in Washington D.C. will stand by their constituents on this one. I would like to think they will, but I have my concerns.

You may be aware that just recently our government effectively banned the use of estriol by compounding pharmacies. Compounding pharmacists play a nice role in integrative medicine, and in fact they are much more akin to how pharmacists operated "back in the day" than our current big pharma conveyor belt model. I'm not even supposed to insinuate that the compounding pharmacists were providing a bio-identical hormone to women, since this association has not been proven by the FDA. All of this helps big pharma, but doesn't do much for women. This all came about when Wyeth used a "citizen's petition" to ask the FDA to ban estriol, which is a part of bio-identical hormone therapy. Why? Was the public in danger again? I'm sure it has nothing to do with the fact that the clinical data on Wyeth's hormone replacement therapy products were damning, and sales plummeted. This is the same Wyeth who hired ghostwriters to make these very same drugs seem so appealing.

You may recall that in 2002 the progestin-estrogen arm of the massive Women's Health Initiative trial was halted. The researchers found that those who took the hormone therapy had a higher risk of breast cancer and cardiovascular events and thus halted the trial in good conscience. The drug used was Wyeth's PremPro, which is a combination of progestin and conjugated equine estrogens. The source of the estrogens is from pregnant horses, and the estrogen only product known as Premarin derives its name from its source (**pre**gnant **mar**e's ur**ine**). Perhaps they were trying to salvage what they could from their sales by going after the handful of compounding pharmacists nationwide.

Unfortunately for Wyeth, the lucky benefactor from these efforts will be another company. Pipex Pharmaceuticals is seeking approval for a drug called Trimesta, which is essentially estriol, the same compound the compounding pharmacists now can't make. Although their goal is in the treatment of multiple sclerosis, doctors can prescribe it for other conditions. I am not knocking hormone replacement therapy at all; I just believe in its proper administration. The transdermal route is more desirable than the oral route, which is why compounding pharmacists were popular with more educated practitioners.

In yet another example of the movement of pharma into natural medicine, a biopharma company named Genelabs effectively got FDA approval for their drug Prestara. Prestara is a "drug" to treat lupus. This drug is a synthetic form of DHEA. DHEA occurs naturally in the body and thus cannot be patented, which is why they made a synthetic version. The extra molecules thrown onto these naturally occurring hormones, however, may not be free of side effects. Their genesis is based on some old Stanford data showing that DHEA helped lupus patients at a dose of 200mg per day. I'll bet you can't guess at what dose Prestara had been studied for lupus. If you didn't know, DHEA is a widely used supplement. As an approved drug, Prestara can be covered and we'll all pay for its exorbitant price instead of the very affordable price at your local health food store.

I am trying to provide a crystal ball to you. Do you see where this is going? It is not a collaboration between providers, pharmaceuticals, nutraceuticals, and your government. This is a financial war in which you'll pay the price in dollars, and maybe even your health. Some providers in integrative medicine already know this data. They have known it years before you'll even see these products come to the market as drugs. I've told several people over the years about DHEA and lupus. I'm sure compounding pharmacists are well aware of the connection of estriol and MS. The pharmaceutical industry is cherry picking from natural medicine and has the money to satisfy the insane system in place as dictated by the system in place. Your health care choices are being threatened, and you don't even know it.

When is the last time you went to Washington D.C. to speak with your congressman? I'll bet the answer for most all is never. Of course you haven't; it's impractical. You have a job, kids, and a house. When you do get your two or three weeks of vacation a year, the last thing on your mind is to argue with some congressman with some potentially serious integrity issues. You want to relax or do something fun, and no one can blame you for it. However, as you well know, large financial interests send very well paid lobbyists there as their profession. You're fighting an unfair fight. It's like you've been challenged to the heavyweight boxing title and no one even told you about it. The sad fact is that it is not likely to change.

The Kaiser Daily Health Policy Report informs us that health care interests spent $445 million on federal lobbying in 2007. Once again, that was $445 million on federal lobbying. This was more than any other sector of the economy for the second consecutive year. Pharmaceutical and medical products companies came in first, while others included health insurance, hospitals and nursing homes, health professionals, and HMOs. The American Medical Association alone as a single spender came in fourth with $22.1 million. What do they all have to say that's so important that they are willing to spend what equates to $831,775 per congressman?

We have a number of large issues looming over our heads, none larger than cost. We cannot maintain this unsustainable increase in health care spending on personal, corporate, and governmental levels. It would be nice if measures can be implemented to give the best quality of care at the most affordable price. This would in part require patients to take on more personal responsibility, and moves between drugs and natural approaches when warranted. It all sounds well and good and is much easier said than done. The intensity to which natural medicine is derided is unjust.

Take, for example, a study on Echinacea, which is one of numerous possible examples. The results from a July 2005 trial published in the *New England Journal of Medicine* went a long way to discrediting this herb. Let's first take a closer look at the trial. Researchers prepared their own Echinacea Augustifolia (one of three main types used) and administered 900 mg per day in divided doses to the treatment group. Both treatment and placebo subjects were sequestered in a hotel room and began taking their pills seven days before exposure to the rhinovirus (common cold). Once exposed, all rated their symptoms. The results showed no difference between the placebo and the Echinacea.

Mark Blumenthal is the founder and executive director of the American Botanical Council, and he explains that the dose wasn't correct. He states that the researchers used the recommended dose for Echinacea pallida established by the German E Commission, which is a FDA-like natural medicine agency. The appropriate dose for the form of Echinacea these researchers used would be 3 grams per day, as recommended by the WHO. As you will read more than once in this book, dose can make a world of difference. Beyond his point, there are other things you can do to markedly reduce your chances of catching a cold.

My successful regimen is a bit more thorough. When the very first symptoms of a cold occur, I make what's called a decoction. I'll take about 2-3 grams of Echinacea (pupurea or augustifolia), licorice root, ginseng, and astragalus. I boil it for about 3-5 minutes, and then let it sit. This should make enough for three generous servings. The boiling draws out of the roots the active principles you are looking for, which are readily absorbed. You don't have to rely on gut absorption from some encapsulated herb, which may have other issues in quality. Other extras that should be incorporated are vitamins A and C, zinc, selenium, and berberine or volatile oil containing herbs. You should avoid sugar, dairy, and iron supplements and foods high in iron, such as meats. As an extra bonus, juicing vegetables, plenty of sleep, and getting your body temperature up from a hot bath or sauna are desirable. For colds, influenza, pneumonia, or most any other condition, you should ensure that your vitamin D levels are in an ideal range year round. I'll put my regimen up against any placebo with any researchers any day of the week.

What is the value of not being sick? Whether it's work, an expensive vacation, a big date, or any other week in your life, being sick is an unwanted outcome. For a little bit of effort and money, you stand a very good chance of avoiding it altogether if you know what to do. This is why these trials that just look at low dose vitamin C on colds are a bust. I can construct any trial to fail. It is unfortunate that those who are less than competent create these backlashes towards this industry that only fuel the already doubtful medical establishment.

As I will say many times in this book, natural medicine has its limitations, which is also true for modern medicine. In addition, natural medicine has as much to do with what you eat, how you exercise, and stress reduction, as it does with supplements and diagnostics. With that said, there are many disease states that can benefit from appropriate care in regards to dose, quality of product, and patient compliance. Americans know there is something to this natural medicine concept, and have become very wary of costly drugs and their potential side effects. Upwards of one third of Americans use alternatives to modern medicine, and many more take supplementation in some form. Their intentions are not entirely misguided; they just need some honest direction. On the flip side are those who are skeptics, and sometimes rightfully so. As one who advocates for stricter quality controls in the manufacturing of natural medicines, I feel there are those who have done damage to this industry in one form or another. One outspoken critic of alternative medicine is Dr. Wallace Sampson, who is the founding editor of the *Scientific Review of Alternative Medicine*. He is also on the board for the National Council Against Health Fraud and is a clinical professor at Stanford University's medical school. He states that alternative treatments are either not proven or disproven and that "Acupuncture is a placebo and Homeopathy is one step above fraud."

I too am a skeptic of many things, and as someone with a firm footing in science I want to see evidence to support anyone's conclusions. I am not an expert in either Acupuncture or Homeopathy, and can't comment as such. However, I do know providers who praise either one for certain conditions. One may have concerns about certain aspects of alternative medicine, but to make blanket statements is irresponsible.

Since the topic of Stanford came up with Dr. Sampson, we should make note of a similar parallel to the events in Washington D.C. It seems that several *Mercury News* stories in 2006 prompted officials at Stanford to look into faculty ties to medical companies as reported by Steve Johnson. Stanford Medical School has not been the only recipient of these gifts. <u>In 2006, drug and medical device companies contributed $1.2 billion to continuing medical education</u>. For Stanford, the value of their contributions from industry sources was about $1.87 million, or 38% of the school's budget for continuing education. It seems that things changed as of August 2008. The companies will no longer be able to designate specifics in how their contributions are to be used, but can make general purpose contributions. Apparently public pressure has urged them to reconsider their conflicts of interest. Others hail the decision, but at the time of the article only five other medical schools had a similar program in place. I guess those pharmaceutical and medical device companies are some serious philanthropists.

Humor may or may not be in good taste here or in other examples within this book, but it beats outrage. The fact is that this quandary we're in is no laughing matter at all. According to the AHRQ the average expenses of a person with any medical expenses in 2006 was $4,078. That's a lot of money. In total there was $1.03 trillion spent on medical care in 2006 not including the institutionalized. Hospital inpatient and all outpatient costs accounted for about a third of costs, while prescribed medicines was about 20%. The average annual medical expenses for someone over the age of 65 was $9,080. If they had supplemental insurance above and beyond their Medicare they spent an average of $10,925! This last fact implies to me that those who have coverage will use it! You can't blame them, can you? The problem is that if we're going to have some form of nationalized health care then we had better come up with a plan to get these costs under control.

This crisis has not gone unnoticed with our politicians, but action may be another matter. In an Orlando Florida conference entitled "America's Health Care at Risk," Irwin Redlener of Columbia University and co-chair of Doctors for Obama said, "There's a true crisis in American health care. We're looking at a financial meltdown." I couldn't agree with him more. In fact, Senator Tom Coburn said that "administrative costs account for more than $700 billion of the $2.3 trillion spent on health care annually and 8% of what's spent is for tests nobody needs." The bloating in health care can be illustrated best in regards to prescription drugs. According to the Kaiser Family Foundation, spending for prescription drugs was $216.7 billion in 2006. The number of prescriptions purchased from 1997 to 2007 increased by 72% while the U.S. population only increased by 11%. That was enough for 12.6 prescriptions for every man, woman, and child in the country in 2007. Of course this is great news for stockholders. From 1995 to 2002 pharmaceutical manufacturers were the nation's most profitable industry when analyzing profits as a percent of revenue.

Employers are the principle source of health insurance in the U.S., which provide coverage for about 59% of us. As you well know, your employer's costs are going up, and as a consequence yours are too. Medicare has exploded and will continue to do so. The Medicare Prescription Drug, Improvement, and Modernization Act of 2003 established a voluntary Medicare outpatient prescription drug benefit (known as part D), which took effect January 1, 2006. This act offers pharmacy benefits to 42 million Medicare beneficiaries nationwide. As we all know, the rapidly rising costs of Medicare are crushing. Not only do we have a massive influx of baby boomers born between 1946 and 1964, but the costs of all medical expenses are escalating too quickly. As you have seen taxes, food, higher education, and fuels steadily increase in costs, the same holds true for medical expenses. Sticking with our pharmaceutical analysis, a recent AARP report informs us that in the 12 months ending in June of 2006, the 193 brand named drugs they followed increased in price by 6.3%. This is compared to an inflation rate for the same time period of only 3.8%. How much did your income go up during that period? I'll speculate that for most of you it was less than inflation, never mind the cost of drugs.

These increases in costs have affected your health plans. Health plans have responded by excluding certain drugs from coverage, increasing deductibles, using quantity dispensing limits, increasing the tiers within the plan, and by increasing the costs to their enrollees. Kaiser informs us that preferred drugs increased in cost by 67% from 2000 to 2007. Now that the economy is not as robust as in recent years, your medical costs are an even greater factor in regards to your household expenses. The simple fact is that Americans are cutting back. According to IMS Health, the number of filled prescriptions is significantly falling. Walgreens Chief Executive said that the U.S. is experiencing the "tightest prescription market" in his 27- year career, as more cash-strapped patients skip their dose or take half doses. This may not be entirely a bad thing since the side effects from some drugs can be worse than the condition, and the use of other drugs such as statins is questionable in many cases.

The number of physician visits has continued to decrease since the end of 2006 when the economy really started to trend down. The National Association of Insurance Commissioners found that 22% of respondents avoided physician visits because of cost concerns. LabCorp, which is the country's second largest clinical lab company, reported that the number of blood tests and other labs for the uninsured fell 8% in the second quarter, which is in contrast to its usual growth.

Prior to these drops, prescription drug taking had become a way of life for many Americans, which is truer for older Americans than younger ones. In a 2003 study out of Tufts, 46% of the Medicare beneficiaries polled took five or more prescription drugs per day. About 25% said they were forgoing medicine because of cost. <u>Many others did not refill prescriptions because they felt the drugs didn't work or the drugs made them feel worse</u>. A more recent *JAMA* study, which polled 3,000 adults aged 57-85 in 2005/2006, found that almost 33% take five or more medications per day. That's a lot of people taking a lot of drugs.

If any of this sounds familiar to you, you are not alone. It is for these reasons that many people are seeking out natural medicine. It is for these reasons and more that I have written this book for you to help guide you through this maze of which you may not be familiar. This book is geared to the following:

- Those who want to try natural medicine for the first time but have their reservations.
- Those who have tried natural medicine before with a practitioner and failed.
- Those who try to treat themselves with supplements.
- Those who take supplements for preventative medicine.
- Those who are fed up with going from doctor to doctor with no success.
- Those who seek some serious guidance on nutrition.
- Those individuals, HMOs, and companies who want to augment their healthcare and save money.
- Those who want the truth.

With that said, I don't pretend to have all of the answers to resolve our healthcare crisis. I will now put forth some concepts; perhaps some will stick, and some won't. In the end take what you will in any measure, small or large, and implement it into your lifestyle. Either way, I think you'll find what I have to say quite interesting, and yes, controversial.

Chapter 2   Natural Medicine

What is natural medicine to you? A recent government study shows that 38% of Americans use some form of alternative medicine. If you recall from the introduction, I defined natural medicine as the use of non-conventional and conventional diagnostic techniques that implement nutritive, mental, and physical aides to allow the body to heal itself, while adapting one's lifestyle to mimic the optimal conditions in health for the human genome. This implies that you have developed a condition that needs treating. One could argue, and successfully so, that preventative medicine through nutrition and natural medicine should be a component as well, and in fact should be the method of preference. In any event, you grasp the concept that there is a lot more to this than taking a pill in a bottle.

Natural medicine has its roots in most of our history across the globe. Whether it's Asia, Europe, North America, or other corners of our planet, the use of botanicals and other facets of natural medicine have endured through the millennia. How could that be? Perhaps there may be some actual value to this "new" rage in medicine.

To begin, the optimal form of natural medicine is preventative medicine. In many disease states it is much better to not get sick in the first place, since in both conventional medicine and natural medicine there may be a lack of highly efficacious "cures". One of the better examples I can think of here is that of the gallstone. Simplified, gallstones form when the bile becomes oversaturated with cholesterol, and it precipitates out to form stones which attract minerals such as calcium. Numerous studies show that your habits play a key role in the development of gallstones. These include exercise, diet, and drugs. For gallstone prevention, probably the most significant dietary modification you could make would be to introduce non-legume water-soluble fiber such as that from fruits, vegetables, and oats. Obesity, animal protein, and refined carbohydrates are other important considerations. Given the list I just provided, and how predominant those food items are in America, it is no surprise that well over a half million gall bladder surgeries are performed each year. There are non-surgical options both in natural medicine and by prescription. They are both based on taking ursodeoxycholic acid which is a bile acid that promotes cholesterol solubility. The problem is that they only work for a certain set of conditions, and they take a long time to do so. Therefore, surgery, which is at a significant cost, is the predominant "treatment".

In the event you do develop some type of condition, then your likely course of action following dealing with the symptoms for a period of time is to go see a provider. You go to the provider hoping for a quick resolution. A quick resolution implies an accurate diagnosis during the initial visit, and a drug that can resolve things. All of this assumes that your all-knowing physician can make those things happen. We all know of someone, perhaps even yourself, who has gone to see a practitioner and received a completely incorrect diagnosis. Why is that? Well, I have news for you: doctors aren't magicians. They can't know all. Even if they did have any magic, I don't think an 8 minute appointment is enough time to conjure up any miracles. They have been put in a difficult spot. Balanced between time constraints through growing operating costs, fear of lawsuits, a plethora of drugs and conditions, having to be coding and business experts, which focuses less time on perfecting the art of medicine, and a tilted education in mainstream medicine, they cannot and do not know all. That is where a different model comes into play. I have more news for you, however. Practitioners of natural medicine are not magicians either. They are confronted with many of the same problems that plague the conventional doctor. They do have a couple of distinct advantages, and they also have a couple of hindrances. So what can you expect from a visit to an alternative practitioner?

We first have to begin with your practitioner options. There are naturopathic doctors, chiropractors, osteopaths, nutritionists, acupuncturists, nurses, nurse practitioners, massage therapists, and M.D.s. Yes, I said M.D.s. Medical Doctor involvement in natural medicine is growing at an amazing rate. Whether this is in response to demand, seeing the light, or something else, it's up to the individual. So let's do a quick review of what they may or may not offer. I will highlight the three main types of practitioners you're likely to see that should be able to provide you with full care, minus any complex referrals.

Naturopathic doctors (NDs) are the only practitioners whose training is solely focused on providing medical care through the various components of natural medicine. Here in the U.S. it is likely that they will have attended one of four schools offering such a program. You can expect your visit in most states to be an all cash affair. In fact, NDs only have licensure in 14 states across the country, and even when licensed, coverage through managed care my not be an option for you. You can expect your first consult to last about 90 minutes, give or take. The cost will run somewhere in the neighborhood of $200-$300, and again this can fluctuate highly on geography. You may even pick an ND who is also an acupuncturist, a nutritionist, or has other qualifications. They will most often carry what is called a dispensary or medicinary, which is basically their natural pharmacy on hand. This dispensary will vary from office to office, but the same themes run true for most all of them. They will likely "prescribe" products to you from this mostly professional line of nutraceuticals to hopefully help you with your condition, for which you will have to pay at the time of service. They may run various non-conventional labs to help in the diagnosis and to monitor progress. These labs may be analyses for heavy metals, pathogens, nutritional status, neurotransmitters, and many more. You will likely be paying for that out of pocket as well. Whether or not you live in an ND-licensed state, you can perform a search online to find an ND near you on naturopath.org. State associations also have their own websites for which you can search. The philosophy of the ND is to find the root cause of your problem, and to treat the body holistically. These are two fantastic beliefs engrained in their training. Does this mean that I am exclusively recommending ND's as your first choice in natural medicine?

Let's cover the M.D. next. For all intents and purposes, M.D.s do not get any training in this field during their schooling. They venture into this field for one of a few reasons. Thus, their expertise is honed over time. Their education is a combination of their medical background, self-education, possible apprenticeships, and organized education through schooling, seminars, etc. As such, which is true for everyone, there is a learning curve. The experienced M.D. who has dedicated his or her practice to natural/integrative medicine over years of experience is a rare bird, but can be a good one. They may require cash for their services as well.

The M.D. who practices natural medicine will do much of the same as the N.D. previously described. They will provide the same set of "unconventional" labs, they will in all liklihood carry a dispensary that looks much the same as that of the N.D., and the time spent with you will also essentially be the same. There really can be little difference in how the two practices are run. The Medical Doctor will have at their disposal a long list of Rx medications that they could prescribe if they so choose. They will usually not want to go down this road, but may very well supplement the natural products with a prescription when necessary. This is not necessarily a terrible thing. Drugs can and do have their place; you just need to see someone who is able to discern when those times are and are not. Some N.D.s, in New Hampshire, for example, do have some prescription rights as well, and they use them selectively.

You may also see the M.D. cross trained in acupuncture, as an N.D., a nutritionist, or another qualification. The alternative/integrative medicine M.D. is possibly closer to the higher goal in healthcare, that of complimentary or integrative medicine, than any other practitioner. Again, "modern medicine" is not all bad. It offers up wonderful diagnostic tools, useful drugs when necessary, and the potentially excellent medical training offered up by our medical schools. To be able to combine the strengths of both worlds provides you, the consumer, with truly the best care available. You can perform searches on sites like ACAMnet.org or Functionalmedicine.org to find the nearest provider to you. Does this mean that I am exclusively recommending MD's as your first choice in natural medicine?

The last potential practitioner I'll address here is the Chiropractor (D.C.). Chiropractors fit into three categories, at least as I see it. In the first, they simply adjust, crack backs. These do not offer up natural medicine, and thus will not be covered. Next we have the chiropractor who mainly adjusts, but also dabbles in natural medicine. They realize that many of their patients are already taking a fish oil, a CoQ10, a probiotic, and so forth, and offer up what may or may not be a higher quality product for you on their shelf. We are not really talking about these folks either. Last we have the chiropractor, who is arguably as heavily invested, if not more so, in providing natural medicine as they are in providing traditional chiropractic care. They will generally run a practice like the two preceding providers listed. They will have the costs, the time, the labs, and the dispensary like the others. They also may be cross-trained in another area of expertise.

If you have already been to see a D.C, you may have been "muscle tested", which is also referred to as applied kinesiology. Although the vast majority of muscle testers are D.C.s, you may find the occasional N.D. or other practitioner using it as well. So, what is muscle testing? It was developed in the 1960s and is a "bioenergetic diagnostic method" based on the premise that your muscle tone will vary as your body is exposed to properties that are either "good" or "bad" for the individual. What does that mean? Typically what occurs is that your arm is raised parallel to the floor. You may be sitting, you may be standing. You may be holding a bottle, a pill, or nothing. You'll provide resistance via your outstretched arm to that being applied by the practitioner. What they are trying to guage is the level of resistance you are able to muster to the pressure applied by the practitioner. Although applied kinesiology is <u>not supported</u> in the clinical literature (1-3), some of these providers are well versed in natural medicine.

So whom should you see? Among the hundreds of practitioners I know and with whom I interact, I find that they are much like everyone else out there in this world. They follow the same bell curve as all others. You remember the bell curve, right? That's where it starts low to the horizontal line, rises in the middle, and goes back down again. You may have been graded on a bell curve in school. Some student got an "F", a couple more got a "D", the average fell around "C" or low "B", and a few got an "A". Just as in life, no matter what your profession, some people are better at what they do than others are. Think about your job. If you don't have a job, think about your life as a stay-at-home parent, or student. You know of what I speak. You can think of others who are better than you, or not as good as you. The same is true for practitioners, and not just in natural medicine, but in all medicine. I'm going to assume you'd rather see someone, and pay the corresponding sums of money to someone who's an "A" rather than someone who's a "D".

Now here's a twist for you. That scale slides as you go through various disease states. In other words, someone who is excellent in caring for one disease may not be as good at another. To further complicate things, those at the top of the list, the "A"s of the world, can be an M.D., N.D., D.C., or anything else. Those at the bottom of the list can also be any of the aforementioned.

I think certifications and degrees are a reasonable guide, but certainly not the sole factor in determining who's competent and who's not. I know many people who do not have a college degree but are smarter, have more common sense and more vision than many who have a college degree. Most times, a degree only proves one thing, and that is that you are capable of learning. That you were fortunate to attend college as compared to another who was unable to do so is another matter. That you can learn is good, but that <u>you can teach yourself, discern fact from bias, put abstract thoughts together, spend your free time honing your skills, and otherwise apply yourself with intense energy and direction to become a visionary is a whole other matter</u>. You want to see someone who "has it" and "gets it". You don't want to see someone who does this because it's cute, because there's good money in supplement sales, who doesn't dedicate themselves in the pursuit of excellence in this industry. This industry is rapidly changing, and requires one to spend vast amounts of time keeping up with the latest information. So let's give you some guidelines to follow to better spend your time and money in the pursuit of optimizing your health.

Many patients who seek out natural medicine are desperate for good care. Whatever their prior medical experience has been, they are still sick, and honestly want help quickly. With desperation and a lack of familiarity with how natural medicine works, the possibility of being "taken for a ride" exists. I don't want that to happen to you. I want your foray into this amazing field to be a success, if that's honestly possible. The unfortunate fact is that there are some practitioners in this field with questionable skills and motives. However, I'm happy to say that the motives are pure for most, and skills will vary between disease states.

I have found that those who best treat a disease are those who have either been a victim of that disease, or have had a loved one under that same circumstance. If a provider, or their child, has been unfortunate enough to come down with a given condition in the past, they may have

36

become a passionate expert on that condition. In fact, I have known many who were initially not providers, but they themselves were ill, or had a sick loved one, and natural medicine either cured them, or helped to significantly manage the disease. They only later went on through formal education to become providers in natural medicine after having "seen the light".

Their quest was the same as many others, and probably you included. It involves going to see multiple doctors in "modern medicine" to no avail. Getting sicker and sicker with the passage of time, and then for some reason, under some set of circumstances, fall into natural medicine. They got lucky, and were helped by someone, or discovered for themselves the keys to their solution. These providers make the best providers for that condition.

Assuming you have a correct diagnosis, then seek out a provider who overcame that same disease. When calling offices for a screening, ask if the provider has any specialties, and inquire as to how he or she chose them. You may hear a long list of specialties from the office staff, but seek specific questions in regards to yours. Some disease states can be tricky to treat, which is why you want someone well versed in your condition. You may find a provider who beat cancer for example, although that's no guarantee that they can help you. Another provider may have overcome CFS/FM, regardless of the cause. One may have had rheumatoid arthritis, or their child may have been ill with digestive disorders or dermatologic issues. Although many of the treatment protocols have consistency across many disease states such as the elimination of certain foods, in conditions such as autism or lyme disease it may be beneficial to find someone who has honed their skills through much repetition.

The fact that many of these practitioners have so many specialties is reflective of the fact that in order to survive financially, they have to take "all-comers". This mostly cash business can be profitable for some, and a struggle for many. When I refer to "all-comers", I am referencing all disease states. Think of your primary care provider (PCP). You go for a visit, and they usually throw a drug at you and tell you to come back in a month or have you call if it doesn't work. At which point they may throw another drug at you. Maybe some labwork was done in there somewhere, maybe not. If the problem still persists, then they refer you to a specialist. The problem has advanced beyond the level of their expertise. This specialist thing is a double-edged sword. On the one hand it exemplifies the fact that there is way too much to know out there. There are too many diseases, too much variability, and too many possibilities. The specialist is there to serve as an expert for your condition when the PCP becomes overwhelmed, but this comes at a price. The specialist treats you, as in your whole body, as if you were a walking kidney, or heart, or stomach. Do you get my point? They lose sight of the fact that if you make a change over here, that something over there may be negatively impacted.

The natural medicine provider will treat you holistically. That too comes at a price. Even though it is a better model, there still exist too many diseases and possibilities for one person to be able to wrap their heads around. There are many intricacies and subtleties in certain conditions. This model exists in order to survive financially. They may very well need every patient who walks in that door or calls on the phone, because the livelihood of their practice depends on it. If you ask the staff if the provider is any good, you'll invariably get the same response from all staff in all offices, and it sounds something like this. "Dr so-and-so is the best." Taking "all-comers" and staff members raving about the expertise of every provider both contribute to varying outcomes across the board in natural medicine. Of course, this is also true of conventional medicine As you will read throughout this book, there is extensive data to support a wide array of natural approaches, but the evidence can be overwhelming.

When looking for a practitioner, use commone sense and consider your source. If you had to lose a significant amount of weight for health reasons, would you go to see someone overweight? If you were losing your hair, would you buy hair re-growth products from a balding provider happy to sell them to you? Do you want advice from a provider who looks like hell, and seems as though he or she may not be around much longer? How about if you're stressed out, and you go to see someone with a crabby personality? Providers come in all shapes, and sizes, and levels of competence. If they appear to be in no better health than you, should you really be spending your money and time with them?

This concept is equally applicable to providers available to you in modern conventional medicine. Is the unhealthy, heavy-breathing M.D. who is providing you with yet another prescription really going to help you? How many medications is he taking? If a provider looks vibrant and healthy, then you might want to listen. If they appear to lack health, peace of mind, and vitality, I would consider another source.

As you probably picked up in the beginning of this chapter, this could be an expensive experience for you, so you'll need to maximize your efforts in all aspects of this care. Seeing a natural/alternative/integrative practitioner is usually a cash pay affair. So, one of the main drawbacks for these providers is that they are pricey. They are unlikely covered by insurance, and not only may the supplements be out of pocket in addition to the consult, but also the labwork will as well. Of course, the flip side is continued ill-health. I'm not so sure about you, but I can't think of anything much more important than that.

Recently, there has been a new positive change in regards to the expense of supplements. It is now quite likely that you can apply the cost of your supplements purchased through your provider, depending on their qualification, through your health savings account or flexible savings account. It requires some minor paperwork on behalf of the provider for your records. If you do have a HSA or FSA, I suggest you do some research and save some money.

With all I've covered thusfar, you might be less likely to go and see any provider in natural medicine. My purpose is certainly not to scare you away from it, but to better educate you and maximize your time and money. Without a doubt, amazing things can happen with these providers. What is your other option? You can keep going to the mainstream medical care, for the same lack of results.

When you have properly screened your provider, and you're now sitting there hoping for a miracle, you must realize that half of the miracle will come from you. You have to be prepared and committed. Show up with your medical history, with your personal notes on symptoms and to what they may be related. Show up having given your condition some serious thought and research. The more information you are able to disclose, the better your results are likely to be. You will have a significant amount of time to discuss your diet, sleeping habits, stress level, family history, labwork, opinions, the drugs you're taking, and much more. Lo and behold, your opinions will count. Your thoughts will not be dismissed. Everything you say, or most everything you say will have value. Be honest. Don't hide facts because you're bashful. You'll likely have too many symptoms and events to recall at that moment, so write down the course of events chronologically, with notes of possible connections.

Solid insight cannot be gathered in an 8-minute appointment with your PCP. Your PCP is not likely to get to the root of the problem. The natural provider will not, or should not try to replace your Rx bottle that treats symptoms, with an OTC one that treats symptoms. Sure, the alleviation of symptomology may be a part of the equation, but getting to the root cause is the goal. Here's a great example. For those who present with GERD/heartburn, your PCP will give you an H2 blocker or PPI to reduce your stomach acidity. That helps with the symptoms, but causes a host of issues downstream. There are issues with absorption of nutrients, and there are issues with pathogens passing further down the GI tract, and even migrating into the stomach. In most cases, the patient is not suffering from too much HCL, but too little. I know it's hard to grasp, but dig into the literature. Most providers in natural medicine will treat as such, and will get results. Keep in mind that dietary and lifestyle changes may and probably should be a part of the solution.

You are half of the equation. Not only are you responsible for finding the right provider for your needs, and then coming prepared to your appointment(s), but you will be required to take responsibility on the tail end as well. You will not be given "magic in a bottle". If you expect to walk out of the office with minimal participation, expecting to feel like twenty again in a day or two, you are setting yourself and natural medicine up for failure. There is a difference between conventional medicine and natural medicine. Drugs work relatively quickly, and usually only address symptoms. Natural medicine on average works slower, but aims to ultimately resolve the underlying problem. It took you a while to get sick, so it may take a while to get better. You should notice gradients of improvement along the way to reassure you that you have done the right thing.

I've said for a long time that a treatment success in this field requires the correct diagnosis, a condition treatable with natural medicine, with the right choice in supplements applicable for the condition, the correct dosing, proper product quality, the correct diet, and a motivated patient. Most disease states can be treated, they may just vary in degree of success.

So maybe you're feeling a little better about trying natural medicine, but you still have some reservations. This is understandable. You've probably heard on a number of occassions that some supplement has been recently shown not to work in clinical trials. As one keeps hearing these reports, anyone would be skeptical. You have to realize that there is an enormous amount of junk science out there. I see it all of the time, and roll my eyes. There are a whole host of variables that need to be controlled for in order to provide the least number of confounding factors, and most valued results. I could take any product, any drug even, and subject it to a clinical trial and construct that trial so that it will fail. It's easy. There are a whole host of variables to consider, such as:

- Does data support that this product even works for this condition?
- Do I have the dose correct?
- Have I provided for a long enough duration to ensure validity?
- Is the product quality such that it has the chance to do its job?
- Is the answer multifactorial, such as a change in diet?
- Is the trial relying on patient recall or other less than desirable controls?

You will also see silly conclusions all of the time. Chocolate is good for your sex life. Caffeine makes you smarter. Green tea makes you taller, and vitamin C extends the life of fruit flies by 50%. Then the next week the research comes out with the opposite conclusion to the above. How can you take natural medicine seriously after all of this nonsense. For example, the Mayo Clinic has an article entitled, "Cholesterol: The top 5 foods to lower your numbers." They state, "A cholesterol-lowering diet in which 20 percent of the calories come from walnuts may reduce LDL cholesterol by as much as 12%." Assuming that the walnuts are not loaded with preservatives, and haven't had their omega-3 fatty acids oxidized, then they are great for you. With that said, no matter how crazy you happen to be for walnuts, no one is going to consume 20% of their calories from walnuts, certainly with no guarantees. There are a million of these examples, but I won't waste your time with them.

Consider this for an analogy. If herbs have the power to kill you, if herbs have the power to be the original source for about half of all drugs, if herbs have been relied upon by people internationally for thousands of years for their ailments, then why can't they work for you? I am implying that the herb is of the appropriate type, quality, and dose for the condition. Let's take one of the analogies.

Belladonna in excess can cause coma. Comfrey root contains substances called "pyrrolizidine alkaloids," which can cause liver damage. Germander can cause liver damage as well. The Chinese herb Aristolochia fangqi has caused deaths in Europe and is consequently banned there and here. Yohimbe overdose can lead to paralysis. I'm sure you remember the ephedra deaths and recall from the market in regards to weight loss products. Ephedra comes from the Chinese herb ma huang. Shakespeare used hemlock to kill MacBeth. Natives used curare on arrowheads to kill as well. You may eat rhubarb as I do, but a high enough dose of the leaves can cause tremors, convulsions, and collapse followed by death in as little as a few minutes. Poison ivy may not kill you, but the actions of this herb are well known. Opium comes from the poppy seed, and dependent on dose may kill you, and at lesser doses will just kill your soul. Foxglove contains cardiac glycosides that have a significant impact on the heart. These glycosides strengthen the force and speed of contraction of the heart, and at the right dose, this too can be fatal.

Don't the attributes of Foxglove sound appealing if they could be controlled? If you needed to "strengthen" your heart, wouldn't you want something that could help. Well, the pharmaceutical industry agreed with you. Its therapeutic role was realized by happenstance in England by a visiting physician many years ago. Do you know the latin name for Foxglove? Digitalis purpurea. Foxglove gives us the drug Digitalis. It is presumed that the glycosides bind to the cardiac membrane, which helps with the pumpimg of sodium and potassium at a cellular level. This in turn decreases oxygen demand, and as we've already stated, increases the contractility of the heart muscle. You see, it all comes down to biochemistry, regardless of the source. Aspirin, as noted earlier, comes from the willow. In the preceeding paragraph we discussed the health dangers of opium, but the drug morphine finds its source there as well. Quinine comes from the cinchona tree, and much of our estrogen in prescriptions comes from the soybean, or even the yam. Reserpine, which is a tranquilizer, comes from the herb snakeroot. Caumadin is a very popular anticoagulant. It is also frequently reffered to as Warfarin. Warfarin was actually the trade name for a rat poison, and Caumadin is the trade name for the prescription anticoagulant. They are both derived from the herb sweet clover. When you subject the phytochemical coumarin to mold, the potent result is called dicoumarol. Dicoumarol interferes with the coagulation affects of vitamin K. I have seen many unsubstantiated claims as to the percentage of drugs that are derived from the natural world. Many will quote 50%, although I have seen no official studies. Whether it's 50% or something less, or something more, the potency of the plant world is a reality. There are, and have been for many years, researchers who travel to remote locations looking for the next great discovery from the plant world, for the profits of the pharmaceutical world. Whether you agree or not with the process, it is a reality, and a testament to the potency of plants.

Again, I ask you, "If herbs have the power to hurt, and they have the potency to become a drug, then isn't it possible that they have the ability to help the body heal in an over-the-counter approach?" Let's reconsider dose. I have harped on dose, and I will in future chapters. Dose can make the difference between a treatment success and a treatment failure. As we have seen with foxglove, it can kill or it can help; it's a matter of getting the dose right. The same was true for warfarin. Dosing guidelines were begun when a man tried to kill himself with the rat poison, but was treated with vitamin K to counteract the effects. Drugs allow for controlled dosing in an otherwise imprecise natural world. You must consider two things, however. In the interest of drug company profits, the natural molecule can be changed such that it's patentable, but also much more toxic. Second, the herbs we're talking about in the practice of natural medicine are not of this potency.

I again refer you to dose. As Aureolus Paraceisus (grandfather of pharmacology) said, "All things are poisons, for there is nothing without

43

poisonous qualities. It is only the dose which makes a thing a poison…" You will likely require at least one herb (or other type of natural product) for your care, whether from the health food store, or given to you by a practitioner. There are hundreds of herbs at your disposal in the world of natural medicine. The same question remains: "Is the herb the right herb for your disease with the appropriate quality and dose?" Just like with drugs, there are many links in the chain to success, or failure. The clinical trials are not always favorable to herbs and other products of natural medicine, because those doing the research often times don't understand the field. You can't take some doctor in some institution who through a grant from the pharmaceutical industry looks over the data from poorly constructed clinical trials and comes to a negative conclusion. I'm not saying natural medicine is the cure for everything. The battles have to be judiciously picked and properly fought. You wouldn't fight tanks with spears, so don't fight a disease with a therapy that's equally bound for failure.

Supplements can be used for several reasons. You can take them for athletic performance or you can take them to alleviate the toxic effects of drugs. Typically, natural medicine products are most often used to treat an active condition, and for preventative medicine.

The supplements that exist to treat a condition are just that. They usually have noticeable results in the form of symptom relief in a reasonable period of time. For whatever reason, genetic, habitual, or otherwise, you and your body have been put in a position of compromised health. The goal of these products is to help your body to heal, and hopefully through dietary measures and so forth, not be revisited. This is a temporary thing, or at least should be. It does not make sense from a financial and logical standpoint to take these products for the rest of your life, assuming you are not addressing the underlying cause. The duration of the road to recovery depends on you and your provider, but in the end it is to be temporary; otherwise, you're treating it like a drug that just treats the symptoms. Let's take IBD for example. You may be taking probiotics, bug killers, mucilage herbs, fish oil, or something else that makes you feel better. But if your labwork has determined that the source of your IBD is a dairy or gluten allergy, and you still continue to eat that food, then you are only using your natural medicine for symptom relief. For the best results, it is best to complete your role in the process.

The second set of available products referred to earlier has to deal with preventative medicine. Realize that I'm making general statements here, which aren't a perfect model, but mostly hold true. These products are more often than not taken on faith. There may be an enormous amount of data to support the product, its mechanism of action, and its use in that state, but if you boil it down, you are still taking it on faith. For example, if you are concerned about developing breast cancer because it runs in your family, notwithstanding the fact that this factor accounts for a very small number of breast cancer cases, then there are products for you to help shuttle out the estrogens from your body. They have sound theories, and some decent data, but in the end you don't know. This is probably most especially true of antioxidants for general use. If you do not have an illness, and are looking for optimal health, antioxidants make great sense based on the data, but they are still ultimately taken on faith. Use natural medicine appropriately to get over or manage a condition, and to intelligently use for preventative medicine based on your lifestyle.

The long-lived Okinawans don't use supplements. But we know they reach their old ages in mostly healthy shape. In an unfair set of circumstances, they are living the ideal set of conditions in accordance with our genome, a set of conditions which few to none of us experience here in America. Use this book to modify your risk factors accordingly. If you live in the northern half of the country, or you otherwise spend a great deal of time inside, then I'd strongly consider vitamin D therapy. If you're a postmenopausal woman concerned about her bone health, and you have recently been diagnosed with osteomalacia, I'd consider a product with the appropriate amounts of vitamin D, vitamin K, and dependent on how far you're willing to adjust your diet, some other nutrients.

The smart utilization of natural medicine does not require you to be on a million products, it requires you to think through your needs. Beyond the supplements, never underestimate the power of good food and exercise. Supplementation can be overwhelming and confusing, which is why I have dedicated a chapter to its service.

The next four chapters are dedicated to conditions where extensive research shows support for the use of natural medicine. I will provide you with many scientific references published in the medical journals, the same journals in which drug studies are published. This is information you don't hear on the nightly news, but should. This is information being gathered at many institutions here in the states and around the globe by many reputable researchers. I am making available information for your consideration. It's up to you to act, if you so choose.

Chapter 3 Inflammatory Bowel Disease (**IBD**)

The intestinal tract is a marvel of evolution. It is designed to reduce nutrients to basic forms to be used by the body while not overburdening the inner workings with a high antigen load from complex proteins. The bacterial load, along with other good and bad bugs in the gut, is enormous. The fine line between an all-out immune assault on these bugs is miniscule. The fully intact gut absorbs what is needed by the body and rejects what is not needed, along with components we're unable to digest, while balancing the immune response. Inflammatory bowel disease (IBD) is a compromise in this balance. The prevalence of IBD is due to a combination of one or more of the components to be discussed. The two disease states that comprise IBD are Crohn's Disease (CD) and Ulcerative Colitis (UC). Although there are minor distinctions between the two diseases from an immunological and histological viewpoint, they owe their origins to the same set of general circumstances. I will break with the medical community and add IBS to this equation. Since IBS does involve inflammation, since it's involvement shares locations with UC and CD, and as it's so commonplace, then it will be included in this review. IBS shares it roots in some of the same seeds as the other two, although IBS owes its symptomology to more of the dietary component, with pathogens playing a role, and little to no genetic compromise as seen with UC and CD.

We must also consider the role of diagnosis. Between practitioners a diagnosis of IBS could be early stage CD or UC. Variability among providers is another reason why IBS must be included. IBS in its truest form, if there even is one, does not present with the extensive tissue destruction as in UC and CD, but does present with inflammation and other shared symptoms. From the viewpoint of the patient, the name of the condition is irrelevant. The patient simply wants to get better. Regardless of the series of events leading to the symptoms, and regardless of what the next set of complications may or may not be, the patient wants to get better, and the underlying factors and downstream complications are shared.

As you will discover, managing IBD through natural medicine is not a quick solution. It does require a patient who has "crossed the line". A patient who is fed up, has tried too many drugs, seen too many doctors, and is willing to do all it takes to tackle their IBD. I am so confident with my regimen that I challenge anyone in the modern medical community to participate in controlled trials comparing treatment protocols. I'm not talking about quick fixes, which can be the benefit of pain or anti-inflammatory drugs; I'm talking about long-term successful management.

Possible Causes

The cause of IBD for all patients is not the result of one single factor. There is no single IBD bacterium, there is no single genetic predisposition, and there is no single food allergy. It is up to the patient, with or without the help of a skilled provider, to identify the one or more factors in each case. This is why the medical community has not been able to encapsulate IBD into a pretty, wrapped package that's easily definable, and can be treated with one class of drugs. They would like it that way for their convenience and yours, but that just isn't in the cards. The practitioner in the world of modern medicine will, in all likelihood, prescribe a drug, usually a corticosteroid, and monitor your progress. This provider is not likely to entertain the concepts here in this chapter, since they don't have the time to perform their own research or don't have the willingness for a variety of reasons. It is up to you, the patient to implement the necessary steps to manage your own health care. The provider cannot help you on your hypoallergenic diet. That responsibility rests on your shoulders. The provider does not live with you day in and day out to gauge your symptoms in response to various possible offenders; it is up to you to evaluate as best you can. You know your body best. It is your health on the line. In the eyes of your practitioner you are but one consult in the course of a busy day, part of a busy week. In the spirit of the "I want it and I want it now" American mentality, they will give you a prescription that will likely relieve your symptoms for the time being, as opposed to the more complex and time-consuming process of getting to the root of the matter. You really can't blame the doctors of modern medicine that much, since they are in business, and they are giving you what you want. If they didn't, they'd be out of work. Symptoms are a roadmap to uncovering the root issue, they are not the root cause themselves. Listen to your body. In my experience, there are many patients who do not want to expend the effort required to uncover the cause of their ill-health, and treat it from a healing aspect, as opposed to a symptom-based modality. Find the cause of your problem, heal yourself, and do the best you can to avoid a recurrence in the future.

Simplistically speaking, there are but two possible causes to most cases of IBD, which assumes we rule out a psychological connection. They are pathogenic in origin, and allergenic/hypersensitivity in origin. There is a third component, that of genetic predisposition, which we'll also uncover. Although the genetic link is crucial for those who develop IBD, it does not explain everything. It's hard to properly estimate the percentage of Americans with IBD, but we know it's certainly not 100%. If dietary factors were the only factors, then accordingly everyone who ate the standard American diet would have IBD. This is clearly not the case. However, we also know that IBD rates are increasing with the "western" diet, but for those who consume a more primitive diet around the globe, which is more in line with our genome, IBD is virtually non-existent. We can assume that as we are the world's "melting pot", the genetic variability between those of us here in the states, as compared to those on "primitive" diets, does not vary substantially. Therefore, although a certain percent of these people will have a genetic predisposition to develop IBD when placed on our diet, they do not on their protective diets. As stated, for those of us here in the States who have gone on to develop IBD, we have a genetic weakness to various allergens, and/or pathogens. Let's take a look at the possible genetic links as we best understand them today.

These are the three pathways to IBD. The first pathway is exclusive to true IBS.

- Patient is born with a genetic compromise in one or more of the following components
- Mucus production
- Antimicrobial defense
- Uncontrolled inflammation (varies slightly between UC and CD)
- A pathogenic load within the GI tract either from acute exposure or lifestyle, which includes antibiotic use, results in pro-inflammatory dysbiosis.

- Inflammation results in tissue destruction, malnutrition, blood loss, pain, etc.
- Allergenicities may also be present at outset, or result from permeability.

Pathway number two mostly excludes genetic compromises of the epithelial cells, but must be considered.

- A food or chemical allergenicity drives an inflammation response.
- Chronic inflammation feeds a state of dysbiosis further complicating matters.
- Inflammation results in tissue destruction, malnutrition, blood loss, pain, etc.

Pathway number three is more of a true IBS, but can share a more benign allergenicity as pathway 2, or could have been misdiagnosed.

- A poor diet and/or pathogenic load within the GI tract either from acute exposure or lifestyle results in a pro-inflammatory condition.
- Inflammation results in diarrhea, constipation, pain, etc.

One of the underlying factors in IBD may be a lack of breast-feeding our infants. This results in the early exposure of complex proteins to an immature GI tract, and/or the chronic exposure to a diet that is not in accordance with our body's genetic make-up. The good news is that management of your IBD is possible if you just consider these problematic proteins. As much complex science that surrounds this field, the solutions are quite simple. They are not found in a pharmacy as evidenced by the fact that primitive diets don't demonstrate IBD prevalence. So what are the general steps?

- Reduce inflammation and work to identify cause of inflammation.
- Eliminate cause of inflammation.
- Kill pathogens.
- Rebuild GI tract during all steps.

- Embrace a diet and lifestyle that reduces chance of recurrence.
- Monitor and re-treat less aggressively as needed.

Now that you have the over-riding principles down, we'll attack each topic individually with proof of validity. This is the most current research in this field. Although future research may highlight some minor corrections, the essence of treatment is here, and it does work. Understandably, I cannot responsibly guarantee that it will work for all people all the time.

Genetic

Defect In Mucin

Mucus in the GI tract is mostly a good thing. We want to separate all the possible pathogens in the gut from the highly charged immune system a fraction of a millimeter away. Without that protective barrier, there would be more direct contact with numerous components of food, which can stimulate the immune system. When stimulated, an immune system increases inflammation. That's simply how it directs other components to actively kill pathogens. However, you don't need excessive stimulation, and its consequent inflammation, on a full time basis. The mucus also helps to move the food along the GI tract. Mucins are a subset of mucus, which are thought to be largely responsible for the viscous and elastic characteristics of mucus. Defects in mucin/mucus production have been observed in many studies.

One particular anomaly related to IBD is an <u>increase</u> in an enzyme that degrades mucus phospholipids which is at the heart of this thin mucus barrier. Several human studies have documented that the activity of this enzyme, called phospholipse A2 (PLA2), is elevated in the intestinal mucosa of patients with IBD. (1) Whether the elevation in this enzyme is caused from chronic inflammation, genes, or nutrient disorders is still unclear. What seems clear, however, is that this PLA2 is up-regulated in quantity, and at its potential sites of synthesis. PLA2 is normally present only in a certain kind of cell called a Paneth cell, but in IBD it seems it can be synthesized from epithelial cells as well. (2) Just as interesting, one of the drugs used to treat IBD, sulfasalazine, is believed to act by inhibiting anti-mucin PLA2 enzyme activity. (3)

Defect In Antimicrobial Defense

You're likely familiar with stem cell research and its controversy. Well, we have stem cells in the lining of our gut. The whole intestinal tract is lined with what's called epithelial cells, which fortunately turn over rapidly, and are derived from these stem cells. Gut stem cells can diverge into one of four epithelial cells. The most common are the columnar cells which are responsible for absorption of the nutrients we ingest. Another type, the goblet cells, produce a mucosal layer that coats the GI tract. Paneth cells, referenced earlier, secrete antimicrobial molecules to keep pathogens at bay. The last of the four, neuroendocrine cells, release hormones. Genetic compromises in the functioning of the goblet cells or in the paneth cells can contribute to the development of CD or UC.

As previously stated, the paneth cells produce antimicrobials for the defense of the gut. Paneth cells are rarely found in the colon, so this aspect would apply mostly to CD of the ileum, which is the end of the small intestine where Crohn's was initially described. In several trials, researchers clearly demonstrated a decreased expression of the antimicrobials produced by paneth cells in Crohn's patients. (4) This compromise in defenses allows pathogens to adhere to and invade the likely compromised intestinal mucosa triggering an inflammation response, which may or may not be controlled.

Another possibility is that the patient isn't making enough of these antimicrobial cells to begin with. If you recall, the stem cells can produce one of four different types of epithelial cells in the gut. There is a cellular signaling process that tells the stem cells how to divide. It has been shown in CD that the signaling pathway that generates Paneth cells from stem cells is reduced.

In the colon, a reduction in different antimicrobial peptides has been shown there by at least two studies. (5) An in vitro analysis showed that the microbial killing capacity from a CD biopsy was significantly lower than that of a UC patient.

In each example given, there seems to be a diminished capacity of the gut of a CD patient to kill potential pathogens. It's feasible that the continual chronic exposure to a pathogen results in chronic unregulated inflammation and tissue destruction. Interestingly, the case seems to be the opposite in UC. The expression of colonic antimicrobial peptides is off the charts compared to CD. It is possible that this increased response, coupled with other factors, results in the more extensive tissue damage frequently seen in UC.

It is uncertain as to the extent of involvement this antimicrobial defect plays in IBD. It is but one of a few possible genetic flaws one could inherit, predisposing one to IBD. Some patients may ultimately have but one, some more than one. The treatment principles are still the same. If your antimicrobial defense is compromised, then it will be supplemented with natural antimicrobials, the mucus layer refurbished, the gut replenished with probiotics, and a focused dietary plan should help to manage the weakness. If an increased antimicrobial response is your curse, as seen in UC, then we'll do exactly the same thing. We'll kill the pathogens naturally, which will reduce the need for your immune system to supply a highly charged inflammation response. We'll then refurbish the mucus layer, rebuild the GI tract and implement an appropriate diet.

Allergens

As I have stated before, and I will state several times in this book, much of natural medicine is the choice you make on which foods to eat and which ones to avoid. The disease manifestations of poor food choices cannot be illustrated any better than in IBD. Much of IBD can be traced to the foods you eat. Yes, I am telling you that it is very possible to treat and manage your IBD by simply avoiding certain foods, many of which you shouldn't be consuming anyhow. The concept that foods play a role in IBD is certainly nothing new. I can find references in the literature as far back as 1942.

One researcher considered that ulcerative colitis was often due to food allergy, giving the figure of at least 66% of the cases. The items he considered most responsible were eggs, wheat, potatoes, oranges, tomatoes, and--by far number one--dairy. He advised the use of special allergy-test diets in order to detect the harmful foods from the benign. (6) Another researcher noticed the allergenicity connection in the GI tract, and also recommended elimination diets. He obtained remissions in 10 out of 14 patients in one small study with these diets. (7) That's it. It's just that simple. If the cause of your IBD is a food allergen, then eliminate it. The likely offenders in descending order are; dairy, wheat, egg, soy, and other miscellaneous to include citrus, tomato, corn, and more. I know you don't believe it can be that simple, so let me show you more proof.

A physician by the name of Dr. Truelove published five very interesting and convincing case studies on the connection to ulcerative colitis and dairy. To summarize, these patients presented with sometimes very severe bloody stools, abdominal pain, and fever. After having noticed a connection to dairy, he excluded dairy from the diets of the patients. After some amount of time, which varied between patients, the colitis was resolved. Upon reintroduction of dairy, severe relapses occurred in every case. As I read his works, I couldn't help but feel the guilt this researcher felt as he re-induced terrible symptoms on these subjects. He didn't expect the relapses to be so severe, and so hard to bring back under control. According to his calculations, the odds of the dairy exclusion, and then inclusion again as a challenge with the associated improvement and consequent devolvement in symptoms were more than 1,000 to one. (8) In other words, according to statistics, his conclusion that dairy was the cause of the IBD would be wrong in one out of a thousand times. Said another way, we can definitively say that dairy was the cause of the IBD for these folks.

He also helped eight other patients, but seemingly did not have the heart to rechallenge with dairy. As cruel as it may seem, it is the rechallenge of the offender that puts the nail in the coffin on that allergen, helping immensely to rule out coincidence. The difficulty is that upon a rechallenge, the symptoms could take days or even weeks to re-appear due to the complexity of the immune system. This can make identification challenging, as many individual food items would have been consumed in that time period.

Numerous other clinical trials have gone on to link IBD with dietary allergens. In an IBS study, a three-week dietary exclusion diet was implemented for 189 subjects. Three weeks is not a long time, considering inflammation could take longer to resolve. In any event, 48% (91 subjects) showed symptomatic improvement. In a subsequent re-challenge of foods, 73 of the 91 responders were able to identify one or more food intolerances, with dairy and grains leading the list. (9) The category of grains includes wheat. The whole anti-gluten fad now is big business because of IBD and other conditions.

In yet another trial, 33 patients with Crohn's disease were studied to see if their symptoms were related to food intolerances. The initial treatments used to produce remission of symptoms were total parental nutrition (feeding tube), elemental diet (powdered food with no proteins) or an elimination diet. 29 of the 33 reported specific food intolerances, with wheat and dairy topping the list. 21 of these subjects remained in remission on diet alone, on average out to 15 months. (10) This further shows you that as I've said, natural medicine has just as much to do with what you ingest as it does with supplements.

As much evidence as there is to implicate food allergens, there is essentially none for chemical allergens. By chemical allergens I am implying preservatives, additives, and other man-made chemical ingredients added to your food. These chemicals serve to help big business sell you more of their products, whether it's via longer shelf life, better taste, addicting taste, or more. You usually hear about these chemicals and their purported effects on the body outside the GI tract, such as neurological function. Although these dermatological, respiratory, and other connections are very real, the chemical connection to IBD has not been addressed.

In this book I want you to walk away with several concepts. I want you to play a larger proactive role in your own healthcare. I want you to optimize your healthcare dollar. I want you to recognize the absolute importance diet plays in your health, and I want you to recognize that natural medicine does offer some excellent treatment options, especially when implemented from a multi-faceted approach. I want the IBD patients to walk away with one very important concept as well. *Although it is not discussed, although it is not in print, there may very well be a chemical connection to your IBD*. You heard it here first. I have been telling people for years of this possible connection. I have seen it in person after person, patient after patient. I am acutely aware of this connection for one special reason: I lived through it. I suffered for years from chemical sensitivities, and I still do. I'll never know if the initial insult to my system was chemical, pathogenic, or allergenic from foods, but the most severe and most recognizable connection to my Crohn's disease was without a doubt in the world, that of chemicals. I just want you to recognize that this connection is possible, and the only treatment for chemical hypersensitivity is avoidance. The best way to approach this obstacle is just like that of the others, and it is a hypoallergenic diet that you prepare from scratch. If you cook with only whole foods, and with processed foods that contain ingredients you can pronounce, you will make marvelous progress.

The only other supporting evidence I can find is a paper from the Inflammatory Bowel Disease Center at Albany Medical College. They state in a paper on treating IBS, published in 2007, that foods and beverages eaten consumed in restaurants will cause problems due to sauces, spices, and hidden ingredients. I couldn't agree more. As an aside, although some spices such as ginger and garlic are anti-inflammatory in nature, and once you're healed should play a role in your diet, in an inflamed state they can be irritating in nature. They go on to list the following items as causes for IBS symptoms.

1. Dairy products
2. Caffeine
3. Alcohol
4. Fruit
5. Spices
6. Sugar free products
7. Fast food and Chinese
8. Fried foods
9. Condiments
10. Breads
11. Extra salad ingredients
12. Corn
13. Gravies
14. Artificial flavors, preservatives, and sweeteners

I like the work they're doing, their conclusions, and their philosophy. As you can see, chemicals are hidden in many of these foods. Your average IBS/IBD patient may only have issues with two or three of these items, but those items can be everywhere. They did not list soy and egg, which are suspects and are ubiquitous in our foods, along with corn and wheat. Chemicals are hidden in almost every processed food, and in many restaurant foods, like chicken, mashed potatoes, beef, and more, that you wouldn't normally associate as processed. That's because most of your restaurants don't have cooks, but have re-heaters of food. The bulk of the foods are processed elsewhere, and the local chain location re-heats many food items to order. A meal regimen which has you preparing as much of your food from scratch as possible is your first step. You must first eliminate the offenders, kill pathogens and then heal the gut. You can slowly rechallenge as described below. You then need to allow months to go by to even consider a re-challenge with the identified offenders to allow the antibodies to be flushed out, particularly for food allergies. In many cases, particularly food chemical allergies, you may always carry that response.

Pathogen

A review paper published in 2008 looked at the relationship between Crohn's and a bacteria you've probably never heard of before, Mycobacterium Avium Paratuberculosis (MAP). Yes, this bug is a member of the tuberculosis genus, but is a bit different. It causes a Crohn's-like disease in cows and other ruminants know as Johne's Disease. There is much more about this in the dairy chapter. After decades of debate as to the connection, we still haven't progressed very far with a final conclusion with which everyone can agree. Of course, it's a rare set of research-birds that can agree on everything. In this paper, the researchers found that there is a strong association between the MAP bacterium and Crohn's disease. (11) Before you run out to get your MAP test done, know that it does not exist commercially, but probably should. Infection from dairy cows is a real issue. However, research has also found that many people without Crohn's (or IBD) have cultured positive for MAP. So this is not a clear-cut scenario.

With this, we find ourselves with evidence to suspect no single pathogen. In fact, other suspected pathogens as causative factors for IBD include E coli, Campylobacter, Clostridium, Salmonella, and many more. In my opinion, non-allergen based IBD is the ramped up immune response gone out of control responding to an invader, or set of invaders. The invaders don't even have to be normally considered highly pathogenic. IBD results from a genetic compromise in the immune functioning of the GI tract, which explains why some MAP positive subjects have IBD, and some don't. The fact that MAP is served up with dairy, the most highly allergic food available is simply a double-whammy on many patients, which is why there is so much evidence against dairy.

Defining the exact residents of the gut, which is a dynamic environment, is possibly a waste of time. Even with today's advanced technology, up to 60% of the gut microbiota has not yet been cultivated in the laboratory. (12) The driving force behind the pathogen-induced inflammation may or may not be due to one bug. It may be the result of a whole colony of bugs, which on average are creating a toxic environment that the genetically compromised IBD patient isn't quite capable of managing. For example, one study looked at E Coli strains in the ileum of Crohn's patients. There are a number of E Coli strains, in addition to the one you associate with food poisoning. It was found that in tissue from controls and CD patients, none of the E Coli strains were of the virulent form. Of the ones they did find, those E Coli strains acted more destructive in the tissue of the Crohn's patient than they did in that of the controls. (13)

In a recent study from 2007, researchers took 190 tissue samples equally from CD and UC patients, and compared them to controls. Their results confirm the results of other studies, as well as general clinical observations. Although they showed a significant difference in the bacterial composition of CD/UC patients as compared to the controls, they failed to identify any one species as a "marker" indicative of the disease. (14) The fact remains, that whether your IBD is primarily caused by a pathogen, or your dysbiosis is a secondary development, there is no "one bug fits all" rule. If you consider the potential virulence of MAP, if infected, then that could be the primary pathogen. If you have suffered from traveler's diarrhea in the past, then that bug could be the primary pathogen. If you acquire another bug from another course, then that could be the primary pathogen. If you have a poor diet, and consequent dysbiosis, then a general pathogenic overload could be the cause. Gut pathogens play a significant role in the development of IBD, regardless of their chronology, and your gut flora must be corrected and likely monitored down the road.

We know the importance of bacteria, specifically from animal data. Animals bred with a disposition to develop IBD fail to develop the disease in a germ-free environment. Studies have also shown that pretreatment with an antibiotic prevents IBD in animals administered a drug to cause the disease. (15) In humans, it has been shown that bacteria that produce a toxin called hydrogen sulphide are seen in larger numbers in UC patients. (16) The significance of this is that this toxin reduces butyrate metabolism in the epithelial cells of the colon. (17). Butyrate is a short chain fatty acid produced from carbohydrate fermentation, and is the primary fuel source for these cells, followed by glucose. In addition, butyrate appears to play a significant role in stimulating mucus production. (18) Putting it all together only makes more sense when you realize that the thickness of the mucus layer is reduced in UC patients. (19) Mucus plays an important role in Crohn's as well. In fact, a defective butyrate metabolism was first proposed as a causal factor in IBD back in 1980. (20) So as you can see from this dense paragraph, pathogenic bacteria can reduce the mucin layer, and also reduce the primary fuel for the cells that line your intestinal tract. This is a bad combination, especially should you have a genetic flaw. We know there is no single factor responsible for IBD, but this particular one may play a role, a role with even more significance in UC specifically.

We know the value of mucus production in the treatment of IBD from a series of supplements. Three different herbs called mucilage or demulcent herbs are used extensively and with great results in IBD. These herbs are marshmallow root, slippery elm, and DGL. The administration of butyric acid itself has shown respectable results. In effect, the fuel is provided to the colonic cells to stimulate the production of mucus. Equally impressive is the administration of phosphatidylcholine, which supplies much of the raw materials needed for the colonocytes to produce the mucus. All are effective, but do not get to the root of the issue, which is an unhealthy imbalance in the intestinal flora. There must be an environmental shift in the flora of the gut, and concomitant supplementation used to coat the inflamed GI tract as well.

Uncontrolled Inflammation

Inflammatory markers are greatly increased in the colon, serum, and stools of patients with IBD. There are many components to inflammation, but the underlying principle is that the immune system is using inflammation to kill a perceived pathogen. Short-term inflammation is not a bad thing; in fact, it's a good thing. When you catch a viral illness, your body responds with a robust immune assault. It is the inflammatory components that in part serve to kill the pathogen. The fever you run from your immune response is a consequence of inflammation. Many people treat a high temperature with pills to bring it down, but that only likely increases the time needed to kill the bug. The body knows how to kill the virus, and you need that high temperature. Unfortunately, in cases of chronic inflammation like rheumatoid arthritis and IBD, the inflammation is destructive. Something has gone wrong. A deficiency, antibiotics, diet, and more can throw off the body's natural processes. Ideally, we want to control inflammation. We want to ramp it up in the first moments we know an illness is upon us to avoid being sick, and conversely we want to minimize it at virtually all other times to delay the aging and deterioration of body processes.

We will focus on compounds known as cytokines. There are many different ones, and I will not torture you with listing them. I will mention a handful, and the importance in controlling them. Cytokines are small proteins mainly produced by the immune cells that are involved in communication, proliferation, and inflammation. There are many immune components present in the GI tract residing the tiniest fraction of an inch away from foods in the gut. A compromise in the mucus layer in the gut can put the immune system in direct contact with bacteria, fungi, and complex proteins you have ingested. A normal immune system will reel in an assault on these "invaders", but in IBD the immune response is not normal. It has been theorized and shown that IBD patients have a ramped-up immune response that is stuck on "go". There is a lack of "braking" being applied by the innate nature of the immune system. It is this out of control inflammation that is responsible for so much tissue damage.

One such proposal is dysfunction of the gp180 glycoprotein. The gp180 is a molecule on normal intestinal cells that appears to play a role in suppressing the immune response. It's basically a parent in the room with kids saying, "enough already". Studies have shown in UC and CD that there are alterations in the capacity of this molecule which leads to a loss in the capacity of the gut to halt inflammation. (20) This defect doesn't cause the disease, but a trigger such as tainted third-world water or another haven for bacteria will start the process. The differences between UC and CD can in part be explained by the fact that the distribution of this defect is different, as it varies between the two conditions, likely from genetic predisposition. The trigger, the compromised mucus, and the lack of control over inflammation are still the same.

In a review of cytokines involved in UC and CD, the researchers broke down the differences in the destructive immune response. Although there were differences, there were also similarities. The reasons behind the differences in cytokine activity can only be speculated upon at this time, but it is likely a genetic component. Fortunately, that doesn't matter too much if you correct the underlying situation. Two cytokines, TNF-alpha and IL-6, were up-regulated in both disease states. (21) This has been observed by other researchers as well. It makes sense, since TNF-alpha exerts its pro-inflammatory effects in part through IL-6. In fact, TNF-alpha is to a large degree the master regulator of the inflammation process. Control TNF-alpha, and you can do a decent job of controlling the downstream inflammation cascade. Corticosteroids only treat one aspect of that downstream cascade, but other drugs are designed to target the TNF-alpha itself.

Anti-TNF therapy has shown some impressive results in the clinical data for both UC and CD. In essence, the inflammation switch has been turned off to a large degree. Remission, steroid discontinuation, and healing of ulcerations occur in relatively quick fashion. However, about 30% of patients have no response to Infliximab, (a prevalent anti-TNF compound) and not all responders have a complete response. (22) The safety of Infliximab also remains a significant concern because of its potential for causing serious adverse events, such as tuberculosis, non-Hodgkin's lymphoma, and other malignancies, as well as death. (23) Anti-TNF therapy has also been used with success in the treatment of rheumatoid arthritis, illustrating the inflammation connection.

Steroids are concerning as well. Before you begin taking steroids for your IBD, or if you're already on them, you should be aware of some of the data, as should your provider. There is data from more than one source showing that in a significant percent of IBD patients treated with steroids, the need to use the drug may accelerate the course to surgery. In one trial, 171 Crohn's patients diagnosed between 1970 and 1993 were followed to determine the progression of the disease. Although only 43% ever took steroids, only a third of those who responded well to the drug still had a positive response at one year. More striking, 38% of those who opted for steroids went on to surgery at one year. (24) For those of you who elect to undergo steroid therapy for IBD, note that it doesn't work for everyone in the short term, and it works for even fewer in longer time intervals. These numbers are also in line with a published Danish study.

It's not that the steroids are necessarily accelerating the disease itself, although I don't rule that out entirely, but that the deterioration in condition "necessitating" their use implies you may have little time to properly treat the underlying cause. In other words, as you mask the symptoms, your actual condition results in more and more tissue destruction as time passes. It's akin to both osteoarthritis and rheumatoid arthritis in regards to the use of NSAIDs. We know NSAIDs reduce the pain temporarily, but they contribute to the disease state in the long run.

This steroid connection also demonstrates that they are not the magic bullet. Although they <u>may</u> be of help for <u>some</u> in the long term, their short-term use may only be warranted when other options have failed. Although there is some data to support their widespread use, and they are used extensively, researchers state in a comprehensive review of vast sums of clinical data on treatment for IBD that, "<u>The overwhelming evidence does not support the use of corticosteroids for maintenance of remission.</u>" (25)

Here is another similar example showing the lack of efficacy and durability of steroids. In patients having no previous history of steroid therapy, 41% achieved remission after 17 weeks, while only 23% had remission at two years. (26) Once again, short-term "success" is higher than long-term. Steroids are limited in their capacity since they only block one of the inflammatory pathways, that of the COX-2. This is the same pathway VIOXX was targeting, but it is still downstream from the master controls.

In addition to the aforementioned corticosteroids and anti-TNF drugs, there are other immuno-modulating drugs available through your provider. These all work by trying to reduce the inflammatory response in one way or another. They have their limitations in success, durability, cost, and side effects. The connection to inflammation in this process is without question, which is why one of the main components of this regimen is to eliminate the cause of the inflammation in the first place. Another one of the goals is to accomplish the anti-inflammatory results through the use of herbs, just as these drugs did, but without the harmful side effects.

As if the IBD patient wasn't aware of a hyped-up inflammation response in the gut, I have more data to connect IBD to inflammation. In another study, 79 patients with CD were given anti-IL12 (another cytokine) therapy versus placebo. The drug group demonstrated a positive response in 75% of the patients, whereas only 25% in the placebo group had such a response. (27) In yet another inflammation connection, patients with active CD were treated with anti-IL-6 therapy. 80% of the patients in the full-dose group responded positively to therapy, while only 31% did so in the placebo group. (28)

Treating inflammation is all well and good, but it's like putting out forest fires after someone has gone around the dry brush with a flamethrower. Let's water the brush instead, and/or take away the flame thrower. That's what this protocol strives to achieve.

It may surprise you that 31% of the patients responded well on placebo in the latter aforementioned trial. For various reasons, IBD patients can go into remission on their own for a period of time.

Temporary remission may not be a hard thing to accomplish for some. The trick is to <u>stay</u> in remission and manage your IBD flawlessly, or as well as possible, and to do that without toxic side effects. That's what this program is geared to do.

IBS

We'll dedicate just a bit to IBS since most of this chapter is dedicated to its more severe cousin, IBD. IBS is characterized by abdominal pain, likely with distension and bowel dysfunction, usually alternating between diarrhea and constipation. IBS is the most common gastrointestinal disorder and represents 30-50% of all referrals to gastroenterologists. (29) Think of IBS as a weaker form of IBD with its roots in the same factors of diet and pathogens. The dietary component likely has two prongs. One is that of allergenicity, and the other of simple diet quality, or lack thereof. For example, one study from 1982 found that specific foods provoked symptoms of IBS in 14 of 21 patients, and 6 were confirmed on re-challenge of the offending food. (30) The allergen may not just be a food, but may also be a chemical. This diet is likely high in sugar, dairy, and low in fiber.

In both cases, inflammation, possible tissue damage, and pathogens must also play a role in the treatment process. Once again a multifaceted approach must be taken. We must identify the root cause, treat, heal, and prevent in the future. In the case of a pathogenic origin, the GI tract can become destabilized and tissue destruction directly via pathogens or by inflammation may result in GI permeability, also known as "leaky gut". Leaky gut allows larger molecules, usually proteins, to bypass the intestinal disassembly process and enter into the bloodstream more or less intact. The systemic immune system figures these foreign bodies to be pathogens, and unleashes an assault, with subsequent antibodies. A result may be the development of a food allergy that may have not initially been present. Acute infections can induce IBS symptoms for as long as nine months and up to a year. (31) The end result is still chronic inflammation where the GI tract has unlikely been given adequate time to heal. In an inflamed state, hypersensitivities to spices, chemicals, and other food constituents may result in pain, cramping, diarrhea, gas and more.

In the case of a food or chemical allergy, the road traveled looks much the same. The allergy causes its inflammation response, with tissue destruction, and likely gut permeability as well. Additional allergenicities can be piled up on top of the first, as well as dysbiosis within the gut. The dysbiosis will feed its own set of inflammatory conditions, create its own toxins, and could also invade the rest of the body. Regardless of the cause, the same set of conditions are quite possible in most IBS patients, depending on how long they've been symptomatic.

The other possible root for IBS is simply non-allergic dietary in nature. We know that sugar slows down intestinal motility, which is the rate at which gut muscles contract to move food through your GI tract. Assuming simple sugars are eaten, which is pretty much the norm here in America, the body reads the instant supply of glucose in the blood and tells the GI tract to "hold up". In fact, white bread, which is a dead fiberless hunk of nothing for food, has been traditionally used to treat diarrhea under that same mechanism. Another component causing constipation is a low fiber diet. Fiber does many things within the GI tract that are of huge benefit to you. One benefit is to create bulk to stimulate GI motility. You don't want your foods to spend too much time inside the body, since toxins are a nature of the beast, and too much exposure is probably a recipe for colon cancer, just to name one possible negative effect.

Traditionally, the most commonly "prescribed" products used for true IBS within the natural world are probiotics and fiber. These are helpful, but only partial in their solution. If in the end you don't change your eating habits, then these products will be treated like drugs in the notion of just treating symptoms. Probiotics are a wonderful thing, so wonderful that I have dedicated a chapter to them. However, if you throw them down the hatch into a difficult environment, you're not giving them a fair chance. It's kind of like fielding a football team with only nine players, and tying lead weights around their ankles. The IBS patient very likely has dysbiosis. The cause could be from an acute infection, or poor dietary habits and antibiotics, which have shifted the gut flora to a more toxic environment. Probiotics will kill some of them, but if the diet is unchanged, the rate at which the "bad guys" can reproduce will be greater than the rate at which your wallet can keep up. You have to kill the bad guys, change the diet, and then repopulate with good guys.

As far as the fiber goes, you have to be concerned about the source. Many people resort to supplemental fiber products. However, if the source is wheat, which is quite likely the case, and if the root of your IBS is a gluten sensitivity, then you're up the creek. Save your money and get your fiber through a proper diet. You'll have plenty of other supplements to buy, so spend your money on your needs not easily filled from regular foods. Get fiber from eating everything you know to be healthy. Fruits and vegetables should comprise a significant portion of your diet, not dairy, fries, and white bread. It sounds like a fast-food avoidance program. Well, it is. Given all the health problems we have in this nation, and the fact that we know fast food to be detrimental to our health, I find it amazing and concerning that in 2008, the year of the great economic slow-down, McDonalds stock ended the year higher than it started.

Just as in the rest of this chapter, antimicrobials, gut restoration, and a hypoallergenic diet should all play roles in your road to recovery from IBS. If I asked you if your heart was more important than your brain to the preservation of your life, you'd tell me that it doesn't matter since the removal of either has the same result. The same is true for this protocol. Unfortunately, many people are willing to take the pills, but not change the diet. With this in mind I'll provide you with a well-phrased excerpt from Richard MacDermott MD, published in 2007 in the journal *Inflammatory Bowel Disease*. This should help to encapsulate much of what I'm trying to relay to you in order to help convince you of the value of this entire protocol.

"The cause of many of the GI symptoms in patients with IBS is food and beverage intolerance. That is, the most important factor in the cause of symptoms in our IBS patients is what and how much they eat and drink. Therefore, the major problem with our current treatment approach is that <u>our therapy for IBS and IBD is based upon using medications to allow our patients to eat and drink what they want</u>. This approach for using medications for illnesses so as to allow patients to eat and drink what they want is not at all unique. We treat patients with statins for hyperlipidemia, we use antihypertensives for hypertension, and we use oral hypoglycemics for diabetes. <u>For all of these illnesses, significant improvement</u> can be achieved by diet, weight loss, and avoiding foods that we unfortunately love to eat, and believe we cannot live without. However, in our patient with IBS, the only thing the medications accomplish is keeping the foods and the beverages in the GI tract longer (referring to anti-diarrheal medications) where the foods and beverages continue to cause symptoms. <u>The stimulation of the GI tract induced by foods and beverages is much more powerful than the medications can overcome.</u>"

As further proof of a dietary connection, another trial from 1985 also looked at foods as a potential causative factor in IBS. They evaluated 24 subjects by means of IgE tests, dietary exclusion, and dietary provocation. In 14 patients, one or more foods or additives were shown to induce the typical symptoms associated with IBS. <u>The authors stressed the importance of finding a possible food causation, and stated that "dramatic clinical improvements can result from the introduction of an adequate exclusion diet.</u>" (32) Of importance to note is that these same researchers found that the presence of candida (yeast) within the intestinal tract seems to be of major importance, which leads us to our next section.

Downstream Problems and Dysbiosis

Antibiotics offer up a different treatment mechanism of action than do the anti-inflammatory drugs, and in fact it is one that is closer to getting to the root cause. As the name implies, antibiotics kill bacteria. They kill bad bacteria, and they kill good bacteria, but they only kill bacteria. So if you're immune system is up-regulated to attack bacterial pathogens, then antibiotics will help, at least temporarily. They will quickly do for the immune system what it's been trying to accomplish through inflammation, assuming the bacterium is not resistant to the chosen drug. However, the changes caused by killing both bad and good bacteria can set the stage for a yeast predominance. Also, if your pathogen is viral, it won't help. Additionally, it will not help to protect the lining of the gut or repair the gut. In time, as dysbiosis predominates, or a new acute ingestion of bacteria (think food poisoning) should occur, we're back to the doctor's office.

There are clinical trials that show a correlation between diets high in sugar, and lower in fruits and vegetables with the development of Crohn's. The consumption of these foods sets the stage in the gut for a poor balance in gut microflora, which is the good bacteria vs the bad. It does this in several ways with the inhibition of detoxification, and the supplying of sugar to fuel the bad guys to predominate. It is this pathogenic imbalance that may increase immune reactivity, ultimately resulting in an inflamed state.

The fecal bacteria of IBD patients has been found to be more pathogenic in nature than that of controls. This is a likely effect of flaws in antimicrobial defenses. If antibiotics are given, yeasts will proliferate, which are otherwise normal GI residents kept in check. Upon discontinuation of the antibiotic, bacteria will again multiply, but the ratio can be determined much by the health, or lack thereof, within the diet. In time, one can sow the seeds for dysbiosis, and in turn the pathogens can produce inflammation through their toxins or their cellular components directly. It is more likely that dysbiosis is the result of IBD, whereas an acute bacterial infection can be the cause. The continual inflammation within the gut, combined with the toll the standard American diet takes on the flora in the gut, will alter its composition. Again, it is likely that these IBD patients will have been prescribed antibiotics to help with the disease, an idea that's not all bad when done appropriately.

Candida cleanses and candidiasis are the hot topics of late. Relatively recent attention and acceptance has brought it into people's consciousness. For example, one possible cause for Chronic Fatigue Syndrome/Fibromyalgia is systemic candidiasis. You don't believe me? In April of 1989 the following was presented at the Chronic Fatigue Syndrome Conference. 1,100 patients presenting with symptoms of Chronic Fatigue, IBS, headaches, allergic disorders, and emotional disturbances were put on an anti-fungal drug with a no-sugar-no-alcohol diet for three to twelve months. 84% of the patients experienced a major reduction in symptoms. The program was so effective that in the beginning stages in September of 1987, 685 of those patients were on disability, whereas a year and one-half later only 12 were. Those little week-long candida-cleanse supplements you may buy won't do the trick. This stuff requires your complete participation.

As you can see, candida is not just limited to the gut, but can impact one systemically. This is due to the fact that candida will release toxins, cause inflammation, and essentially bore through the GI lining while also causing gut permeability, which creates food allergies. Depending on whom you reference, candida is capable of producing around 50 or more substances that our bodies find toxic. This is why the common symptoms of a systemic candida infection are not just digestive disturbances, but also include fatigue, allergies, immune dysfunction, depression, and chemical sensitivities. So how did this normal bowel resident become so pathogenic? We've previously touched on it in part.

The use, and likely overuse of antibiotics plays a significant role in shifting the populations around in the gut. Antibiotics do not kill yeasts. All of the organisms in the gut compete for residence at the mucosal epithelium, and for your nutrition. If you do away with bacteria, both good and bad, yeasts gain free reign. We've also mentioned sugar. Sugar is the primary fuel source for yeasts. Simple sugars dominate the standard American diet. Other causes give us insight into why women are eight times more likely to have candidiasis. Not only do they use more antibiotics than men, but their endogenous estrogen and the use of birth control pills are promoters of candida.

Beyond the fatigue and other previously mentioned symptoms, some more direct indicators can be considered. If you have thrush (yeast in the mouth), intestinal cramps, rectal itching, gas, yeast or bladder infections, or dermatological yeasts in the groin, armpits, or between the toes, then you might be a yeast hotel. If you have used a lot of antibiotics, birth control pills, or steroid drugs, then I'd think the same. I find it very interesting that IBD patients are likely to have been treated with both antibiotics and steroids, both of which contribute immensely to yeast issues. Another possible drug the IBD crowd may have been prescribed is anti-ulcer or anti-GERD medication. This too is a bad idea since the decrease in HCL in the stomach reduces one of the factors that keeps pathogens at bay. In fact, patients on anti-ulcer drugs such as Tagamet and Zantac actually develop candida overgrowth in the stomach. (33) As you can see this is all a viscous circle, which is why seeing the "modern" doctor can be of limited use since you'll receive a drug to treat one symptom, while causing another problem elsewhere. The body needs to be viewed holistically, and the root cause of the problem needs to be found and addressed.

Other considerations are foods high in yeast (although controversial), alcohol, and allergenic foods. Foods high in yeast, such as mushrooms, although perhaps not carrying candida albicans itself, may still contribute to a yeast dominant environment and have a synergistic effect. Alcohol, which is also a yeast product, further feeds the yeast. Dairy products are the best example of foods to not ingest with candidiasis. Lactose is the sugar in milk, and it is broken down into simpler sugars that can feed candida. Also, milk is a common food allergen that can create an inflammatory environment on its own. Milk may have trace levels of antibiotics, which can alter the bacteria balance, or, conversely, could have pathogens in it which could cause an acute case or contribute to dysbiosis. In addition, milk may have trace levels of estrogens, which are administered to the cows for production. All of these contaminants and more have been identified in milk.

So how do we treat dysbiosis, and candida specifically? Again, follow this regimen, and the dietary recommendations in the book. You can attempt to kill the candida with drugs or natural products, but if you do not change your dietary habits, then your success will be temporary. Luckily, the antimicrobials listed later will not only kill bacteria, but also yeasts. I recommend utilizing several different ones since there may be a resistance to one at some level. You will not totally eliminate candida from your body, but you can control it. The killing-off may take quite some time, and you may need to boost your immune system, but not before you've reduced inflammation in the gut by reconstituting the mucin layer. While killing the bad guys, you'll also need to rebuild the GI tract. This would involve probiotics, but not taken near the antimicrobials during the day. In addition, supplementing with HCL and/or digestive enzymes can help. The diet used to starve and kill the candida should be the same diet you use from then on to keep them at bay.

Treatment

Chronic inflammation, dysbiosis, bleeding within the GI tract, possible decreased food intake, frequent stools, and a poor diet will all likely lead to some level of malnutrition. Many nutritional issues complicate the care of an IBD patient. Malnutrition can weaken you in the form of anemia, reduce your immune system from a lack of zinc or other nutrients, contribute to fatigue from a magnesium deficiency, or more. The GI tract, as you are well aware, is responsible for absorbing the nutrients necessary for the body to function. It sounds simple enough, but when you complicate that with possible pathogens, inflammation, and more it becomes a challenge. Deficiencies in protein, fats, iron, calcium, potassium, B vitamins, zinc, vitamin C, vitamin A, vitamin K, and vitamin D have all been reported in hospitalized IBD patients. In the beginning of your treatment, you'll need some kind of nutrient supplementation, but even though iron deficiency anemia is likely, I recommend you gradually get that from the foods you eat, since non-heme iron is pro-inflammatory. The main goal at the outset is to eliminate the agent causing inflammation, and begin the healing process of the inflamed tissues. We do not want to pour gas onto the fire by introducing supplements prematurely.

I cannot emphasize the hypoallergenic diet enough. This is the primary key in the success of treating IBD. Hypoallergenic means a diet low in things likely to cause an allergenicity. This without a doubt includes chemicals as much as it includes foods.

Steps in the Hypoallergenic Diet

- Eliminate all dairy, wheat, corn, citrus, tomato, soy, and egg from your diet. This should cover most cases of food allergy. Look for these foods or components thereof, many of which are routinely hidden in other foods. However, we'll resolve that with the next step.
- MAKE YOUR OWN FOOD. Said another way, eliminate pre-made foods. This includes restaurant food too. The only way you can control for chemicals and food allergens in your food is to have control over it entirely. Prepare your foods ahead of time, such as for work, etc.
- Take a food allergy panel from a provider of natural medicine. This is not a fail-safe approach, but it could make the process clearer and quicker.

- Begin to add foods back one at a time at four to six week intervals, the longer the better. Begin with the least likely offenders such as citrus, tomato, and corn. Ultimately there's no need for corn, dairy, wheat, and soy in your diet anyhow.
- DO NOT EAT PREMADE FOODS AT ANY TIME IN THIS PROCESS! Although you will likely feel better between the food avoidance and the supplementation, you are not "cured". Don't think in terms of cure, think management.
- As time passes, you can begin to eat out. Avoid chain restaurants, as these foods are usually loaded with chemicals, since the people that "cook" the food for you are not cooks in the true sense; they are "re-heaters of food". Avoid soups, sauces, and anything complex (usually most appetizers) and you'll go a long way to controlling what goes into your mouth. If you do have a chemical sensitivity, you will learn which foods to avoid the hard way. Make a mental note and avoid that, and like foods in the future.

So what can you eat? I realize that dairy, wheat, and even corn and soy dominate the American diet. It is an unfortunate thing since we weren't even designed to eat those foods, as evidenced by our nation of sick people. They dominate our plates due to their economies of scale on many levels. There are still plenty of things for you to eat. Refer to the chapter on "Our Ideal Diet" and you will find a nutritious mostly hypoallergenic diet. Also, consider that although oatmeal does not cause gluten-based allergenicity, it can be cross-contaminated in a plant that processes gluten containing foods, which are wheat, rye, and barley.

Natural anti-inflammatory agents

Boswellia

Also known as frankincense, this tree is found in India, northern Africa, and the Middle East. Boswellia is an anti-inflammatory herb with good data in its support. Among other mechanisms, it specifically inhibits the 5-lipoxygenase pathway, which is a particulary inflammatory cascade of events in your body.

In one clinical trial in patients suffering from ulcerative colitis, the effects of a boswellia preparation at 350mg three times a day for six weeks was compared to sulfasalazine at 1 gram three times a day. 82% of the boswellia-treated patients went into remission as compared to 75% of the drug treated patients. (34) Sulfasalazine is one of several drugs in first line therapy for IBD, and although it can be effective for pain relief, it does have a number of side effects.

In another similar study, thirty patients with chronic colitis were split into one of two groups. Twenty were given a boswellia preparation at 300mg three times a day for six weeks, and ten were given sulfasalazine at 1 gram three times a day. 90% of the boswellia patients showed improvement in various parameters, while only 60% of the drug treatment group showed improvement in those same parameters. In fact 70% went into remission in the boswellia group, while only 40% did so in the drug group. (35)

In yet another trial, Crohn's disease was studied comparing a boswellia preparation to a drug called mesalazine. Mesalazine has fewer side effects reportedly than sulfasalazine. 44 patients were treated in the boswellia arm, while 39 patients received mesalazine. Results were determined by the Crohn's Disease Activity Index (CDAI), where a value of under 150 is considered a better prognosis. In the boswellia group, the CDAI decreased by an average of 90, while the mesalazine only reduced the score by an average of 53. (36) The authors concluded, "Considering both safety and efficacy, boswellia appears to be superior over mesalazine in the benefit-risk evaluation."

Fish Oil

One way to help reduce inflammation is to change the fatty acid consumption of your cells. The fats you eat get incorporated into the cell walls and other components of the body. You can alter your inflammatory response for the better by moving away from fats that increase the inflammatory response, such as from meats, dairy, and vegetable oils, and move to lesser inflammatory fats from cold-water fish and flax. This is one of the primary reasons why fish oil is good for us, and why it's so popular. Many disease states are associated with inflammation, and since fish oil can reduce that systemically, it had many applications.

Based on this premise, one trial from 1998 looked at the use of fish oil in the treatment of inflammation of the colon. Nine patients received fish oil and nine got placebo for six months. The researchers found that there was a significant reduction in the scores they used to determine inflammation and tissue damage between the two groups. (37) In fairness, I should note that the amount of fish oil used was a bit more than people are usually willing to take.

In another trial, 39 Crohn's patients were given 2.7 grams of fish oil per day for one year and compared to placebo. Just to let you know, 2.7 grams of total fish oil is very easy to achieve. After the year, 59% of the patients in the fish oil group remained in remission as compared to only 26% in the placebo group. (38) It should be noted that this marked difference was likely due to the fact that the fish oil was enterically coated. Much like you will read below for phosphatidylcholine, the goal here is to prevent their absorption in the upper GI, for use in the lower GI. In other studies, we do know that the fatty acids from the fish oil get incorporated into the mucosa phospholipids at the expense of the more inflammatory omega-6 fatty acids. (39)

In yet another trial, 18 patients with active ulcerative colitis finished a 9-month cross-over study. Cross-over means that they took turns being on placebo and fish oil. For the first four months half were on each, then they all took a month off (referred to as a wash-out period) and then "crossed over" to take the other pills for the next four months. The pill burden (the amount of pills taken per day) was fairy substantial. The fish oil group experienced huge drops in one marker of inflammation of the rectum, significant improvements in histology (tissue damage under a microscope), experienced significant weight gain, and were able to cut the dose of steroid therapy in half. None of these results were seen when on the placebo arm. (40)

In the spirit of full disclosure, I must inform you that not all trials on fish oil and IBD show impressive results. The bulk of the data calls into question the use of fish oil as a therapy for IBD. (41) It's not that fish oil made things worse; it's that in certain cases it may not have produced significantly better results. Honestly, I don't find this hard to believe. It's not that I don't think that it has a place in the treatment of IBD, but that its place is not near the number one position, and it may not have been used properly in the trials. My first point is that although stable fish oil has numerous anti-inflammatory benefits, its focus is on "downstream" agents such as some of the leukotrienes, prostaglandins, and thromboxanes. I'm sure that means nothing to you, so take from this that its effects are good, but it's only one piece of the puzzle. Second, as seen with the enterically coated trial, it must get to the lower GI to really be incorporated into the local matrix as opposed to being absorbed and used elsewhere in the body. Third, the dose may not have been high enough. Lastly, the oil may have been unstable, and thus oxidized. I really think the main points are the first two.

To take the fish oil correctly for IBD, several considerations have to be factored in. One, a mixed tocopherol vitamin E product should be taken at the same time. I don't care how stable someone tells you their fish oil is, it's still fish oil in a bottle. Fish is meant to be caught and eaten within a very close time frame. Those oils oxidize very easily under heat, light, and air. A timed-release oil would be better for IBD. I know of at least one that exists in the market, but I cannot speak to its stability. Seemingly the dose of total fish oil should be between 3-6 grams a day, which possibly offers up a lot of oxidized oil. Lastly, an added benefit would be to take phosphatidylcholine along with the fish oil to facilitate the incorporation of the omega-3 fatty acids into the cells of the GI tract. Speaking of phosphatidylcholine…..

Phoshatidyl Choline & Mucilage Herbs

The use of phosphatidylcholine (PC) is based on the premise that there is a dysfunction in the mucosal layer of the colon, particularly in UC, and that administration of PC would supply the raw materials needed to up-regulate mucus production. This dysfunction could arise from a genetic, pathogenic, or dietary factor. This premise is based on several supportive studies. Two such studies show that the mucus layer in IBD is thinner than that of healthy individuals. (42) This thinner layer of mucus combined with higher counts of pathogenic bacteria would create an inflammatory environment as the host's immune system up-regulates to do battle with the bugs in close contact, and who aren't dislodged by mucus flow. Further evidence is shown in another study that found anti-mucin antibodies in 18% of UC patients. (43) Yet more data in animals show that the administration of phospolipids (PC is a phospholipid) prevents mucosal damage induced by acids, NSAIDS, or bile salts in the stomach and small intestine. (44) Furthermore, PC itself has been shown to inhibit inflammation in induced colitis in other animal models.

The rationale behind the use of PC is that it is the main constituent found in mucus. It is of extreme importance that there is some mechanism to protect the epithelium in such a manner. In yet more proof of a connection, it has been found that both CD and UC patients have increased activity of an enzyme that can "break apart" the phospholipids. (45) The increase in these enzymes may come from bacteria in the gut. Just as H pylori (the bacteria that causes most gastric ulcers) has these enzymes, which in part allows it to nest itself in the lining of the stomach, so may other intestinal pathogens. This would easily explain why more bacteria are found in the epithelial cells of UC patients than in controls. The bacteria may likely use the stolen components of the phospholipids to build their own protective coating.

In a recent study from 2007, researchers looked to the use of phosphatidylcholine (PC) in the treatment of ulcerative colitis. 60 patients were assessed for 12 weeks, half took PC at 2 grams per day, half took a placebo. It was shown that 50% of the PC patients had clinical success as defined by the researchers as compared to only 10% in the placebo group. In fact the success was so impressive that 80% of the 30 patients receiving PC were able to discontinue their steroid therapy. They illustrated how their numbers were much better than those seen for the TNF-alpha inhibitor drug. (46)

A previous study in 2005 by some of the same researchers used a very similar format. 60 UC patients were studied; PC and placebo were given. The dose of PC was 6 grams per day this time, and the study lasted for 3 months. Significant clinical improvement was seen in 90% in the PC group as compared to only 10% in the placebo. The results were so profound that clinical remission was attained in 16 of the 29 PC patients.

In what matters most to the UC patient, improvement in quality of life was reported in 16 of 29 in the PC group as compared to only 2 in the placebo. (47) The factor in this equation, which lends itself to such an impressive success rate, is that the PC was encapsulated in a timed-release formula, such as used with other drugs. This prevents early absorption in the upper small intestine. We want the PC to be intact and make its way all the way down to the colon. Although standard PC does have its value, I am unfortunately unaware of any timed-release PC product here in the states. I theorize that encapsulating butyric acid in the same fashion administered concomitantly with PC would help in the epithelial uptake and production of much-needed mucus.

A later in-vitro (think test tube) study looked at PC and inflammation markers. Once again, TNF-alpha was in the spotlight. It's a good marker to analyze since we know that TNF-alpha is elevated in IBD and causes profound gut changes, such as increased GI permeability, decreased absorption, gene expression, and other damaging effects. Their results clearly showed that the administration of PC inhibited the inflammatory cascade of events triggered by TNF-alpha. (48) Beyond the timed-release consideration, there's another component to be factored. The data from this trial show that although PC inhibits inflammation, by its very anti-inflammatory nature it may decrease the body's effectiveness at killing microbes. Do not construe this to mean I'm disqualifying PC. This simply furthers my point that there must be a concomitant "bug killing" component to a regimen.

While discussing the usefulness of PC, I should mention its use for those who've had their gallbladder removed. Instead of possibly flirting with chronic diarrhea, you can use PC as well as enzymes and bile salts to aid in your absorption of dietary fats. It is akin to using enzymes to help with lactose for those who are intolerant. It's yet another example of how natural medicine can improve your quality of life, and perhaps save you some money in doctor's visits as well.

Three mucilage herbs are used extensively in natural medicine to accomplish much the same thing as the administration of PC. These herbs are DGL (a modified licorice root), marshmallow root, and slippery elm. Their use is well established, and quite successful. They may be used as a part of a larger regimen, or may be needed on a more permanent basis. For example, if your IBD is actually from a food allergen, then assuming you eliminate the allergen(s) from your diet, you may only need these herbs until you've reduced the inflammation and healed your GI tract. If your UC is caused by a genetic defect in mucus production then the need for supplementation may be more permanent in nature. These herbs accomplish much the same thing as mucus. In fact, if you were to take one of these herbs dry, and mix it with water, you'd find what for all intents and purposes is mucus. These herbs have wonderful soothing properties indicated for inflamed and irritated mucus membranes. These herbs are a must for IBD therapy in the inflamed state.

Curcumin

Inflammation reduction is important for IBD and more, as many conditions are caused by dysregulated inflammation. (49) Inflammation can be initiated by a variety of stimuli to include free radicals, mechanical injury, UV radiation, and more. We have discussed the pro-inflammatory cytokine TNF-alpha, which has implications beyond the GI tract. TNF-alpha activated other mediators of inflammation and degradation in other locations as well, such as joints. The resultant damage is lost cartilage, and potentially the development of or worsening of osteoarthritis (OA). As in IBD, anti-TNF drugs have been used in OA with some success, but serious side effects and a lack of complete response make these drugs less than ideal.

One of the common downstream targets mediated by TNF-alpha is an intracellular signaling agent known as nuclear factor kappa-beta (NFKB). (50) Upon activation, this NFKB goes to the nucleus of the cell and induces the expression of more than 200 genes shown to feed factors involved in inflammation and cancer. (51) The activated form of NFKB is so important because it has been found to mediate cancer, atherosclerosis, heart attack, diabetes, allergy, asthma, arthritis, Crohn's, MS, Alzheimer's, osteoporosis, psoriasis, septic shock, and others. (52) Curcumin (turmeric) has been shown in several studies to inhibit the intracellular enzyme that activated the NFKB. Curcumin and its connection to NFKB is so important, that to date over 1,900 papers have been published on curcumin. (53) Studies to date have suggested possible benefits in the prevention or treatment of atherosclerosis, cancer, neurodegenerative diseases such as Alzheimer's, pancreatitis, and rheumatoid arthritis. (54) In IBD, a number of mouse and rodent models show support as well. There are two published human trials that lend additional support.

In one study from 2005, researchers administered curcumin to five patients with UC and five patients with Crohn's. Nine of the ten patients reported improvement at the end of only one month, and four of the five UC patients were able to decrease or eliminate their medications. (55) In a larger trial, 43 UC patients without disease activity received curcumin at two grams a day plus a drug, while 39 control patients received a drug without curcumin. Only 5% of those in the curcumin group had disease relapse over six months while 21% of the controls had a relapse. (56) With curcumin's excellent effects on this inflammatory mediator, it is being reviewed for drug development, and in such dosing and tolerability trials data shows us that it is safe in oral doses up to eight grams per day. (57)

Relying on one medicine, whether natural or pharmaceutical in origin, is probably not your best recipe for success. If you trust just a fish oil, just curcumin, or just something else to resolve your IBD, then you may wind up disappointed. These solutions require a multi-factorial approach. The clinical trials will most often utilize just one compound because they are trying to control for multiple variables, and sometimes sponsor a given product. If a manufacturer is pushing a trial, they will try to demonstrate success with their one product, and success in clinical trials equals success in the bank. However, in these trials you will not usually see exceedingly high levels of success, just levels that are significantly higher than the control arm. In the real world, we don't care about anyone's profits, but are concerned about healing as many patients as possible. We'll use what we can at our disposal regardless of manufacturer. As a part of your protocol for IBD, or most any other disease, or for preventative medicine, I would think curcumin would be an effective and inexpensive addition worthy of your consideration.

Probiotics

Probiotics are of such value to the treatment of IBD and overall health in general, I have dedicated a chapter to its use. Enough said for now.

Vitamin A

Vitamin A plays a critical role in GI health. It's wide array of other benefits are unknown to most. In fact, it has undeservedly gotten such a bad reputation, that we go out of our way to avoid it. I have dedicated an entire chapter to vitamin A.

Bug Killers

To me, there are two herbal families of antimicrobials that stand out above the rest. One is that of the berberines, most notably barberry, goldenseal, and Oregon grape. The other family is considered a volatile oil. The most notable in this group are the volatile oils of oregano, peppermint, and thyme. The clinical data is packed with various uses for the volatile oils in food preservation and disease. Volatile oils have been studied extensively in their effects on pathogens such as staphylococcus, listeria, MAP, clostridium, candida, E. coli, salmonella, and more, in both human disease and food preservation. If its antimicrobial properties weren't of value, then why has it been studied in the preservation of chicken breast, sausage, ground beef, wine marinade, swordfish, and more?

When I say antimicrobial, I am referring to both antifungal and antibacterial properties in particular. There are many ingredients you may see on the back of products used for gut health. These all pale in comparison to the potency of concentrated volatile oils. One of the many beauties of having broad-spectrum antimicrobial properties is that unlike an antibiotic, which leaves behind pathogenic yeast, these guys take out everything. Yes, they are likely also taking out most of the good bugs as well. This is why timing is important in taking probiotics and volatile oils.

In a trial from Germany published in 1996, 39 IBS patients who all reported moderate to severe pain at the start of the trial were split into two groups. 19 received a peppermint/caraway oil pill while 20 received a placebo. After four weeks of treatment 90% of those in the peppermint oil group reported improvement in pain as compared to 45% in the placebo group. (58) The theorized mechanism of action was a combined positive impact on the smooth muscles that line the GI tract making them "less spastic," with an antimicrobial effect as well. Peppermint oils have a long history of use in IBS. Remember, there is likely a microbial issue in IBS, given a variety of dietary, drug, toxin, and allergen issues. These herbs are key in restoring gut health.

Berberine is a plant alkaloid with a long history of use in both Chinese medicine and Ayervedia (Indian medicine). Much like volatile oils, it has demonstrated its use against bacteria, viruses, fungi, protozoans, helminths (worms), and chlamydia. Its mechanisms of action include inhibition of bacterial enterotoxin, inhibition of intestinal fluid accumulation, inhibition of smooth muscle contraction, reduction of inflammation, and stimulation of bile. (59) All of these qualities make the use of a berberine product very valuable in the treatment of IBD. One could argue the merits and detriments of a stimulation of bile, since bile can irritate the lining of the GI. I dismiss this, as it will help with nutrient absorption, dose can be adjusted, it will kill pathogens, and the concominant use of PC or mucilage herbs should render any extra bile innocuous.

If you do not use one or both of the products in your treatment of IBD, I cannot guarantee your failure, however, I'd put your odds of success at significantly less than what they could have been. There are other natural based ingredients that have been shown to be antimicrobial, such as caprylic acid, garlic, Pau D'Arco bark, undecylenic acid, grape fruit extract and others. In my experience, and in accordance with the data, berberines and the volatile oils of oregano in particular have the most potency.

Others

Research has shown us that there are a number of natural compounds that can modulate inflammation. Products that utilize milk thistle, chamomile, quercetin, vitamin C, and ginger may be wonderful options or add-ons to your therapy. Butyric acid may be of mucin benefit. There are certain enzymes that degrade candida cell walls, thus more mildly killing off the yeast. Although there is data to support the use of garlic, ginger, and ginseng as anti-inflammatory herbs, I am hesitant in their use in IBD when symptoms are severe, and some data shows that they may up-regulate the immune system. The best example of the three for this unwanted immune up-regulation is probably ginseng, which is great as an immune boosting product, in addition to several other great qualities. I would side with caution in its use with anyone with a possible "autoimmune" connection, at least until symptoms are under control. Particularly since there are several other excellent options.

Green tea is another herb to consider in IBD, and for many other conditions. Resveratrol has some interesting data, which go beyond its famous life extension role. Resveratrol has been found in over 70 plant species, but is most famously known for its presence in the skin of red grapes. Although hundreds of papers have been published on diseases such as cardiovascular, cancer, and immunomodulation, none to date have been conducted in humans with IBD. (60) In actuality, most if not all of its benefits could be centered around its immunomodulation, which would control inflammation. Cardiovascular disease, cancer, and longevity all have inflammation in common as causation. So when we talk resveratrol for inflammation, we can infer its use in IBD. Several animal studies show significant promise for resveratrol in the treatment of IBD. Although I think animal studies can have some benefit, I like to reference them only as an adjunct to human data to further illustrate a point. You will not find a resveratrol product in the marketplace made exclusively from grape skin, as the cost would be prohibitive. It will usually be sourced from a member of the knotweed species.

Vitamin D is so important it gets its own chapter in this book. However, I'd be remiss if I did not mention it briefly here under inflammation and IBD. In numerous studies, the supplementation of vitamin D has been shown to have positive effects on inflammation. In one study, 2,000 IU of vitamin D per day for nine months was able to increase concentrations of the anti-inflammatory cytokine IL-10 and prevent increases in serum concentrations of TNF-alpha. (61) This is good stuff here, because we know the value of increasing IL-10 which acts sort of like breaks on the inflammation process, and we know the damage from long-term high TNF-alpha levels. It has been shown that a vitamin D analogue (think a vitamin D product that someone's trying to patent) was shown to inhibit TNF-alpha and its cascade of inflammatory markers in Crohn's patients. (62) In yet another Crohn's trial, vitamin D was shown to again increase the "good" IL-10 level significantly while down-regulating other inflammatory markers in an in-vitro study. (63)

In essence, we have covered 5 different "diseases" under the unifying title of IBD.

- Ulcerative colitis, which is likely caused by pathogenic dysbiosis in close contact through a compromised mucus layer, with a GI immune response showing a reduced capacity to halt its own inflammation.
- Crohn's disease, which is likely caused by much the same mileau of circumstances, just focused in a slightly different location. Its tissue damage varies from UC and is likely related to genetic factors.
- A food allergy, which causes inflammation, dysbiosis, and possible tissue damage resembling Crohn's or IBD.
- A chemical sensitivity, which can mimic a food allergy.
- IBS, which is more dietary in origin, has little to no history of genetic compromise, is less destructive than UC or Crohn's, and may be related to or caused by food or chemical allergies.

In this protocol, there is no reliance on a single component, whether it's an herb, a dietary exclusion, or a pathogen killer. They all work together for the best results possible, in the quickest fashion. These supplements should probably be a component of yours to help reduce inflammation, rebuild a healthy GI tract, and kill pathogens. Depending on the true cause of your IBD, you may have only so much time at your disposal. If you have IBD in its truest sense, with the uncontrolled immune response dominating tissue damage, then consider the following. It appears that the disease location essentially remains stable over time, yet the disease behavior evolves, such that <u>after 20 years at least 80% of patients with originally non-complicating disease progress to complication, either penetrating or stricturing in nature</u>. (64) In other words, if you don't so something to resolve your condition (masking the symptoms with drugs doesn't count), then you are likely headed for some serious issues. It's a matter of time. Should you go down the surgery path at this point, your odds of decent disease management and even quality of life diminish.

Natural medicine is perfectly suited to treat IBD. Considering that in many cases the initial cause is dietary in nature, then why wouldn't it be? In my opinion, modern medicine has little to no role in the treatment of IBD. The diagnostics and labs can be of great use, but I do not consider the drugs to be of long-term value, and they do not address or resolve the underlying cause. It then becomes a long battle of inflammation verses anti-inflammatory drugs. In the end, the drugs will lose. I repeat, natural medicine is perfectly suited to treat IBD. If you get into a car accident, do not see a practitioner of natural medicine; go to the hospital. This sounds so simple that it's stupid to mention, but then why is it that when the opposite is true, it doesn't seem like such a simple decision. Modern medicine continues to bring many life saving and improving qualities to our world, and we owe sincere gratitude to those who have brought us those technologies over the decades. But, like anything else in life, you've got to know your limitations.

Chapter 4   Bone Health

Typically here in America, we have this "mono-nutrient fixation" which hits us, by definition, one at a time. Currently you could argue that vitamin D or resveratrol are the big thing. A year or so ago it was the acai berry. In the coming years we can only guess. These single nutrient trends are a blend of science and marketing. Sometimes the science is reasonably valid, sometimes not, but there's always someone looking to make a buck from the perceived benefit.

As Americans, we adopt these mono-nutrient fixations and hope that by taking the next new thing we'll feel better, look better, and live longer. These fixations are easier and cleaner because the real truth is very complex and filled with debate. We are not single nutrient mammals; our bodies operate in a complex way that we still do not fully comprehend, with a complex interplay of ALL nutrients, and other factors as well. My hope is that you will come to appreciate this in reading this book, and be able to take in the information for yourself with an open mind, and come to your own conclusions.

There is no other single mono-nutrient fixation that can hold a candle to that of calcium. We have been immersed in the calcium trend for DECADES. We still are. In fact, calcium was the first nutrient approved by the FDA for the prevention of a specific disease. Calcium is the single most recommended and used supplement to this day. Why? Because it's the most prevalent mineral in your bones, and in your whole body for that matter, and by extension of reason, it should be able to prevent or at least curb osteoporosis. Right? Wrong.

If this were true, then after decades of taking calcium pills, and at the same time buying into the dairy craze, we should have next to no osteoporosis in this country. Well, guess what? We are no better today than we were decades ago. In fact, if you look around the globe at the nations with the highest consumption rates for dairy products, they do not have the lowest rates of osteoporosis; they have the highest. How can this be?

Osteoporosis

First, let's briefly look at the primary reason for calcium supplementation. Although calcium is required for such vital functions as muscle contraction, blood vessel expansion and contraction, blood clotting, secretion of hormones and enzymes, and transmitting impulses throughout the nervous system, and more, we typically solely focus on bone health. So let's do that.

At the time of this writing, here is some information presented on the National Osteoporosis Foundation's website.

We are familiar with the definition of osteoporosis, which is a disease characterized by low bone mass and structural deterioration of bone tissue, leading to bone fragility and an increased susceptibility to fractures, especially of the hip, spine and wrist, although any bone can be affected. In simpler terms, osteoporosis is a condition in which the bones become weak and can break from a minor fall or, in serious cases, from a simple action such as a sneeze.

Osteoporosis is a major public health threat for an estimated 44 million Americans, or 55 percent of people 50 years of age and older. In the U.S. today, 10 million individuals are estimated to already have the disease and almost 34 million more are estimated to have low bone mass, placing them at increased risk for osteoporosis. 80% of those who suffer from osteoporosis are women, which doesn't leave men off the hook, as by default 20% are men.

So let's discuss cost, since that's the gist of this book. On a national level, in 2005, osteoporosis-related fractures were responsible for an estimated $19 billion in costs. By 2025, experts predict that these costs will rise to approximately $25.3 billion. What's the personal cost in money, and in suffering? So let's get the real truth behind bone health, and uncover where we're going wrong.

Supplements

Bone health is a complex scenario. Like the other body functions we have seen, it is not resolved by just throwing one nutrient at the situation. Although the question of supplement is important, keep in mind that this is only one aspect to consider.

There can be a number of reasons why your chosen supplement is part of the problem. As any average consumer, you are not an expert in natural medicine. Guess what? The vast majority of doctors that tell you to go to the store and buy calcium pills are no more an expert than you. When in the store, many opt for the least expensive product, some settle in the middle, and few pick the most expensive. When it comes to the manufacturing of natural products, given that there is very modest oversight for this industry, cost may or may not be a good beacon.

One question to consider is whether the product breaks apart within the GI tract so that the active ingredient, whatever it happens to be, is ultimately absorbed. Good manufacturers will perform what's called dissolution tests on their products to test for just that. If you take a product with certain binders and other ingredients, it can potentially make this more challenging, which could mean you may not be absorbing the nutrient.

Another factor to consider is the form of calcium. For example, the cheapest form of calcium is calcium carbonate. This is also the same form used to temporarily "treat" heartburn in whichever antacid product you so choose. The upside for calcium carbonate is that by weight, it contains more of what's called elemental calcium than the other forms. So what does this mean? Well, if you somehow were able to extract all the other ingredients from the product, and were left with a mound of powdered calcium carbonate, 100% of that mound is not calcium. Only 40% is elemental calcium. The molecular structure of calcium carbonate is $CaCO_3$. So for every calcium molecule, there is one carbon, and three oxygens as well. When you look at the dietary guidelines for your age and gender, those guidelines are referring to elemental calcium. From this viewpoint alone, you may not be ingesting enough calcium, as the label may or may not distinguish between the two.

To complicate matters even more, there are other forms of calcium on the market in addition to calcium carbonate. Calcium citrate is perhaps the most popular of the other forms. Whether it's citrate, malate, or something else, the process is simply applying an acid, in this case citric acid, to calcium, and using that new complex. The upside is that you have a more absorbable form of calcium pill, which is very useful for certain people who we'll discuss in a second. The downside, other than cost, is that there is less elemental calcium per unit of weight, which will increase your pill size, or more likely your pill burden (the number of pills taken).

So it boils down to you understanding yourself. If you're older, and you take PPI's or H2 blockers (drugs that cut down on stomach acid for GERD/heartburn), then you may want to consider the calcium citrate form, as proper stomach acid is necessary to "activate" calcium carbonate. Another problem I continually see is that many bone formulations on the market are very limited, which can in part explain why we're no closer to a solution to osteoporosis after decades of calcium ingestion. Products may contain alone or in combination: calcium, magnesium, zinc, manganese, copper, vitamin C, and more. Bone requires many nutrients to be made. There are many nutritional co-factors (necessary assistants) needed to form bone faster than it is broken down as per the needs of the whole body. Many will argue magnesium is as important as calcium, especially as our standard American diet (SAD) supplies so little of it. Well, let me ask you: Which is more important to your survival, your heart or your brain?

More recently you'll see vitamin D added to formulations. Obviously vitamin D has received much attention of late, and I have an entire chapter dedicated to it, but let's not lose perspective on the whole body. Vitamin D enhances calcium absorption from the gut and increases the synthesis of osteocalcin. Osteocalcin is a protein that lays down bone matrix. Both of these attributes of vitamin D are very good for bone health, but possibly at the expense of calcifying your soft tissue. You'll be surprised to know that vitamin D is used in some rat studies to INDUCE soft tissue calcification. So let's not get too crazy with just vitamin D and calcium, as you may be helping your bone, at the expense of calcifying your soft tissue.

Calcium Exchange

Calcium balance in the blood is extremely crucial to our survival. The range in which it occurs is a narrow one, indicating fine control measures so levels aren't too high or too low. Some 99% or so of your calcium is in your bones. So bones serve multiple purposes beyond structural, and marrow, but also as a reservoir of sorts for your serum calcium levels. Through higher control mechanisms, osteoblasts (bone builders) and osteoclasts (bone destroyers) directly take or add calcium to and from bone for the rest of the body. There are a variety of factors, some debated, some accepted, that cause this bone remodeling to move in one direction or the other. It is these factors, following the development of peak bone mineral density in early adulthood, that result in a slow decline in bone health later in life. We'll briefly touch on sex-hormone balance and exercise; both have accepted bone health merits. We'll end by spending more time within the topic of nutrient intake as it relates to calcium balance. This is fairly hotly debated, where much confusion exists, and where special interests serve themselves at your expense.

Sex Hormone Balance

The reason that 80% of osteoporosis patients are women is that there is a clear link to bone remodeling and estrogen. Men have estrogen as well, and as men age, hormonal production will wane. Testosterone, which leads to muscle and bone strength when younger, is a fraction of what it once was. Progesterone, again made by both genders, is also significantly lower. But since most patients are women, and there is a clear increased risk after menopause, that's what gets the focus.

If you recall, many menopausal female patients have in the past, and less so today, been prescribed hormone replacement therapy in the hopes of preventing osteoporosis. Unfortunately, cancer and cardiovascular problems trump the prevention of osteoporosis, and this practice has been discouraged. It's unfortunate, as the drugs used in the trials were patentable hormones and thus more synthetic in nature. There are many who argue that what's referred to as bio-identical hormones, especially those that are administered transdermally, offer up vastly superior qualities. The sad fact is as these are not patentable, so you will see no long-term clinical trials to verify this, as trials are very costly, and there's no profit if you can't patent.

Within the world of medicine there are other "hormonal" options for you, as we know full well the benefit that estrogen has, especially for women. Some of these products target estrogen receptors, while another class goes right to the heart of the matter. As a loss of estrogen seems to activate osteoclasts, biophosphonates target those pesky bone-destroyers. According to the package insert for one of these drugs, the product works by inhibiting osteoclast activity. It makes sense; you inhibit the culprit responsible for breaking down bone. There's plenty of data to show that it does what it's supposed to do.

Here's where we enter into the world of trying to outsmart the human body with logic based on the limited information at hand with synthetic patentable products, which yield huge dividends. There are now lawsuits in motion as at least some of these drugs have been linked to avascular necrosis of the jaw, or what's more commonly being called "dead jaw". The whys and wherefores of dose, duration, mechanism, dental history, and more still need to be worked out, but my guess is that it has something to do with upsetting the fine balance of calcium deposition and removal to and from the serum. If you're taking them, or have only recently discontinued, you may not be able to get certain dental procedures done, depending on the dentist, so call ahead.

More natural approaches center around phytoestrogens. Phytoestrogens are plant based molecules that are able to connect to the estrogen receptors, but don't have the same power as endogenous estrogen. So when you hear of Japanese women breezing through menopause or suffering significantly less osteoporosis than their American counterparts, it may very well be IN PART due to their MODEST phytoestrogen ingestion. I say modest, as they do consume soy-based products, but they don't partake in the over-the-top soy craze with cheaply made, highly processed soy crap that we buy here in the states. Their quantity is lower, although this is debated as well, and their quality is higher. For more on soy and phytoestrogens I refer you to Kaayla Daniel's book, *The Whole Soy Story*.

I think it is quite reasonable to assume that you can find fine natural products based on phytoestrogens, whether from soy or another herb, at a dose that is reasonable, healthy, and efficacious. This can be done if you are health-savvy, or through a practitioner of natural medicine who specializes in women's health care (not hard to find), and who knows of what they are speaking (harder to find). You would be wise to consider your options, as there is plenty of data to show that phytoestrogens support bone health in post-menopausal women. Furthermore, they can do more than just help bone health; there are other great reasons, sexual and otherwise, to consider their use.

You have even more options with pregnenolone, DHEA, and the aforementioned bio-identical hormones. Some practitioners will gladly provide these, and some get cautious with them. If you choose estrogen therapy of some sort, it would be worth your while to research transdermal progesterone creams, which are sold over the counter and in my experience work very nicely. This serves to offset the estrogen induced cellular growth, which was first uncovered many years ago when estrogen only HRT was given to fully intact menopausal women and the incidence of uterine cancer went through the roof.

Exercise

This is the only section in this book dedicated to exercise. Not because it's of little importance, but for several reasons. First, everyone knows exercise is good for you, but even with this indisputable evidence, few people do it regularly. Why? Because it's hard work. It's easier to do most anything else other than exercise. This is why I often get questions pertaining to weight loss products. My response is usually, "Focus on exercise and eating right." Sure there are products that can assist the process, there are various diets that may work temporarily, but the human body is designed to eat a certain diet and get plenty of rest and exercise. Second, this book has become large, and although I'd love to add a chapter on exercise, I am reserving space for the third reason. Third, I assume you want to hear about research and facts that you have not seen anywhere else. You already know that exercise is good for you, but you probably have never heard very much about what I discuss in this book.

Since you want to learn about natural medicine, that's what I will present to you.

With that said, there is no doubt that exercise helps to build and maintain bone mass. Ideally you got plenty of exercise and a healthy diet as a child, so your peak bone mineral density is at its highest possible level, and you continue to exercise to maintain that bone health for the remainder of your long, happy, healthy life. There is much clinical data to support exercise's benefit on bone health. Ideally, your exercise program will include a weight-bearing regimen, but do what you can do, as much as you can do it.

Nutritional Intake (Calcium, Acid/Base Balance, Oxalates, and Vitamin K)

Calcium

You see the ads all the time. The milk mustache, the calcium added to everything, and even antacids advertising the benefits of calcium. We blindly believe these ads, and consume calcium at a phenomenal pace. One would reasonably think that we must be winning the war on osteoporosis, but we are not. Even though we consume high quantities of dairy, calcium fortified foods, and calcium supplements we are no closer to reducing the suffering and costs of osteoporosis than before all of this began. It only serves to line the pockets of people with a vested interest in how you spend your money. The striking fact is that if you look around the globe at nations, some of which are "third world", they have healthier bones than we do with much lower rates of calcium consumption. So honestly ask yourself this question: "Is there more than just calcium to this bone health equation?"

You've now read about exercise, hormones, and the variability in calcium supplements and how they relate to bone health. Immediately you can see that there's more than just calcium to the health of your bones. Yet, many researchers continue to look at calcium exclusively, determined to show its benefit. Some researchers control for such factors as hormones, protein, exercise, and more, while trying to either prove or disprove that calcium alone at certain intake levels is an independent factor in bone health. We need calcium for our health, but at what level, and with what other nutrients?

That's the multi-million dollar question. As there are so many complicated factors behind bone remodeling, it's very difficult to control for all of them in these trials. We'll look into a good many trials, and show results in both directions, which leads to the general confusion about this topic. Just keep in mind that from a simplistic biochemical view (acid/base balance) and from a larger epidemiological view (our national bone ill-health), what we are currently doing is not working.

We'll begin the debate with a look at milk intake and bone fractures in women. This makes sense, as women are targeted for higher calcium intakes, and the primary marketing message comes from the milk people. In fact, that was the basis of this trial. The authors state, "We focused our investigation on milk and dietary sources of calcium, rather than the use of calcium supplements, in order to examine the validity of public health messages and advertisements that advise women to increase their milk consumption for the prevention of osteoporosis." (1) Over 12 years they studied the dietary intake through 3 questionaires in 77,761 women who had never taken calcium supplements. They looked for fractures of the proximal femur (upper leg) and distal radius (lower arm). What they found was that women who drank two or more glasses of milk per day had about 1 ½ times the risk of hip fracture as compared to those who drank one glass or less per week, and a modest increase in risk for forearm fracture. They concluded, "These data do not support the hypothesis that higher consumption of milk or other food sources of calcium by adult women protects against hip or forearm fracture."

Food frequency questionnaires are frought with possible errors, but milk consumption is fairly straightforward, and that's the message to which we've been subjected. Also of note, calcium from all food sources was not a factor in bone health, whether the consumption was more than 900 mg per day, or less than 450 mg per day. I'm not advocating a no-calcium diet--it's clearly important to our health and well-being--my point is simply that calcium alone doesn't work. There are many other factors at play, and we need to be cognizant of them all. The reason why milk may have caused more fractures will be addressed in the acid-base subsection.

It's even theorized that calcium alone can increase the risk of cardiovascular disease (CVD). There's conflicting data on this point, with some studies showing that calcium may benefit those with CVD. With this in mind, New Zealand researchers in a recently published trial took 1,471 women with an average age of 74, and placed them on a calcium or placebo regimen for five years. (2) We're looking at a study with a large population taking place over a fairly significant length of time, a study built to look at cardiovascular variables. In their conclusion they state, "Calcium supplementation in healthy postmenopausal women is associated with upward trends in cardiovascular event rates." In plain English, calcium supplements increased the risk of CVD, as evidenced by more than twice the risk of heart attack and almost 1 ½ times the risk for stroke in the calcium group.

They make an important note in comparison to other short-term trials, which saw a reduced risk for CVD in calcium supplementation. What they say is that in the short term, roughly the first three years of calcium therapy, there's no obvious risk in CVD because it takes time to develop, whereas the longer you go on therapy, and the more compliant you are, the greater your risk for calcifying your soft tissue, notably your vasculature. The mechanism they note is how calcium supplements acutely, albeit temporarily, raise serum calcium levels, which can in theory imbed themselves in soft tissue. It's a reason to consider taking them with food, and with vitamin K in particular, as you will read later.

Instead of looking at individual trials, we'll now look at a few reviews or meta-analyses. These are research articles where investigators looked at as many relevant individual trials as possible to try to determine if there is a trend one way or another in the data. So in one meta-analysis published in 2006, the researchers looked at 19 studies they determined to be relevant for calcium supplementation in healthy children aged 3-18. These studies encompassed 2,859 children, who were given one of several calcium supplements, or placebo. Looking at bone health in children is important because this goes a long way to determining your peak bone mass, which is essentially a "start line" for you theoretical gradual decline throughout life. The more bone mass you pack on until the age of roughly 20-30, the better your starting position. Based on their extensive review of the data they selected, they state in the first line of their discussion that,

94

"Calcium supplementation has little effect on bone mineral density." (3) That's right, a review of 19 studies yields that finding. Surprising, isn't it? Just consider that we're looking at calcium alone.

In another review, published in the *American Journal of Clinical Nutrition* in 2000, two researchers looked at 57 papers that analyzed the intake of dairy and bone health. They state many times, as do many other researchers, that there are far too many variables to control for in any given study, particularly dietary analyses. For example, the food you eat may or may not vary by day, week, or month, as may your exercise, drinking of alcohol, salt intake, smoking, etc. They state the unequivocal truth that dairy foods have NOT been part of the diets of adults for most of human evolution, which is a simple common sense application to this whole equation. What they did find was that young white women may derive some benefit, but in a bit of contradiction they state, "The body of scientific evidence appears inadequate to support a recommendation for daily intake of dairy foods to promote bone health in the general U.S. population." (4)

In yet another review, an even larger one I might add, researchers again looked at bone health as it related to age groups where you'd hope to see peak BMD development. These researchers looked at the relationship between dairy products or calcium intake as compared to BMD or fracture risk in those aged 1-25. They conducted this review for reasons I will quote directly from their paper.

"However, because the level of dairy product consumption in the U.S. is among the highest in the world, accounting for 72% of dietary calcium intake, and osteoporosis and fracture rates are simultaneously high, numerous researchers have called into question the effectiveness of nutrition policies aimed at osteoporosis prevention through dairy consumption. Findings from recent epidemiological and prospective studies in women, children, and adolescents also have raised questions about the efficacy of the use of dairy products and other calcium containing foods for the promotion of bone health." (5)

They looked at 58 studies, controlling for factors that could skew the results. What did they find? They state, "Currently, available evidence does not support nutrition guidelines focused specifically on increasing milk or other dairy product intake for promoting child and adolescent bone mineralization." This trial was published in 2005 by a PhD, and PhD/nutritionist, and an M.D. in the journal *Pediatrics*, not some goofball radical publication. They found that physical activity seemed to them to be the PRIMARY modifiable stimulus for increased bone growth and development in adolescents, as many other researchers universally emphasize.

Their research seemed to point to low calcium intakes, roughly less than 400 mg per day, may not be advisable for bone health, but that intentionally increasing that to more than say 400-500 mg per day through dairy or calcium supplements in no way guarantees bone health either. They also "found no evidence to support the notion that milk is a preferred source of calcium," and that "calcium in dairy products is not as well absorbed as that in many dark green leafy vegetables."

That's the catch, isn't it? How many people eat calcium-rich green leafy vegetables, and other calcium-rich foods like broccoli? I'm not talking about one piece of nutritionally devoid iceburg lettuce grown on chemicals and wedged in between your hamburger and cheese, I'm talking about Romaine lettuce, kale, turnip greens, plus nuts, beans, and broccoli. These are the types of foods we evolved eating. The fact that we eat so few calcium-laden whole foods is in part why Dr. Robert Heaney advocates dairy consumption.

He qualifies his position with the relative fact that, "At a total diet level, it is worth recalling that the primitive human diet, the one that prevailed during the millenniums of hominid evolution, and to which our physiologies were adapted, had a high calcium density." Roughly 1,500 mg for a 2,000 calorie per day diet, which is fairly high. Of course this is estimated, as I'm pretty sure there weren't any dietary recall forms back then. The sources he references are vegetable ones predominantly, and bones and insects as well. But one also has to consider that a very large portion of the diet was meat based, and as you will learn in the acid/base section, that would require a lot of calcium to offset the acidity.

So he goes on to summarize that as we moved more towards and through the agricultural revolution, we left behind these dietary habits from which we evolved, which is also true. In fact, if you look at our ancient recorded history over the past 10,000 years, you'll be amazed at how small these people were in comparison to us, and to our Paleolithic ancestors. In any event, he also presents the caveat that we now generally eat low-nutrient foods, and we are essentially physically lazy, as we have machines to do our work for us, also all true.

His general premise is that since we do not consume the high calcium foods with which we evolved, our bodies require calcium from some source, and as dairy foods are high in calcium, that's the preferred source. In an attempt to justify this view, he reviewed 139 trials looking at the relationship between calcium and bone health. As I read through many of the papers he referenced, I found that a number cannot be counted as calcium-only trials as they were confounded with estrogen, exercise, and vitamin D intake. Still, that leaves many other trials to try to prove his point, just not 139.

One of his referenced studies with postmenopausal women showed that 1 gram of calcium a day only slowed bone loss as compared to placebo. (6) When this study was extended out another 2 years, the results were the same. (7) As seen in many trials, much of the benefit is seen early on, and then lost. A 2008 study in men increased BMD at 1,200 mg per day (8). This was the same research group referenced earlier who mentioned increased risks for CVD in those receiving calcium therapy, and who stated in one trial that "the potentially detrimental effects (CVD) of calcium supplementation should be balanced against the likely benefits on bone."

In another of his referenced trials, 80 white girls with an average age of 12 drank their normal milk consumption, or an additional pint per day for 18 months. (9) Both groups gained in BMD (9.6% vs 8.5%). It is of interest to note that serum IGF-1 (insulin-like growth factor) increased in the high milk-consumption group by 35%, and in the low milk-consumption group by 25%. By the way, the low milk group wound up consuming more milk than when they started, which may explain their significant rise in IGF-1 as well. As the authors state, "IGF-1 has a potent anabolic (growth) effect on growing skeletal tissue." A high IGF-1 may not always be such a desirable thing, as you will read in the chapter on dairy.

In the last one of the references for the argument that calcium alone can help with BMD, we'll look at a twin study, which brings an interesting new twist to things. Twin studies are helpful, as they help to rule out genetic variability. In 42 pairs, with an average age of 14, 1 gram of calcium or placebo was given for 18 months. As is seen in many other trials, there was an initial increase in BMD of about 1.5% above the placebo group, which was maintained, but no additional beneficial increase was seen after 6 months. (10)

In general, there can be some benefit in calcium-only trials, usually temporary. Other lackluster trials yielded similar results. A slowing of bone loss is good, but at what expense. What if you could increase BMD?

Bone health is much more complicated than just calcium intake. There are a whole host of variables to consider, everything from exercise, hormones/age, other dietary factors, and more. Most of the data pertains to females, and at best, increasing dairy or calcium via supplements in adolescent females may help, and in the case of dairy, partly by increasing IGF-1 levels, which may have far reaching undesirable effects. The simple fact is that today we know much more about bone remodeling than we did when many of these studies were done, but the sad fact is that this knowledge has not made its way to you, the community at large. The majority of researchers I've found, as per their own statements, see little to no value in calcium-only therapy, have concerns about high dose calcium ingestion, and soft tissue calcification from spikes in serum calcium.

In all fairness, it should also be noted that Dr. Heaney has had financial relationships with a number of companies. For example, General Mills and The National Dairy Council have given him grants for research, and he has worked for General Mills as an advisor/consultant as well. I think it's safe to say that these groups have something to gain by sending out a pro-dairy message.

When you hear conflicting nutrition and/or supplement news-clips from supposed experts in the media, they are just reciting one paper. Your information is only as good as your source. Researchers can cut and skew data, and build trials to sway one way or another to shoot for a desired outcome. I'm not implying any of the aforementioned researchers did this, as I don't know first hand, but I'm urging you to use common sense and consider your source. Don't abandon common sense because some ad tells you one thing or another. It's the old fallacy: "If you hear it enough, then it must be true." My friends, that's called marketing. To bolster your common sense with science, consider these next three very important sub-sections.

Acid/Base Balance

I know you will find this shocking, but there is plenty of debate within the scientific community as to the optimum acid/base balance in your body, how it may or may not relate to your bone health and other conditions, and which foods contribute to this balance. A number of culprits have been identified to play a role in your acid/base balance. They include protein (to include dairy), salt, soda, caffeine, alcohol, grains, and more. So what does this acid/base balance mean anyhow? In essence, you consume foods that result in a net acidic load within the environment in your body, and your body compensates by primarily releasing calcium from the bone in order to neutralize that acid load, as the body has to run within a reasonably narrow pH range.

What I will do is present what appears to be the bulk of the consensus on this topic, not to say that you can't find those who'll disagree. I happen to believe that protein and salt in particular weigh heavily on our pH balance, and there's an enormous amount of data and basic biochemistry to support this statement. Let's first consider our Paleolithic ancestors for a moment. The topic of what our distant ancestors consumed has been brought to our attention through the work of Loren Cordain. As she mentions in her book, *The Paleo Diet*, these people consumed wild meats, fruits, vegetables, nuts and seeds. They did not eat dairy, grains, salt, and many other constituents of our current diet. In theory, the amount of fruits and vegetables offered enough buffer to counter the acidity of an otherwise high protein diet.

What we seem to know is as follows. We need animal protein. We need it for a variety of reasons. There are simply some nutrients we cannot get enough of without it. One of many problems today is that the quality of our protein is horrific, but that's another topic. When it comes to bone health, much like many other things in life, animal protein is good, but in moderation.

One of many researchers goes on to state, "Western diets are also high in protein, especially animal protein. The international epidemiologic data show an association between protein consumption and osteoporotic fractures. The aciduria (acidic urine) caused by such diets promotes urinary calcium loss." (11) Proteins are made from amino acids. There are two types of amino acids that contain sulfur, cysteine/cystine and methionine. The sulfate from these two amino acids causes calcium to be excreted in the urine. Many studies have shown a clear link between protein ingestion and calcium excretion.

In one review paper from 1999, the authors state from references that doubling protein intake results in a 50% increase in urinary calcium, and that the effect of dietary protein on calcium balance is a well-documented phenomenon. (12) They then make the very important statement, "As a result, recommended intakes of dietary calcium are influenced by the protein intake of the population for which they are set. This largely explains why recommended calcium intakes for the U.S. population are higher than those for populations in other, less-industrialized nations." So as you can see, our high calcium RDA/RDI is derived from the fact that we consume so much protein. The conclusion is that one can either eat less protein, or eat more calcium. As it is unlikely that your average American will eat less protein, then they conclude dairy is the best high-calcium food to fit the equation.

The problem with this logic is that it isn't working. One reason it fails to work is because milk, and other dairy products, especially cheese, are high in animal protein, and thus high in sulfur, and phosphorus for that matter. Other foods such as nuts and seeds may have a high sulfur content as well, but we consume them in very minor quantities. I don't often see someone ordering a 16-ounce plate of seeds, medium rare. Milk has actually been referred to as "liquid protein". Other dairy products are higher in protein, and at times salt as well, because the water content of the product has been markedly reduced, and you're left with a much higher ratio of protein per serving size.

This is why other researchers look at the argument for dairy to conserve bone mass, and question its value. In one paper it's stated, "Even with the calciuric effect of protein and sodium, dairy product consumption should result in a positive calcium balance and, presumably, a positive effect on bone mineralization. <u>However, in clinical, longitudinal, retrospective, and cross-sectional studies, neither increased consumption of dairy products, specifically, nor total dietary calcium consumption has shown even a modest consistent benefit, for child or adolescent bone health</u>." (13)

To confirm this entire concept, researchers conducted a novel trial. They took 15 subjects and put them on three different diets for 12 days each, and then monitored for acid/base balance. The diets were otherwise equal as far as calcium, sodium, calories, phosphorus, and total protein. The only difference was the type of protein. They progressed the patients from a purely vegetable-based protein, to an ovo-vegetarian, to an animal protein source. They stated. "In our study, switching from vegetarian, to ovo-vegetarian, to animal protein diets caused a progressive increase in urinary sulfate and net acid excretion, which was accompanied by a rise in urinary calcium excretion. <u>Our results suggest that the major calciuric (calcium in the urine) factor during animal protein ingestion is bone resorption in response to the acid load</u>." (14)

Many other researchers have substantiated this link. Upon assay, it has been found that the content of the sulfur amino acids methionine and cysteine in animal derived proteins is 2-5 times higher than in grains and beans. (15) In one study, which looked exclusively at methionine, it was found that the ingestion of 6 grams of methionine raised urinary calcium excretion by 80 mg in 24 hours. (16) That's a lot of calcium when you consider that much more than 80 mg of dietary calcium is needed to replace that, given absorption.

You will probably find it interesting that calcium excretion in the urine can be reduced by giving buffers to subjects. It has been shown many times that a diet high in fruits and vegetables, which are metabolized to bicarbonate, have a bone sparing effect. It has been speculated and shown by some that the high potassium content in the diet is largely responsible for this effect. It is widely documented that potassium ingestion increases sodium excretion, which is certainly one mechanism to conserve bone. But in regards to protein consumption, the value of potassium likely still holds some truth, but this has not been shown repeatedly. It may be that the bicarbonate is the more effective participant in this equation.

With this in mind, 171 men and women over 50 received either placebo, potassium bicarbonate, sodium bicarbonate, or potassium chloride for three months. All of the subjects got 600 mg of calcium per day and 525 IU of vitamin D3 daily. They found that the bicarbonate groups had favorable effects on calcium excretion and bone resorption markers, while potassium on its own did not have these effects. (17) This study was replicated in 2009. This would imply that they've taken into consideration previous trial biases and flaws, to build a more refined answer.

Years earlier, other researchers took a look at just bicarbonate use and markers of bone health. Nine healthy volunteers were administered bicarbonate in a controlled setting. They found that the acid excretion (urine) decreased very significantly. In their words, "Urinary calcium excretion decreased immediately, reversibly, and significantly during bicarbonate administration and remained decreased throughout the seven day period, resulting in significant cumulative calcium retention. (18)

In this same study, another important consideration must be noted as well. Based on studies linking cortisol levels to bone loss, and the known association between corticosteroid drugs and osteoporosis, these researchers looked at cortisol levels among other hormones. They referred to the acidic condition in the body as chronic metabolic acidosis (CMA). They go on to reinforce what we already know about sulfur, pH levels, our high protein western diet, and calcium loss. They proudly state that, "These results furnish the first evidence that a very mild western diet-induced chronic metabolic acidosis results in a state of increased cortisol excretion and plasma concentration, and provides several novel findings in humans regarding the possible causality of the western diet in the etiology of osteoporsosis."

By now, I'm sure you've heard of cortisol, and how it can be detrimental in excess. These changes are subtle, but the lifetime accumulation can have significant consequences. This acidosis-induced increase in cortisol secretion is but one aspect. It has also been shown that this acidic environment inhibits osteoblasts, and increases osteoclast activity. (19) This makes sense, and further proves the point that the body needs to mobilize calcium to neutralize the acid.

Add to all of this that as we age, there is a decline in kidney function as well. In one review, researchers noted a 6-7% increase in blood hydrogen (acidic), and a 12-16% decline in plasma bicarbonate (buffer) between 20 and 80 years of age, with most of the decline occurring after the age of 50. (20) So as you can see, there are a great many things going on inside the body that can contribute to osteoporosis, and even more, as you will read. The abundance of data would seem to point towards a modest protein diet. This means more protein in your youth, but less as we age. For some reason, probably hormonal mostly, children are able to put on bone mass, despite diets in some cases that would not be very helpful for adults. Again, we do need some protein for bone mass. A modest rise in IGF-1 is just one aspect. However, it may mostly boil down to eating your fruits and vegetables, which isn't rocket science, just not routinely practiced.

If we again take a look at our distant ancestors, people who had hardy bones, we can use it to help come to some conclusions. First, these people had plenty of exercise, far more than we have on average today. As we know, exercise is the most influential single factor in bone health. We know they didn't endure the 24-hour stresses we do, and thus had lower 24-hour cortisol levels. We know they consumed a lot of animal protein, as well as brains, marrow, and other organs, which may have affected their pH. We also know they consumed more vegetable matter, which could help offset the acidity of the protein. What we don't know is, had they lived to an old age, as we do, what would their health have looked like?

As our average lifespan closes in on 80, we have to look at epidemiological data that is relevant now. This is a limitation of both the Paleolithic model and Weston Price's observations on isolated races with their historical diets as compared to their relatives sickened by the western diet.

One last note on acid/base balance. It is widely known that sodium plays a major role in calcium balance. In one study, the authors state that, "Urinary sodium was found to be one of the most important determinants of urinary calcium excretion." (21) Other researchers who gave postmenopausal women modest doses of sodium speculated that if those levels were maintained over the long term, that 7.5-10% of calcium stores could be mobilized over 10 years. (22) That's a lot of bone. Of course salt is not an entirely bad thing either. The phrase, "worth your weight in salt" came from somewhere, somewhere hot, I'm sure. Again, it comes down to moderation and balance.

The fact is that I could bore you with many, many more studies showing the clear association to both sodium intake and animal protein, and their roles in bone demineralization. I think by now you have an understanding that calcium alone is not the solution, and there are some other aspects of your diet that play a role in bone health. With that said, we'll look at oxalates and "the new calcium" pill, vitamin K.

Oxalates

Perhaps you may have heard the term oxalate. You may even know that spinach is high in oxalic acid, and may not be as good as Popeye advertised. So why are we even discussing oxalates? Well, they play a role in your serum calcium balance, dictate when you should take your calcium supplements, if you choose to take them, and are the overwhelming contributor to kidney stones. They have also been linked with several other disease states you would not think have a correlation, such as vulvodynia, chronic fatigue/fibromyalgia, and autism. So, in the context of preventative medicine, please consider oxalates.

Many foods contain oxalates, or oxalic acid. The only difference is that when oxalic acid is bound to a metal, it becomes an oxalate. There are so many foods that contain them that you simply will not be able to avoid them all, but you may want to become cognizent of the top offenders. Peanuts, spinach, strawberries, chocolate, teas, rhubarb, nuts, wheat bran, beets, swiss chard, turnip and beet greens, and soy are the top offenders from the diet. About 50% of oxalates come from the diet, and the other half come from your body's metabolism.

During digestion, the oxalic acid that is liberated from your food can go down one of two routes. It can be absorbed into the bloodstream, or it can be bound and excreted in the feces. As oxalic acid is very negatively charged, it's more than happy to find a positive partner, and the most likely partner of choice is calcium. If it binds with calcium, or another in the GI tract, it's simply excreted, but if absorbed into the serum alone, then it still looks to bind, but now it's in your tightly regulated environment. Calcium still remains the partner of choice, and as you can guess, it removes the calcium from your pool, and thus you have to free up more from your reservoir, the bone. As a bonus, as it leaves your body via the urine, its water insolubility may result in kidney stones.

Depending on whom you reference, kidney stones affect about 12% of the population. As with most everything else, it is multi-factorial in nature, which we will discuss. Most kidney stones are derived from calcium oxalate. There are other types, but due to general relevance we will discuss this type, as some 80% or more of stones originate here. It was initially thought that since the urine of kidney stones sufferers is high in calcium, and since the stones are comprised of calcium, then to avoid more stones in the future, of which the recurrence rates are high, patients should go on low calcium diets. This sounds like solid reasoning, but it's unfortunately not the only time the medical community was wrong. It did not take into consideration the other component of the stone, the oxalic acid. Thus, at this point in time, we have considerable evidence to show that a higher calcium diet is protective for stones. Sounds contradictory, but let's look at some evidence.

In a study done in 1993, 45,619 men from the ages of 40-75 who had no history of kidney stones were evaluated via food questionnaire, and followed for 4 years. They found that the risk for developing a stone for those consuming the most calcium was about half that of those consuming the least. (23) They also found that the intake of animal protein was directly associated with the risk of stone formation. This should make sense, as you'll recall protein consumption requires calcium to retain serum pH values at the expense of bone.

These same researchers quoted numerous other trials and state, "Calcium restriction increases the absorption of oxalate in the GI tract of normal subjects, and in patients with kidney stones, leading to an increase of 16 -56% in urinary oxalate excretion." They go on to discuss the role of fat malabsorption, and how dietary fats not absorbed by the GI tract can bind up calcium. This is something to consider for those of you who've had your gallbladder removed, as it's the storage site for bile, which is released during digestion, part of which aids in fat absorption. Thus, if you don't digest your fats properly, you will absorb less of your dietary calcium, as it will be bound to them.

They go on to quote more researchers and state, "Urinary oxalate may be more important than urinary calcium for stone formation, because calcium oxalate saturation of urine increases rapidly with small increases in the oxalate concentration." In other words, because calcium oxalate is so water insoluble, small increases in oxalate, which will ultimately mostly bind with calcium, are more detrimental than similar increases in just calcium in the urine.

Many other trials have shown similar results. For example, when calcium was given with oral oxalates, urinary oxalate excretion decreased by 50% in several patient types. (24) In 2009, the *Cleveland Clinic Journal of Medicine* stated that, "Calcium restriction can put the patient into a negative calcium balance." (25) Essentially, as the patient excretes calcium, they need to replace lost calcium store to maintain bone mass. They also go on to quote a number of other researchers to say that the less dietary calcium there is in the gut, the less that can bind to oxalic acid for excretion, and more oxalates in the serum, which can increase the urinary oxalates to the point of "supersaturation". Furthermore, they state that several studies show that the more calcium consumed, the better the subjects fared. One of these referenced trials is the following Italian study.

In a study published in 2002 in the *New England Journal of Medicine*, 120 men with recurrent calcium stones and high urine calcium were placed on two separate diets for 5 years. One diet was low in calcium, the other had normal calcium intake with reduced animal protein and salt. Those on the low calcium diet had twice the risk for a recurrence of kidney stones. (26) They blame the low calcium diet in the one group for being unable to bind and excrete oxalate in the GI tract, resulting in higher calcium loss in the urine. They noted that urinary oxalates and urinary calcium both decreased in the normal calcium, low salt and animal protein group. They credit the low salt and low protein diet with sparing calcium excretion by the same mechanisms we saw previously in the acid-base balance section of this chapter.

Another easy measure one could take to reduce the likelihood of kidney stones is to simply drink more water. You often hear this advice, but may not always follow it. The mechanism works by just diluting the concentration of the urine. For example, in one such study, 199 patients following their first stone were either put on a high fluid intake or on no regimen. After 5 years, only 12% of the patients on the high fluid diet got another stone, whereas more than twice that (27%) in the other group had a recurrence. (27)

The only caveat here is to consider your source of drink. Preferably it's water, but from a clean source. In a shocking recent report by the Associated Press, a vast array of <u>pharmaceuticals were found in the drinking water affecting at least 41 million Americans</u>. In areas tested all across the country, molecular residue from medicines for pain, infection, cholesterol, asthma, epilepsy, mental illness, and more were found. Philadelphia ranked the worst as they discovered 56 pharmaceuticals or their by-products in their treated drinking water. Bottled waters are often simply run from taps, and these drugs and other toxins permeate deep down into our aquifers as well. Even though supposedly pesticides, lead, and PCBs are monitored, I have to wonder about everything else out there in addition to drugs, to include other heavy metals, herbicides, fungicides, fluoride (which is a whole other topic), solvents, fuel residue, chlorine and more. By the way, chlorine has data to show that it magnifies the affects of the drugs. Lab research shows detrimental effects on human cells, and feminized fish are found when exposed in the environment. The sad fact of our fast-paced, highly synthetic, overpopulated world is that we are rapidly jeopardizing our future. So get clean water and drink it. Back to oxalates.

The data on calcium oxalate kidney stones in particular has become so accepted that you will see similar recommendations today from various sources. In a review in the *British Medical Journal,* for example, they support many of the main points of this chapter. They state as part of a regimen to prevent recurrent stone formation, and by extension of reason, first time formation, you should:

- Increase your fluid intake.
- Decrease your intake of animal protein, as it will lower your ACID INDUCED CALCIUM EXCRETION.
- Avoid low calcium diets as they increase urinary oxalate excretion.
- Decrease dietary oxalate.

If this sounds like natural medicine to you, it is. If you'll recall, I have stated in this book that half of medicine is simply your food choices. It's what you put in your mouth that can have enormous ramifications for your health. To further support natural medicine, this *British Medical Journal* article also recommends the use of calcium supplements, probiotics treatment (a mechanism we didn't discuss), and the use of vitamin B6. (28)

Let's just consider one more aspect of the natural medicine approach to the prevention of kidney stones. As stated previously, vitamin B6 is commonly recommended. Curiously, it has been well-recognized for many years that pharmacological doses of vitamin B-6 can be very effective at arresting disease progression in 10-30% of patients, long before we became aware of a genetic flaw discovered in 1986. (29) Note that this statement is made for disease progression, those already with a stone diagnosis, which has a high recurrence rate of 30-50% within 5 years. (30) No long-term preventative study has been conducted to my knowledge, and with no financial gains to be had, probably won't happen. So what is this genetic flaw thing?

As discussed in other chapters of this book, we all possess genetic flaws. These flaws correlate to how long, and how healthy we will live. As we continue to understand more about our genome through the remarkable gene work of the past 20 years or so, we will hopefully one day incorporate this into preventative medicine. It's a combination of your genes and your lifestyle that dictates your morbidity and mortality. This is why one guy can smoke and drink and live to 90, and another drops dead of a heart attack at 45. Genes!

In this instance, there are at least two main defects, the GRHPR gene, and the other is the AGXT gene. We'll discuss AGXT, as it has more data. To complicate things even further, there are now at least 146 mutations that have been found for this one particular AGXT gene. (31) So what does this gene do? The protein that is supposed to be made is an enzyme in the liver called AGT. This AGT enzyme is a part of a metabolic pathway that degrades oxalic acid into the amino acid glycine. In the presence of this flaw, more oxalate is formed from this equation. As we already know, oxalate can only be excreted via the urine, and its insoluble nature, combined with other common factors, may result in kidney deposition. The frequency of this flaw varies from rare (whatever that means), to 20%. (32,33)

From a genetic viewpoint, your calcium oxalate kidney stone risk is dependent on the quantity and strength of any flaws you may possess. Vitamin B6 helps, as it is the cofactor for this AGT enzyme. Giving supraphysiological doses has a proven track record. This is in part what natural medicine is. We *push* certain pathways with high doses to compensate for a shortcoming. The theory is that if your genetic flaw is 80% useless, then if we take your synthesis of flawed protein and double or triple it by pushing the pathway, then we've upped your total production of valid protein, even though in total it's still 80% useless.

So, if you have a family history of kidney stones, if your urethra hurts following a spinach binge, if you have had a kidney stone, then it may be wise for you to consider taking calcium citrate with your meals, vitamin B6, increasing your water consumption, limiting your salt and animal protein intake, and reducing your dietary oxalate intake. You may save yourself money, time, and pain in the process.

Vitamin K

What in the world does vitamin K do? There are four fat-soluble vitamins, A,D,E, and K. Vitamin K is probably the least known, while our other chapter on A will show it's probably the most misunderstood. Some of you may be aware of vitamin K's role in clotting, but you probably don't have the full picture even on this. So why is it in our chapter on bone health? For very good reasons, as you will soon discover.

Vitamin K essentially exists in two forms. There is the form found in vegetables called phylloquinone (K1), and a form made from bacteria called menaquinone (K2). You will also see vitamin K on supplement labels called phytonadione, which is made commercially, but is identical to phylloquinone. Vitamin K does only one thing, but its affects are far-reaching. It is the only nutrient that works for one single enzyme, which ultimately results in the activation (carboxylation) of what's referred to as a Gla protein. To date, there have been about 15 Gla proteins discovered, but researchers think that as many as 100 may eventually be found. (34) It is the activation of these proteins by vitamin K that allows them to "do their thing". This is critical to the understanding of how vitamin K works.

Vitamin K is typically known for its role in blood coagulation. There are several Gla proteins responsible for blood coagulation, which is a necessary thing to prevent blood loss. What's less known is that there are several other K-dependent Gla proteins that prevent excess clotting. When the prospect of vitamin K supplementation comes up, some people get concerned about excess clotting. There have been numerous studies done on multiple doses of vitamin K, and I did not find one incidence of clotting anywhere in the literature. In fact, time and again, the literature states that it is generally accepted that even in high doses, supplementation with K1 or K2 has not produced adverse effects. (35) In fact, the Institute for Medicine at the National Academy of Sciences chose not to set a Tolerable Upper Limit for K in 2000 when it revisited the topic of vitamin K. There is only one group of people who have a theoretical risk of taking too much vitamin K, and that's those on oral anticoagulants. These drugs specifically work by inhibiting vitamin K's ability to activate Gla proteins. Well dive into this more in the chapter on vascular health.

K1 is highest is kale, parsley, green cabbage, and spinach, respectively. Of note, parsley and spinach are high in oxalates. Broccoli tops, brussel sprouts, lettuce, water cress, canola and soybean oil round out the rest of the top sources. (36) Consider that during the processing of these K1-rich oils, trans-fats are likely created, which at the least nullify the activity of K. The values for these vegetables were taken raw, and data when cooked is scarce. Also, the K content will vary within a plant based on where grown, plant maturation, and more.

The ability to absorb K1 is compromised by the need to break down the plant constituents to get at the vitamin K built into its matrix. Therefore, the absorption of K1 from plants, although debated, is not particularly high. In those with compromised digestion, particularly in regards to fat absorption, the rate is likely less. What is much higher, is the rate of absorption for oral supplemental K1, as it's in its free form, and thus does not have to be extracted from its matrix. It's estimated that in a healthy adult, about 80% of supplemental K1 is absorbed. (37)

In addition to all of this, K1 has a relatively short half life, and has no real storage sites. So K1 needs to be continually replenished via the diet. The clearance of K1 is continual, and calls for a diet high in green leafy vegetables. Consequently, this is theoretically the diet from which we evolved. Interestingly, dietary vitamin K is abundant in the healthiest and longest lived people on the planet, the Japanese.

As you can see, the foods high in vitamin K, especially in raw form, are not a staple of the American diet. Pizza, soda, candy, doughnuts, and other fast foods are not high in K. We somehow consume enough vitamin K to maintain clotting integrity, but as many researchers argue very well, we do not consume enough to prevent soft tissue calcification, and promote bone calcification outside of the liver.

The second form of vitamin K is that of K2, which is structurally just a little different, but this small difference has a big impact. This form is made by bacteria. The bacteria in your gut make some from K1, but it's not possible to measure, and relatively negligible. Cheese is a reasonably good source, as are some other fermented foods. By far, the richest source of K2 is the fermented soybean product called natto, which contains more than 100 times more K2 than various kinds of cheese. (38) This stinky food is consumed widely in Japan, and with its very high K2 content is likely one of the primary reasons for the notorious good health and longevity of the Japanese. However, here in the U.S. our K2 primarily comes from dairy and eggs. Although K2 comprises only about 10-20% of our dietary K, because of its superior absorption, it is thought that it comprises about half of the K that is absorbed. (39)

Shockingly, the first indications that vitamin K-dependent proteins were involved in bone metabolism was found in the mid-1970s, when serious bone malformations were observed in children born to women who had been treated with vitamin K antagonists (drugs that counteract vitamin K) during the first trimester of pregnancy. (40) The RDA/RDI for K ranges from 75-120 micrograms in adults based on gender and pregnancy. Many researchers feel this number is entirely too low as it is based on the liver K requirements to meet basic blood clotting requirements, and it is not adequate to maintain healthy Gla proteins outside of the liver, notably for bone health in this case. (41)

The best marker for vitamin K status is to look at circulating undercarboxylated osteocalcin (ucOC) alone or relevant to osteocalcin, which is not done routinely. The whole role of vitamin K is to carboxylate, or activate Gla proteins. One such protein is osteocalcin, which can't work unless K activates it. Once activated, osteocalcin is able to grab calcium and build it into the bone matrix. So, undercarboxylated osteocalcin is simply an inactive pro-bone protein awaiting vitamin K to turn it on to do its job. Currently, K status is usually measured as it pertains to blood clotting. Numerous studies show a STRONGLY INCREASED FRACTURE RISK, and low bone mineral density in those with elevated ucOC. (42,43)

For example, in a study with 359 women, increased levels of undercarboxylated (inactive) osteocalcin were associated with about twice the rate of hip fracture. (44) In addition, a series of reports in elderly women showed an extremely high correlation between inactive serum osteocalcin levels and risk of hip fracture. In fact, those women with abnormally high inactive osteocalcin levels were between 3 and 6 times more likely to suffer a hip fracture. (45) These are just two of many such studies.

There is mounting data to support the use of vitamin K in other conditions, such as cardiovascular health, cancer, brain health, diabetes, and more. Although very interesting, we will soley focus on its marked effects on bone health in this chapter. Vitamin K activates Gla proteins, and one of these identified proteins is osteocalcin, as we discussed previously. Osteocalcin is made by osteoblasts (bone building cells), which, when activated, have the ability to bind (chelate) calcium into the bone matrix. So remember back to the calcium-only studies on bone. One of the concerns was to have too much free calcium with no direction in the body. So in simple terms, vitamin K tells that calcium to go to the bone, which directs it from the vasculature or kidneys.

The most studied form of K2 is what's known as MK-4 or menatetranone. It has a short half-life in vivo (in the body), of only 1-2 hours, and thus it is given three times per day, as it is biochemically similar to K1, and its in vivo characteristics are similar. Another form of K2 called MK-7 has a much longer half-life, of about 3 days, and is therefore able to perform its function days after a dose, while traveling to tissue throughout the body.

In a study looking at the pharmacokinetics of K1 versus MK-7, the researchers noted several important advantages of MK-7, the kind of K2 found in natto. (46) First, as both were given in supplement form, they were both absorbed well, both peaking in the blood at about 4 hours after ingestion. The K1 returned to baseline within hours, whereas the MK-7 was still detectable four days later. This difference in availability in the blood is due to the chemical differences between the two forms of K, and thus the more lipophilic, longer chained MK-7 survives longer in the body. As all clotting factors for blood reside in the liver, and in the healthy population these clotting Gla proteins are fully carboxylated, then the K2 provides more benefit as it is able to help carboxylate other Gla proteins outside of the liver, such as osteocalcin in the bone. (47)

I know this is a bit confusing, so let's consider it in simpler terms. Given its absorption and consumption issues, K1 is still present enough in

113

the liver to adequately affect blood clotting, so that your average person need not worry about having to clot. K1 is cleared quickly by the body, so regular intake is optimal. A good balance of bacteria in your gut, which few Americans have, combined with certain K-rich foods, will help you to make and absorb certain amounts of K2. K2 is absorbed better, is transported outside the liver easily, has a much longer lifetime in the blood, and is more potent in its ability to activate the Gla proteins. These Gla proteins outside the liver, in this case osteocalcin, are not fully active in the average healthy person. When K2 is given in supplemental fashion, the amount of activated osteocalcin rapidly increases. The reason why clotting is not an issue is because when the clotting Gla proteins are fully active, you can't make them more active. Think of filling a glass with water. When it's full, you can't pour in more water because it can't hold more. The fact that the clotting Gla proteins are fully active given our low intakes of K just shows you how vital clotting is to human survival. From an evolutionary viewpoint, the body deems it much more important than calcifying bone, and decalcifying soft tissue.

So let's take a look at some of the data when vitamin K was used alone for bone health. In one 3-year study, 325 postmenopausal non-osteoporotic women received either a placebo or 45 mg/day of K2. Hipbone strength remained unchanged during the trial in the K group while it decreased significantly in the placebo group. (48) Unchanged is not always a bad thing, as you would normally see reduced bone mineral density (BMD) in postmenopausal women as was shown in the placebo group. Thus K prevented the decline.

In another trial, 241 osteoporotic patients in a 2-year study were put on K2 or no treatment. The incidence of new fractures was higher in the no treatment group as compared to the K group, and the differences between lumbar BMD were significantly different as well. (49) The authors go on to state, "These findings suggest that vitamin K2 effectively prevents the occurrence of new fractures."

A Japanese trial studied patients with osteoporosis induced by corticosteroid use for 2 years. Yes, corticosteroids are well known to reduce BMD. The incidence of vertebral fractures in the control group was 41%, while that of the K group was 13%. (50)

A number of Japanese studies show variable effects of K2 used alone in bone health, but substantial benefit when combined with vitamin D. (51) As we will see in a later chapter, Vitamin D has significant impact on bone health as well. It increases absorption of calcium within the GI tract, it reduces serum parathyroid hormone, which is responsible for breaking down bone to supply the blood, and it causes more osteocalcin to be made. (52)

In consideration of this, we'll look at a re-cut of the Nurses Health Study. Dietary assessments through questionaires are not particularly good trials, but they can shed light on trends. We know, for example, that the Japanese have a different diet from our own, and yet when they move to America and adopt our dietary practices, they succumb in time to the same conditions as Americans. This would be epidemiological data. Both types of studies have many variables, but in the end are examinations of dietary variability. With that said, in this trial there were 72,327 women aged 38-63, who were asked in the beginning to keep a dietary history over 10 years. Interested in a link between vitamin K intake and hip fractures based on the fact that vitamin K supplementation has been shown to activate previously inactive osteocalcin and reduce urinary calcium excretion, they analyzed the data for K consumption. As lettuce is the primary source of K in the U.S. diet, they used this as a marker and found that women who consumed lettuce one or more times per day had a 45% lower risk of hip fracture than those who consumed it once or less per week. (53)

Their observed inverse association between K intake and hip fracture supports their statement that the inactive serum osteocalcin marker may be a more sensitive measure of vitamin K status than the traditional blood coagulation tests. Interestingly, women with low K but high vitamin D intake had a high risk of fracture. As is one of the themes of this book, we are not one nutrient mammals. Clearly vitamins D and K work together in calcium status. Vitamin D upregulates osteocalcin production, but it serves little use if inactive, which is the role of vitamin K. With the help of both vitamins, which are really more like hormones, the bone is able to lay down more matrix.

In light of the need to assess the discrepancies in efficacy of vitamin D alone or in combination with calcium in support of bone health, researchers undertook a review of 13 trials looking at vitamin K in 2006. They state that vitamin K is associated with increased bone mineral density and reduced fracture incidence, with a striking 80% reduction in hip fractures. (54)

One of the trials reviewed was a Japanese trial of two years in length, which was nicely done. Why? Because it had 4 well chosen groups, a vitamin D group, a vitamin K group, a D and K group, and a calcium group. So what did these 92 osteoporotic women show? In this case, D or K therapy alone increased bone mineral density (BMD) of the lumbar spine. BMD decreased in the calcium-only group! The combination of D and K significantly increased lumbar BMD beyond that of D or K alone, and it did so much quicker. (55) This supports other data these authors quote, in that K has better results in those with higher vitamin D levels. Of note, on average, the results seem to be better for those with osteoporosis as compared to non-osteoporotic individuals. This makes sense and is a good thing. In contrast to what some doctors may tell you, that supplementation can at best only slow bone loss and not add bone, there are numerous trials that prove them WRONG.

In a similar trial, 172 postmenopausal women were either put on vitamin K, vitamin D, K and D, or no treatment. After 2 years, the K and D group had markedly increased BMD of 5%, which doesn't sound like much, but is quite good. The K-only group barely increased BMD, which itself isn't bad as you'd normally see a decline, which was seen with the control group. (56) In the combined D and K group, most of the progress was made in the first 6-12 months.

Vitamin K has been approved in Japan for the treatment of osteoporosis since 1995. They clearly see the value in the clinical use of this vitamin. As great as it may be, it's even better in combination with vitamin D. A varied diet, which includes other essential minerals such as magnesium, that is adequate in calcium content, controlled for oxalates, higher in fluid intake, and modest in animal protein, salt, and acids helps even more. Exercise and hormonal consideration are an added benefit. This is the equation for adequate bone health. You can listen to people pushing one nutrient, or you can take all the factors into consideration. You may now want to reconsider any bone-health products you are currently taking. In the end, the use of supplements in bone health has a realistic need for at least vitamins D and K. The other factors mostly come down to lifestyle choices. Now that you are armed with the most unbiased, up to date clinical information, you can make a choice.

Chapter 5   Methylation

This book exposes you to a wide array of issues. My 25 years of research is unfolded here for your review and consideration. I will present you with as many facts and figures as I can to back up my case, but you have to make the ultimate decision. I wrote this book in a fashion that would appeal to me as a reader. I'm not just going to say "take this" or "try that" and assume you'll comply. There are many other considerations that need to be measured, which is why it may be helpful to see a qualified practitioner of natural medicine.

I am hesitant to put more emphasis on any one aspect of natural medicine over another, as it would violate of the holistic principles of natural medicine. If there's any one aspect of natural medicine emphasized most consistently, it would be the health of the GI tract. Methylation wouldn't make the top ten, as most providers are unfamiliar with it. However, in going beyond the discussion of what goes down the gullet, how well it is absorbed, and any other dysfunction of the GI tract as it relates to overall health, I would be remiss if I did not expose you to methylation.

What is methylation? Please bear with me through the technical babble, because it's the best way to explain to you how this omnipresent function in the body is crucial to your health and wellness. The vast majority of readers are unfamiliar with this process, but I have to tell you that the majority of natural medicine providers don't know much about it either, nor does your conventional medicine provider. You can't entirely blame them, as they have numerous other items on their agenda than to spend the countless hours researching these things.

I bring this and all information to you free of endorsements. If you haven't noticed by now, I have not endorsed a single product, line, or manufacturer. Whenever I read someone else's work, and they endorse a product, a little red flag goes up in my head. I usually disregard the endorsement and focus on the research. I have the luxury of knowing what goes on in this industry, while you do not. In order to come across as upfront and unbiased as possible, I have endorsed nothing. I have, on the other hand, recommended a number of books, as there are many fine books in circulation that can expose you to the truth behind America's failing health. These books aren't written by fringe granola chewing, tree hugging, pot-smoking, unshaven goofballs. These books are written by highly educated visionaries with conviction and motivation to bring you their version of the truth, which is a whole lot closer to the truth than you'll get from the "got milk?" campaign. These people are experienced and educated MDs, NDs, PhDs, nutritionists, dentists, and many others.

So don't be a lemming; perform your own due diligence. Give everything I say and what others say some honest reflection. You can continue down the conventional path of ill-health with the vast majority of Americans, as our crooked politicians on both sides wage an us-versus-them war over healthcare, or you can take charge of your own healthcare, and keep clear of a system that by all reasonable accounts is at least the 3rd leading cause of death in the United States today.

So, why am I excited about methylation, and what is it? To begin, it is but one aspect of disease and degeneration. In my opinion, the cornerstones of aging and disease within the human body are inflammation, glycosylation, hormonal reduction, oxidation, and metabolic inadequacies, of which methylation is one. This book addresses all of these aspects of health and degeneration to some degree. Methylation is both extremely important, and poorly understood.

A methyl group is a carbon with three hydrogens attached. Methylation is the act of having this little group of four attached to something else. What needs methylation? Everything. Do you take CoQ10? Methylation is involved in its synthesis. CoQ10 is called ubiquinone, from the word ubiquitous, which means everywhere. So just from the very aspect of CoQ10 use, you can see that methylation is involved in everything in your body. Do you take MSM? MSM is used with some success for arthritic conditions. The first M in MSM stands for methyl, which needs to be methylated to work. How about melatonin, phosphatidlycholine, or carnitine? They all require methylation. DNA requires methylation in order to eventually properly produce proteins that have effects everywhere in the body. Whether it's the lining of your GI tract, the enzymes made by your pancreas, the lining of your nerves, the collagen of your joints, or the receding gums in your mouth, methylation has a role in everything.

As we age, our ability to methylate declines. Combine that with a gradual accumulation of toxins from fish, plastics, cleaners, and innumerable other sources, and you have an aging person. Now throw into the equation a poor diet, which does not supply the nutrients needed to properly methylate, as well as other foodstuffs, such as trans-fats, which interfere with virtually every body process, and you have a sick nation. Take away exercise, which stimulates methylation, and add a genetic flaw or two, which is much more common than anyone would like to admit, and here we are. As the Okinawan Centurian study states, "Okinawan elders, and centagenarians in particular, have experienced a slower age-related decline and markedly delayed or avoided entirely the chronic diseases of aging, such as Alzheimer's Disease, cardiovascular disease, and cancer." One of their many healthy habits is that they eat healthy protein, but not much. So they avoid a lifetime accumulation of iron, which we know to be a pro-oxidant, and they also keep in check their homocysteine levels. Homocysteine is a toxic by-product of metabolism. The source of homocysteine is the amino acid methionine, which is present in foods but more so in animal proteins. This implies animal proteins are bad. However, methionine is an essential amino acid, and we need animal proteins for a variety of key bodily functions, to include vitamin B12. B12, in turn, is one of several nutrients that metabolizes homocysteine. So what does this mean?

If you're a strict vegan, then you'd better take your B12 supplements, as being a vegan is not in harmony with our genetic needs. In response to this statement, vegan fans will state that on average a vegetarian lives longer and healthier than the average American. This is true. However, the reason why being a vegan seems like a healthier choice is that they've picked a poor standard of comparison. Anyone can look good against a sick population. Set the bar higher, pick a fight with the Okinawan's.

One factor in this protein-methione-homocysteine connection is the total intake of methionine. Research shows that the greater the methionine intake (think animal protein), the more homocysteine gets shuffled out of the body. Whereas, the less methionine ingested, the more the methylation cycle spins efficiently. (1) So you would infer from this that one could eat all the animal protein they want, as the body will compensate by processing the homocysteine faster. However, you have to consider that as time passes, the body's ability to methylate diminishes, and as a result, homocysteine accumulates. The other important take-away from the previous statement is that as one consumes less protein, one creates more of a substance called SAMe (s-adenosyl-methionine), which then methylates more throughout the body. This is a very good thing. We want to make the methionine-homocysteine cycle run as much as possible to produce this all-important SAMe. Also, as you consume less protein, and the ravages of time and toxins take their toll on your ability to methylate, you accumulate less homocysteine and SAH, which in turn inhibits this cycle from running.

This transitions us into another interesting point. We have known for some time that caloric restriction in animals and humans is the best way to increase life span. Many studies attest to this fact. The theories have usually centered around the concept that although food and oxygen are critical to life, their metabolism is also pro-oxidative. This is in part likely to be true. Studies show that the rate of generation of what's referred to as mitochondrial reactive oxygen species (MROS) is lower in long lived animals. MROS are free radicals inside the energy centers of our cells. The pro-oxidant free radical generators damage DNA and proteins, but some researchers have done some interesting studies of late. So longer lived animals have fewer of these damaging radicals.

Many studies have consistently shown that caloric restriction decreases MROS generation, but the dietary component for this change was unknown. (2) A recent study interestingly showed that protein restriction without a strong caloric restriction decreased MROS, while neither lipid not carbohydrate restriction had the same effect. (3) So this tells us that some component of proteins is a main driver in reducing life expectancy, and carbohydrates and fats do not posses this feature. Based in part on the fact that protein methionine content is inversely related to maximal life span in mammals, these researchers focused on methionine. What they showed was that methionine restriction, in similar fashion to previous research on both protein and caloric restriction, reduced cellular pro-oxidants and their associated damage. (4) In their conclusion, they state:

"This suggests that the decrease in methionine ingestion can be the single molecular component responsible for the decrease in MROS generation and oxidative stress that occurs during caloric restriction, and thus for part of the decrease in aging rate elicited by this dietary manipulation, although a role for other dietary amino acids cannot be discarded without further investigation."

Keep in mind that this is important stuff but is not the total answer. Lipids do play a role, as well as many other features of our health. In fact other research shows us that although methionine restriction without controlling for calories increases maximum lifespan in rats and mice, the effect of caloric restriction has a larger impact. So there is more to this story than just methionine-homocyteine-methylation, but this is still big news.

We can be fairly certain that most Americans aren't going to give up their animal protein. We love it. When someone asks "What's for dinner?" the reply usually isn't "Broccoli." We center our meal around protein as it is coded into us. Unfortunately, the protein we eat today is far inferior to that of out distant ancestors, but that's another matter. This does give us some guidance. We can reduce total protein intake. We can take certain supplements to better process the toxic effects of methionine. We can also take other supplements and eat better in general to cope with the components of aging. As we've done in this book before, we'll take a look at disease states relevant to our current topic, that of methylation.

Alzheimer's

Anyone with exposure to Alzheimer's Disease (AD) knows full well how horrific and debilitating this terrible disease can be. It robs the victim of their true self, their brain. Alzheimer's accounts for 60-70% of progressive cognitive impairment in elderly patients, and while about 360,000 patients are diagnosed each year with it, it is forecasted that our aging population will quadruple its occurrence during the next 50 years. (5) To add to this terrible story, two epidemiological studies found that the median survival rates for these patients is only 3-4 years. (6) This is less time than stated by the Alzheimer's Research and Prevention Foundation. However, they both go on to tell us that it is the third most costly disease in the United States, while most insurance does not cover the long-term needs. As you combine the skyrocketing cases and costs of Alzheimer's with that of diabetes, and virtually every other condition known to medicine, you see we have a recipe for financial disaster.

I won't take the complex dive into the pathology of Alzheimer's, discussing beta-amyloid plaques, neurofibrillary tangles, and the like. We'll all get lost in what is literally brain surgery. I am not proposing a cure for Alzheimer's, but merely offering information about a disease that has modern medicine in confusion. Once again, prevention is clearly the best solution, as the treatments are clearly not working.

You have likely heard of a theoretical connection of aluminum to AD. In fact this connection has been well researched. So what's the conclusion? As with anything in research, there is no consensus. So what do we know? We know that aluminum is a neurotoxin; we've known this for over 100 years. We know that in many cases there are increased aluminum concentrations in the brains of AD victims. We know our environment, our food, our medicines, and our water are contaminated from decades of aluminum production and use, which is ubiquitous in our way of life. We know that Alzheimers's (AD) is NOT a normal part of aging, according to the Alzheimer's Research and Prevention Foundation and others. Like every condition known, there is a biochemical explanation. For example, as we consider another condition, that of cardiovascular disease, we know that many factors play a role in atherosclerosis, which revolve around inflammation through the interplay of nutrition, genetics, and toxicity. We also know that in IBD, insults to the GI tract primarily through pathogens and/or allergens, initiate a sequence of detrimental events, and should you have a genetic compromise, the extent of disease is more severe. These are biochemical explanations. Your insomnia, your ulcer, your "you-name-it" are the result of your biochemistry being out of whack.

What we can say is that neurotoxins such as aluminum, mercury, and fluoride have no role in our bodies, yet we accumulate them as time goes on. Fish is virtually unsafe to eat now because of mercury and a host of other toxins. Fluoride is one of the most abundant elements on the Earth's crust, but science cannot find any use for it in the human body, despite what many dentists will tell you. Although these elements don't belong in us, they are in some part playing a role in a host of human tragedies. Mercury has been investigated in its potential role in AD. Once again, the results are mixed. It becomes a matter of how one does research, which varies wildly at times. But we do know that it's a neurotoxin. Even a well balanced paper on metals and AD states that regardless of the contradictory evidence, studies in both humans and test tubes continue to suggest that mercury plays a role in AD. (7) In yet another review of metals and AD, the authors state that "the use of antioxidants and iron chelators, which are also aluminum chelators, have shown some effectiveness in the treatment of AD. (8) This same author also goes on to comment about the mercury connection as well. You may be surprised to learn that there is some connection, which is even more vague, to essential minerals such as zinc, iron, and copper.

Now that we've briefly touched on the vaguary of exogenous toxins, let's look at an endogenous toxin with more evidence. I'm referring to the homocysteine connection. Homocysteine is a free radical amino acid formed from the metabolism of methionine. With proper nutrition, its levels are kept in check with adequate vitamins B6, B12, and folate. There is extensive data correlating homocysteine levels to the occurrence of vascular disease, as you'll read in the next chapter. However, homocysteine does not only affect the vasculature, but the central nervous system (CNS) as well. In fact, one could make an effective argument, which I'll try to do, to highlight the fact that homocysteine has a greater impact on the CNS proportionately than it does on the rest of the body. Why is that? Of the three pathways present in the body that metabolize toxic homocysteine and its toxic precursor SAH, only one predominates in the brain. The effective TMG pathway does not exist in the brain. The B6 pathway does exist in the brain, and depending on whom you reference, has some degree of lesser capacity in the brain than it does outside the CNS. That leaves one primary pathway in the CNS to reduce homocysteine, the methionine synthase pathway.

Methionine synthase is a two-part reaction that takes a methyl group from active folate (MTHF), gives it to cobalamin to make methylcobalamin, which then gives the methyl group to homocysteine to make methionine. We want to make methionine again, because from this amino acid we make SAMe, which is the body's major methyl donor. SAMe donates methyl groups to DNA so you can make the various proteins throughout the body essential to life. More SAMe is a very good thing. One of the many things that SAMe donates a methyl group to is the lining of nerves. Without an intact lining, compromised nerves lose functionality. This has obvious importance in neurological conditions like Alzheimer's.

So what can go wrong with this essential methionine synthase pathway in the CNS? Well, you could have a genetic flaw in either your ability to make active folate, or you can have a genetic flaw to take the methyl group from active folate to donate it to cobalamin, which in turn donates it to homocysteine. Whether you have the flaw or not, a build-up of both homocysteine and SAH reduces your ability to methylate. This build-up "freezes" the homocysteine-methionine-methylation cycle, which is crucial for health. So as you can see, it's a self-feeding downward spiral that must be broken.

With this knowledge of biochemistry, numerous researchers have looked at B6, B12, folate, and homocysteine status in those with dementia. In study after study, several key findings are repeatedly shown.

- The elderly on average have reduced B12, folate, and B6 status, which has been linked to cognitive decline and other neuropsychiatric disorders. (9) B12 is particularly obvious and important as stomach acid production declines with age. You need adequate HCL to activate the intrinsic factor to absorb B12. Perhaps you should reconsider your acid blocking medications for your GERD.
- Among the measured factors, <u>total plasma homocysteine appears to be the most consistent marker of tissue deficiencies as well as cognitive performance</u>. (10)

- In a number of studies measuring cognitive function as assessed by various testing protocols and homocysteine levels, high homocysteine correlated with the lowest scores.

In one study, homocysteine levels were significantly higher in AD patients, while these same AD patients had significantly lower folate and B12 levels. (11) In fact, the patients in the top third, whose homocysteine levels were 14 or more, had 4.5 times the risk for AD as those with a homocysteine score of 11 or less. Having reviewed hundred of trials in my time, this is a strong correlation and should be taken seriously. In addition, a score of 11 for homocysteine isn't exactly a desirable score. The lower the better, and 11 is NOT low. So if you were to find controls with serum levels say below 6, then what would the result show? Beyond all of this, keep in mind that serum homocysteine is only an indicator of CNS homocysteine, where the affects of a high body homocysteine may be great, but reflective of an even more toxic CNS environment.

For example, one paper discussed CSF (cerebrospinalfluid)/CNS homocysteine, which isn't exactly a readily available lab for your use. The CSF levels of homocysteine were 131% higher in AD patients than in non-AD controls. When the actual brain tissue was analyzed, the level of homocysteine was almost double that of controls. (12) We have so little CSF/CNS data on homocysteine that we do not know if there is some line in the sand that tips the scales to AD.

A study published in the *New England Journal of Medicine* assessed plasma homocysteine at a baseline, and eight years later in 1,092 elderly subjects. (13) They found high levels of plasma homocysteine more often in those who later developed AD. In those with a homocysteine level over 14, the risk doubled. They concluded that, "An increased plasma homocysteine level is a strong, independent risk factor for the development of dementia and Alzheimer's disease." I have to reiterate, "A STRONG, INDEPENDENT RISK FACTOR". This wasn't published in Bob's pot-smokin' tree-huggin' journal, this was published in the *New England Journal of Medicine* seven years ago. So why haven't you heard about this? Why isn't this a part of healthcare reform? There are many reasons, an inept media, money and power in Washington DC, doctors who don't have the time for research, doctors who won't stray from common medical practice for fear of being sued, and the symptoms-drug method of medicine which is taught and practiced today.

The literature is full of this information. Let's look at another example. An Australian study measured levels of homocysteine, B12, and folate in the plasma and cerebrospinal fluid of those with AD as compared to controls. (14) This well-designed research study looked at several key parameters and included tests of the cerebrospinal fluid (CSF). So what did these researchers find? The concentrations of homocysteine were significantly higher in the CSF of Alzheimer's patients than in the control subjects. There was also a significant positive correlation between the plasma concentration of homocysteine and the CSF concentrations of homocysteine. In other words, the more homocysteine in the blood, the more in the brain. They went on to state that, "These results demonstrate that there is a relationship between increased homocysteine concentrations and in Alzheimer's Disease."

We could do this all day long, so instead let's focus on why. There is a great deal of evidence that both homocysteine and its precursor SAH cause CNS damage by a variety of mechanisms. Whether it's degeneration of blood supply to the brain, oxidative destruction, neuronal DNA damage, facilitation of the characteristic AD beta-amyloid toxicity, neurotoxicity, cell death, or neural excitation, they all spell bad news for you and your brain. Again remember, there is only one primary way to metabolize homocysteine in the brain, and also remember as time goes on, homocysteine and SAH accumulate more and more, and they inhibit the very methylation reactions designed to detoxify them and keep your brain healthy. If you throw in poor dietary habits, drugs, toxins, and bad genes, you have a recipe for the third most costly disease in America.

If we return to the subject of metal toxicity, we've found that they can inhibit methylation in the liver, which would in turn raise body homocysteine, which would in time raise CNS homocysteine. All tissues possess the methionine cycle with active folate as the methyl donor, but only the liver, kidney, pancreas, intestine, and brain contain the transsulfurtion pathway. (15) This transsulfuration pathway is the vitamin B6 (CBS enzyme) pathway that metabolizes homocysteine out of the methionine cycle and into other useful intermediaries. So if you make the liver and kidneys toxic with metals and the like, you reduce this important pathway. Likewise, the valuable TMG pathway only exists in the liver, kidney, and optic lens, although the latter is not of systemic significance. So again, a toxic liver and kidney markedly reduce your ability to both methylate and clear high homocysteine levels, which are both interrelated.

Science and medicine do not have all the answers, but we just might know enough to do some good. A methylcobalamin series of shots is not the magic bullet. Neither is taking active folate, active B6, TMG, or heavy metal chelation. Together, in conjunction with other steps, it's possible to alleviate the torture experienced by so many, and at the same time reduce our expenses.

Let's take a closer look at vitamin B12, which is another unheralded key player here. To reiterate, B12 in its active form of methylcobalamin is essential in the methylation process. In fact, it plays THE central role in the brain. In this next study, a couple of key points are highlighted. The researchers took 141 patients with neuropsychiatric disorders due to cobalamin (B12) deficiency, and found that 28% had no anemia and macrocystosis. (16) What does this mean? We know that a B12 deficiency causes neurological problems, and these folks were diagnosed as such. However, it is a common perception that if you're sufficiently B12 deficient to have neurological problems, it will show up in your blood much earlier. This study proves that's not true. How does this affect you? It's easy. When you go to the doctor and explain your symptoms, but the blood tests don't confirm your symptoms (which happens all the time), then you're usually told it's in your head, or something to that affect. This is why a provider needs more than 7-9 minutes for a patient, where symptoms are at least equally as important as diagnostics in getting to the root of the problem. In this study, EVERY patient in this group benefited from cobalamin therapy, which included improvement in neuropsychiatric abnormalities. These findings were also published in the *New England Journal of Medicine*.

Other studies show some improvements with B12 therapy, but in some cognition is not positively affected. So here are a few considerations where a researcher or provider may go wrong. Cyanocobalamin cannot be used under these conditions if you expect clinical success.

Methylcobalamin must be used instead. Why? Again, the body needs to methylate dietary cobalamin to turn it into the active form of methylcobalamin. If the body is not methylating well, as in the case in a number of conditions, then you will not be doing as much good. It could be that the patient has genetic flaws in methionine synthase, or high cerebral SAH and homocysteine. I repeat methylation is impaired. So, the ability of the patient to methylate dietary cobalamin to its neurologically active form is highly compromised, which is why you must administer methylcobalamin.

Second, there comes a point of no return, so to speak. Said a different way, the good that can be done through natural medicine is much less after crossing this point than what could have been done before. In this case we are referring to extensive CNS destruction, but this could be equally true for many other conditions. For example, in IBD, if you've had parts of the GI tract removed, the good I could do for you is compromised more so than prior to surgery. In cardiovascular disease, the introduction of a stent changes the equation. So when you see limited success in trials for AD patients with severe disease progression, it comes as no surprise. Perhaps instead of using alternative medicine as a last option, which happens all the time, it should be the first option when more/most/all health can be returned.

There are scarce successful case reports with the use of methylcobalamin in the treatment of Alzheimer's, but here I offer up one study that looked at its value. I will quote the abstract word for word from the researchers.

"The efficacy of intravenous methylcobalamin in the treatment of Alzheimer-type dementia was evaluated in ten patients using several rating scales. Vitamin B12 levels and unsaturated binding capacities were also measured and compared to the evaluated intellectual function scores. Methylcobalamin was shown to improve intellectual functions, such as memory, emotional functions, and communication with other people. Improvements in cognitive functions were relatively constant when the vitamin B12 levels in the cerebrospinal fluid were high. Improvements in communication functions were seen when a certain level of vitamin B12 was maintained for a longer period. There were no side effects attributable to methylcobalamin. We conclude that methylcobalamin is a safe and effective treatment for psychiatric disorders in patients with Alzheimer-type dementia."(17)

Glutamate

Glutamate is the body's major excitatory neurotransmitter. This is a good thing if you're taking a test or playing a game of football. However, it's not a good thing 24 hours a day. Let's begin with a brief definition of a neurotransmitter (NT). An NT is an amino acid or something structurally very similar that allows the nervous system to communicate. They can be excitatory or inhibitory. For example, serotonin is a neurotransmitter synthesized in the body from tryptophan, and even more immediately 5-HTP. If you take SSRI's for anxiety, they work by keeping the serotonin in the synapse of the neurons longer. In other words, you get more of the relaxing feeling, as serotonin is a calming NT that now remains active longer. If you've taken recreational drugs such as marijuana, cocaine, amphetamines, PCP, or others, they also work by modulating neurotransmitters. Even alcohol, MSG, and all of those adrenaline-spiking drinks do the same.

So let's discuss MSG just a bit. MSG stands for monosodium glutamate. As you can see from its name, it is the sodium salt of glutamic acid (glutamate = glutamic acid). MSG is added to an enormous amount of our food, and may come under different names, such as hydrolyzed vegetable protein, natural flavor, yeast extract, and more. So much for truth in labeling. MSG provides the body with an elevated level of glutamate, which works its way to the brain. Do you know why it's added? To make you want to eat more food, as it stimulates the taste center. As I've said, it all comes down to money and power. I may sound like a conspiracy theorist, but the more you educate yourself, the more you realize it's true.

Glutamate transmission plays roles in cognition, memory, movement, sight, hearing, and taste. Glutamate doesn't even have to cross the blood-brain barrier to affect the hypothalamus, posterior pituitary gland, the pineal gland, and several other parts of the brain. If we just take the hypothalamus alone, we're talking everything in the body. The hypothalamus is the true master gland in the body. And glutamate is the principle NT of the hypothalamus, making it very sensitive to glutamate neurotoxicity. So the more glutamate you eat, the more you expose key parts of the brain to its toxicity.

Why do I mention all of this? Because glutamate, as well as aspartate (another amino acid), which is a part of aspartame (Nutrasweet), are both major excitatory neurotoxins. So how do these fractionated synthetic bolus-dose amino acids affect our brains? There are 4 main classes of glutamate receptor, but we'll just hit the most common in the brain, what's called the NMDA receptor. When glutamate (or aspartate for that matter) attaches to this NMDA receptor, sodium and calcium flow in, while potassium flows out. This causes the neuron to "do its thing". After the neuron has "fired," these tiny pumps send the excess sodium and calcium back out of the cell. This is good if you want to do something like sleep. However, these pumps require fuel and tools in order to do their job. They need ATP (cellular energy), B vitamins, CoQ10, and more. If they don't have one or more of these needs met, then excess calcium builds up inside and causes chronic firing of the neuron. In an interplay between glutamate, intracellular calcium, free radical production, inflammation, and DNA destruction, the neuron eventually dies. Unfortunately the story doesn't end here.

When the neuron dies, it releases its contents, and glutamate is a part of the contents. It has to go somewhere. The brain has mechanisms in place to store up the free glutamate so it doesn't cause more excitotoxicity. One place the excess glutamate can go is into what's called glial cells, which protect and nourish neurons. There are factors such as low cellular energy and free radicals that can hinder this protective process as well.

So what can we take from this brain science? Glutamate, aspartate, and homocysteine are toxic excitatory neurochemicals that can act together, creating a snowball effect within the brain for neurodegeneration. In a dense paper published in 2009, the authors stated, "Homocysteine interferes in a complex way with NMDA receptors, activating the glutamate binding site…" (18) Essentially what they are saying is that both of these excitatory neurotoxins work together.

This downward spiral ultimately results in noticeable destruction of CNS function, and in the end, possibly death. These authors are by no means alone.

I am going to quote several statements from a great paper, and try to summarize them for you. The paper is entitled, "Increase of Total Homocysteine Concentration in Cerebrospinal Fluid in Patients with Alzheimer's Disease and Parkinson's Disease," by Chiaki Isobe and others, published in 2005 in *Life Sciences*. You can gather the format of the study clearly from the title.

"In the present study, the total homocysteine concentration in the CSF was significantly higher in untreated AD and untreated PD subjects, while no correlation between the disease duration and severity was observed."

Translation – Parkinson's and Alzheimer's patients had high homocysteine in the CSF, which is in accordance with my biochemically based theory. As the disease progressed, the level of homocysteine did not go up. This implies a set "trigger point" if you will, at which a slow degenerative process ensues.

Their next quote.

"Selley (another researcher) recently examined the CSF of 8 patients with AD, and found that total homocysteine in the CSF was high in the AD patients and that a positive correlation existed between total homocysteine concentration and the concentration of 4-hydroxy-2-neonal, which is a biochemical marker of neurotoxic products of lipid peroxidation."

Translation – A researcher who took the time to look in the right place, the cerebrospinal fluid, found high homocysteine levels, and as it's a pro-oxidant, a marker for oxidation was found to support the theory that homocysteine works by oxidative damage at the least.

Next.

"Total homocysteine is metabolized to various products, including homocysteic acid, which has a structure similar to that of glutamate, which is itself an excitatory neurotransmitter. Studies have shown that homocysteine metabolites such as homocysteic acid activate the excitatory NMDA receptor and induce apoptosis (cell death). The cytotoxicity of glutamate causes cell damage from excitotoxicity via the receptor, and from competitive inhibition of cysteine transport by an increase in glutamate concentration. The latter causes a deficiency in intracellular glutathione, and consequently, neurons succumb to apoptosis due to oxidative stress."

Translation – This basically reaffirms a previous study that stated that homocysteine and glutamate seem to work in conjunction to induce neural excitotoxicity and neuron cell death. To further back up previous works, they speculate that this is at least in part done by reducing glutathione, which is the body's main antioxidant.

A quote from a different study is as follows:

"The main mechanism of homocysteine-induced neurotoxicity in this chronic in vitro model of excitotoxicty is, as in our previous acute experiments, mediated by both NDMA receptors and group I mGluR's." (19)

Translation – You'll recall the NMDA receptors are the main glutamate receptors to initiate excitation. mGluRs are just another type of glutamate receptor. Once again, from separate researchers, we are shown that homocysteine works in conjunction with glutamate, and in fact, when these receptors are blocked, protection is provided.

In yet another study, this one out of UMASS Lowell, another in vitro study verifies our previous findings. (20) Among the many excellent statements from the paper, we have:

"These findings and those of earlier reports suggest that homocysteine may exert deleterious effects on neurons hypersensitive to excitotoxicity."

"Homocysteine is a potent neurotoxin."

"B12 deficiencies are common among psychogeriatric populations."

"B12 deficiency correlates with AD and senile dementia of the Alzheimer type."

"Homocysteine is toxic to human and murine (mouse) neuronal cells in vitro in part through overstimulation of NMDA receptors and resultant calcium influx."

"Homocysteine potentiates glutamate toxicity."

"Homocysteine-induced NMDA channel activation might ultimately lead to neuronal degeneration via glutamate excitotoxicity."

I hope from this you've gained an appreciation of the connection between glutamate, homocysteine, and your brain. Glutamate, aspartate, as well as a host of other neurotoxic chemicals are omnipresent in our society. Perhaps you'll think twice about the highly processed food you're about to buy for yourself, or even worse, for your children. High homocysteine doesn't come directly from food, but is a function of diet, genetics, and nutrient availability. If you have a loved one with some type of neurological condition, you may want to consider the information in this chapter. Methylation, or the lack thereof, ties into this entire equation, and plays a possible key role in recovery.

Supplements with these fractionated amino acids are not recommended for someone with a neurotoxic condition, or propensity. You can take glutamine for certain conditions, but be aware that the body easily converts it to glutamate. In my experience, doses of glutamine worsen a pre-existing excitatory neurological state.

Supplementation to consider for a wide array of CNS issues include CoQ10, lipoic acid, ginkgo, vitamin E, vitamin C, acetyl-l-carnitine, ribose, B-vitamins, curcumin, and magnesium. Ginkgo may work via the fact that it is a glutamate antagonist, which means it competes with the glutamate receptor sites, thereby reducing the excitation via those receptors. CoQ10 works by helping energy production for those pumps, and as an antioxidant for the often referenced pro-oxidative damage. Lipoic acid does the same. Vitamins E and C work as antioxidants in this equation. Acetyl-l-carnitine and ribose work from the energy production viewpoint. In fact, ribose is the rate limiting component of ATP production, and acetyl-l-carnitine has its own data in cognitive impairment and Alzheimer's. In fact, in one meta-analysis of 21 studies encompassing 1,204 patients, the authors state, "There is an extensive body of studies suggesting the efficacy for ALC in improving cognitive deficits or delaying the progressive decline of AD patients..." (21) Each one of these individual components is only a part of a larger solution. Although it may not be good science to incorporate too many variables into one study, it may be good medicine.

Curcumin, ginger, and other herbs act from an anti-inflammatory viewpoint. Magnesium works via energy production, and has the important role of blocking the NMDA channel. However, under certain conditions, this block can be overcome. Using any one of these natural supplements to treat Alzheimer's or Parkinson's for example, is asking for failure, or at best only partial success. For example, in a study using 1,200 mg of CoQ10, the progression of Parkinson's disease was slowed by about 44%. (22) CoQ10 is expensive, and 1,200 mg is a LOT of CoQ10. Although the results were OK, it just slowed progression, it did not stop it, or what we hopefully can do, reverse it.

The real champions here are the B vitamins in concert with TMG. They have extensive roles in energy production as well, but as you already know, folate, B12, and B6 play key roles in the homocysteine cycle. In the right forms, at the correct doses, and in compliment with one another, we can only then hope for better results.

The inevitable reduction in methylation from age, homocysteine, and other factors, both in the CNS and without, dictates that one must consider methylcobalamin over standard cyanocobalamin. For example, in yet another in vitro study, SAMe and methylcobalamin were researched in reducing glutamate induced neurotoxicity. The researchers concluded, "These results indicate that chronic exposure to methylcobalamin protects cortical neurons against NMDA receptor-mediated glutamate cytotoxicity." (23)

At some point a practitioner might measure your MMA levels. MMA is a metabolite of a B12 driven enzyme. MMA is a fantastic marker for a frank cobalamin deficiency, since serum cobalamin is a relatively poor marker. In one study of 402 patients with B12 deficiency, the researchers found that of the 434 episodes of cobalamin deficiency, serum MMA was predictive for 98.4%. (24) In other words, probably the best marker to diagnose a cobalamin deficiency is MMA. But, there's a catch, and very few people know this. MMA needs the other active form of B12 to work, known as adenosylcobalamin. This is a different story then, needing methylcobalamin for the CNS and more. The body can make adenosylcobalamin from dietary or supplemental cobalamin, yet cannot make enough methylacobalam. In my opinion, adenosylcobalamin is not reflective of methylcobalamin stores, especially in the CNS. As such, MMA levels are not an adequate marker for these neurological conditions.

So when some study says that serum cobalamin or MMA were not indicators of AD, or some other neurological condition, and they discount the role of B12 for said condition, then you're now armed to contradict their conclusion. Researchers are wrong a lot of the time, which is why you're so damn confused as to what's good for you, and what's not. So most people figure, "What the hell, I've gotta go somehow, so I might as well go happy," and they go on to pollute their body and live out a great many years sickly and on drugs. My goal is to give you the best facts available anywhere to properly parse out the reality from the fiction.

TMG

Use of trimethylglycine, (TMG) also known as betaine, is the most effective way to reduce your stores of homocysteine outside the CNS. For those with some background in biochemistry, all you have to do is look at the pathways. As established, there are three ways to metabolize the harmful homocysteine, and its precursor SAH. The B6 pathway helps shuttle it out of the system altogether to be made into other amino acids. The methionine synthase pathway is a good "full time" system, as it donates a methyl group to homocysteine to reform methionine. I say "full time" because the TMG pathway is mostly based on dietary intake, while in comparison, folate has a reasonable serum half-life, and B12 is plenty available in the long term in an adequately nourished person. TMG, as I said, is a dietary feature. It can come from a number of sources, but the best is sugar beets, which is how the name betaine is derived. Betaine/TMG can also come from the oxidation of choline, of which the egg is a good source. But as this requires a couple of extra steps, TMG as a supplement is better.

If one wants to methylate homocysteine, and assuming there's plenty to be methylated, then you need an adequate dose. Remember, dose can be everything. You can take in folate of around 1 mg or so, and the same is true for B12, but with TMG you can easily take in hundreds and thousands of milligrams. Granting that the molecular size of B12, folate, and TMG are not the same, and a one-to-one comparison by weight cannot be made, you can still donate over 100 times more methyl groups with TMG as you can with B12 or folate. Not that the B vitamins aren't necessary, as they are, but for quicker and deeper results, TMG is the way to go.

TMG will do the trick to "unfreeze" the homocysteine/methionine cycle, which was all but stopped through SAH/homocysteine inhibition. Once you get the cycle going again, some interesting things will happen. Results will depend on how much homocysteine stores you have, how much TMG you take, empty/full stomach, how poorly your methylation has been, and your stores of other essential nutrients in this pathway, such as zinc and magnesium.

You may also feel relaxed. This comes from the huge release of adenosine in this cycle. As SAH (S-adenosyl homocysteine) is metabolized in homocysteine, it releases the adenosyl portion of its name in the form of adenonsine. Adenosine is one of the body's major calming neurotransmitters.

TMG has so many far-reaching effects because it kicks off methylation everywhere--just think DNA and proteins. DNA plays a role in everything in your body. Your body has been behind the curve in methylating a wide variety of needs, and combined with your genetic flaws, your needs may be different than those of another.

The real data behind TMG has been in the pursuit of lowering homocysteine. The two--methylation and homocysteine--are intricately linked, so really we're discussing one and the same. Let's look at some studies and quotes in regards to its use.

In a study where each group of 12 subjects received 6 grams of TMG, 800 micrograms of folic acid, or placebo for 6 weeks, TMG was found to be superior. (25) The authors went on to state, "In conclusion, betaine appears to be highly effective in preventing a rise in plasma homocysteine concentration after methionine intake in subjects with mildly elevated homocysteine. It is not known whether this potential of betaine to "stabilize" circulating homocysteine concentrations lowers the risk of cardiovascular disease."

Another trial with 42 subjects found that 6 grams/day of betaine given for 12 weeks reduced homocysteine by 9%. (26) These results aren't terribly impressive, but I include them in the interests of full disclosure. Remember, there are many variables.

In a 2003 study published in the *Journal of Nutrition*, groups of 19 healthy subjects ingested various doses of TMG or placebo daily for six weeks. (27) For those who took 3 grams per day, their homocysteine was reduced by 15%; for those who took six grams per day, their homocysteine was reduced by 20%. This was in just six weeks, which is not too shabby.

In yet another example, we reference a trial from the *British Journal of Nutrition* in 2004. They had an interesting twist on things. Thirty-four healthy men and women were given 1 gram of betaine in week one, 3 grams in week 2, 6 grams in week 3, and 6 grams betaine plus 1 mg of folic acid in week 4. (28) The 1 gram had no statistical change, the 3 grams showed a 10% drop, 6 grams showed a 14% drop, and the addition of folic acid to the 6 grams dropped homocysteine by an additional 5%.

Other researchers in a recent review of the data quote, "Recent studies have demonstrated that plasma betaine is a stronger determinant of post-methionine load (think - eat a lot of protein) homocysteine than are B6 and folate." (29) This is not to imply that only TMG should be the sole savior of high homocysteine. Folate, B12, B6, zinc, and magnesium all have their place, at a minimum. For example, in one trial with healthy women aged 18-40, a dose of 500 micrograms of folic acid for four weeks reduced homocysteine by 22%. That's impressive, since it only took 4 weeks, it is just one vitamin in the cycle, and the dose of folate really wasn't that high. Again, results will vary by person dependent on genetics, dietary deficiencies, age, and general health. While discussing folate and healthy women of reproductive age, let's touch on pregnancy. Do you know why women who are trying to conceive and have conceived are told to take folate? It's primarily to prevent neural tube defects, which, by the way, has been working, although not 100%. Neural tube defects are a neurological shortcoming, because as you now know, folate is a part of the homocysteine-methionine cycle, which makes more SAMe to donate its methyl groups to all body parts, to include a developing fetus.

Ideally you want to have as much zinc and magnesium on board as possible. The enzyme (BHMT), which we'll refer to as the TMG enzyme, requires zinc to do its job. No zinc, no getting that homocysteine/methionine cycle flying. Likewise, magnesium is needed to convert methionine into SAMe, which, as you may recall, is the body's major methyl donor. No magnesium, and you get a build-up of methionine, which is not ideal either. So when you look at studies with good intentions but only reasonable design, consider this. How much better could the results have been if all biochemical needs were addressed?

We also have to consider the dose and half-life of any therapy. There are many research authors with questionable motivations. I too could construct a clinical trial to fail for just about any natural medicine. Betaine is no different, so we should build a protocol properly. Not only do we need the other nutrients on board, but we also ought to consider the pharmacodynamic of betaine. Data from a dose-response study tells us that regardless of the amount ingested, betaine peaks in serum in about 30-40 minutes, and much is cleared in about 200-400 minutes. (30) Spreading out the dose over the day, with most at night, given the effects of adenosine, seems to make the most sense. A total daily dose of about 6 grams seems in order as well. In fact, you can find homocysteine management formulas on the market with a blend of ingredients, but the betaine may only be a gram or so. This same study tells us that 1 gram did not lower homocysteine. Build your own protocol for success.

I have to add in this last piece because I find it so interesting. Betaine has been used for decades as a dietary feed supplement to animals for a number of reasons. In pigs, it has been shown to reduce the amount of body fat. (31) Before you run out to buy some for weight loss, you should know that in obese middle-aged humans, 6 grams a day did not affect body weight. (32) Betaine is also used to improve growth efficiency. (33) In other words, through the mechanism of methylation, likely via an improved digestive tract and an efficient methylation process for protein synthesis, less food is needed to raise chicks and pigs, and probably salmon too, as it's used there. Like all things it comes down to money, and so here the use of betaine means it will cost less money in feed to bring the same animal to market. Maybe it will make you a more efficient eater.

TMG Side Effects

Are there any side effects with the use of betaine? Six grams a day seems like a large dose. First you have to consider that the daily dietary intake of betaine is estimated to be about .5-2 grams per day. (34) Also, the body is able to synthesize betaine from choline.

Some researchers will note that betaine administration may adversely affect lipid concentrations, particularly an increase in LDL. They state that these changes may offset the positive changes in homocysteine management in terms of cardiovascular risk. (35) It is true that this has been seen in studies, but you have to appreciate the full situation. As methylation begins to rapidly return to the unhealthy burdened liver from years of abuse, the natural result is a "cleansing" of the organ. One aspect of methylation in the liver produces phosphatidylcholine, which is integral in transporting fat <u>from</u> the liver. (36) Higher blood lipids is a temporary artifact of this process. In fact, this is precisely why SAMe is used to treat liver disorders. One researcher comments that:

"Of all the therapeutic modalities available, betaine has been shown to be the safest, least expensive and most effective in attenuating ethanol-induced liver injury. Betaine, by virtue of aiding in the remethylation of homocysteine, removes both toxic metabolites (homocysteine and S-adenosylhomocysteine), restores S-adenosylmethionine level, and reverses hepatic steatosis, apoptosis, and damaged proteins accumulation. In conclusion, betaine appears to be a promising therapeutic   agent   in relieving the methylation and other defects associated with alcoholic abuse." (37)

A long-term study should look at the levels of LDL with betaine supplementation, as time should show that LDL will be equalized, if not improved.

Of last note, you should take vitamin B6 along with your betaine. I know I've said over and again that all nutrients should be taken for full benefits, but there are those who may just focus on one. The B6 is necessary to shuttle the homocysteine out of the cycle. As homocysteine is metabolized to methionine within the cycle, we want to avoid excessive methionine levels, as methionine itself has a toxic potential. To further ensure best results, you should cut down on animal proteins, as they are high in methionine.

SAMe

SAMe is available as a supplement in the market, and has been for years. Since SAMe is the champion of methyl donation, then why not take it instead? I think I've clearly made the case to reduce homocysteine within and without the CNS, and the other nutrients will get the cycle going to do just that, and in the process make plenty of SAMe. Granted, the data does show that the ingestion of SAMe will get the ball rolling, but I suspect not nearly as much. In addition, it seems logical to not take in any extra methione (SAMe = S-adenosyl-methionine), as we are trying to metabolize methionine out of the system. Don't forget, as soon as SAMe donates its methyl group it becomes SAH and then homocysteine, the very things we're trying to get rid of. So the more methionine you take in, the more homocysteine you'll make. In time, when homocysteine has plummeted, taking SAMe is perfectly warranted, in my opinion. But then again, you have to consider cost as well, as SAMe is not cheap. Some even question its exogenous absorption. As one researcher states, "Because of its high molecular weight and its difficulty in crossing membranes, it has very low bioavailability if given orally or parenterally." (38)

Make no doubt about it, SAMe is the superstar on this stage. We just go about a different way of sending its production into warp speed. Among the many methylating benefits it has, it also inhibits an enzyme known as demethylase, which is expressed in some or most cells in the body. (39) This demthylase, as the name implies, demethylates DNA, which is a bad thing. The integrity of DNA is necessary for protein production and the prevention of cancer. At this point I'm not going to go into methylation and cancer, as it's a whole new can of worms. Just consider that there is a lot of research in this area, and SAMe does seem to have benefit in DNA integrity and whole health in the pre-cancerous condition.

We want to keep an active state of methylation as long as possible. Again, consider those Okinawans. A low calorie, highly active, whole foods, low toxin life style goes a long way. Granted there are many factors to their health, but many can be tied to methylation. A diet with low protein has more methylation per gram of food ingested than a high protein diet. It also will result in a lower homocysteine load, which is integrally tied to the cycling of methylation.

There are a number of factors that can reduce methylation as well, such as smoking, alcohol, high fat diets, many prescription drugs, and the factors behind aging previously discussed. Since the liver is the primary site of methylation, and the liver processes fats, inhibition of methylation at the liver can occur, especially if the fats are unhealthy ones. In fact, SAMe has been well researched in the treatment of fatty acid steatosis in alcoholics with some success. Methylation is so broad-based, it could be researched in just about any condition you can pick. Depression is another area of study, as SAMe influences the metabolism of neurotransmitters in the brain. One study showed that 66% of the patients treated with SAMe showed significant clinical improvement in depressive symptoms compared to only 22% given an antidepressant drug. Like most other natural medicines, the side effects profile is a fraction of that of the drug. In fact, SAMe is sold in Europe for the treatment of depression and liver disease!

In a review of 11 studies, researchers looked at the use of SAMe in comparison to NSAIDS in the treatment of osteoarthritis. In their conclusion, they state, "SAMe appears to be as effective as NSAIDs in reducing pain and improving functional limitation in patients with OA without the adverse effects often associated with NSAID therapies." (40) Sure NSAIDs help reduce the pain temporarily, but as we've discussed in this book, they contribute to more tissue destruction. SAMe (i.e., methylation) goes to the root of the matter, and helps to synthesize new tissue to repair the damage. This is at the core of holistic/integrative/alternative/natural medicine: to find the cause and treat the cause of the symptoms. Some practitioners are better than others, like anything in life, but you owe it to yourself to seek out other options.

Genetics

As I have stated previously, our genetic predispositions can play a large role in our potential for illness, depending on the disease. For example, breast cancer is often thought to have a large genetic component, but contrary to what your perceptions may be, genes may account for only 2-5% of breast cancer incidence. (41) However, other conditions have a higher degree of genetic association. It's no wonder that a man who lost his father at a young age to heart disease, may suffer the same consequences. These alterations in how our DNA codes proteins are at the heart of the variability of disease. Why does one child who is assaulted with batteries of inoculations in the first years of life develop autistic traits, while most others tolerate them without noticeable problems? We all have some weakness, and it would be a great help to know what that weakness might be. This is the ultimate in preventative medicine, and it could possibly be the future as well.

Unfortunately, many people get very concerned about an HMO knowing that they have some genetic high-risk flaw. Can they get coverage, and if so, at what price? These are legitimate questions, and until they get resolved, if they ever do, then being in charge of your own healthcare is in your best interest.

There are a number of labs that offer up a variety of tests to look at what's merely a handful of possible genes out of many. With that said, labs have chosen some of the key genes about which we have knowledge to date, in disease prevention. This implies that some other great diagnostic genetic tests may become the norm down the road, but we have to work with the information we have today. We are actually at a very interesting point in history. With pretty much the exception of the last 100 years, man has had to eke out a living with minimal food selection (dependent on region), high risk, and no trauma care. Of course, genetics would have been a foreign concept to them. At this point in time, especially here in America, we have access to a variety of healthy foods on a year-round basis, quite good medical care when properly used, a supplement industry with tons of biochemical knowledge in the hopes of alleviating disease and making a profit, and the ability to look at our individual genetic code. With all of this knowledge, most still choose to eat pizza, french fries, doughnuts, rarely exercise, and throw a multitude of drugs and OTC (over-the-counter) products at symptoms without addressing the underlying cause in many cases.

There are several reasons why this is the case, but you have to ask yourself, "What's my reason?" Sure, there's a lot of confusion over diseases, proper nutrition, symptoms, and supplements. I hope I have addressed them adequately for you. However, it is time for the average healthcare consumer to take a larger role in their care. Be your own primary care doctor. Do your research. The old fallacy of the doctor being the next closest thing to God is rapidly disappearing. Doctors don't know all, and can't reasonably be expected to. The system in which they operate is a flawed one, and greed on many levels distorts it even more. In this healthcare debate, some pundits rave about the American healthcare system. Well, depending on which need you examine, the results may vary. If you simply look at life expectancy, we rank very poorly. If you throw into that equation that we also have the most expensive healthcare system in the world, then we're even worse. Many "third world" countries have a longer life expectancy than we do, and the last years of life are on average healthier ones at that. Using this as an indicator of the system, I think we

145

can do better. The powers that be, whether it's the clowns in Washington DC, the pharmaceutical industry, or the AMA, will not allow significant change that will help you, the average American taxpayer. Do you have a personal lobbyist in D.C.? In an *American Chronicle* article published on September 18, 2009, the author states that there are now 34,750 registered Washington lobbyists. I think you're outgunned. Be proactive in your own healthcare.

So let's get back on track to what we currently know about genetics and homocysteine management. From here, you can make your own decisions. In review, we need the active form of folate (5-MTHF), one of the two active forms of B12 (methycobalamin), and the active form of pyridoxine (P5P) in the metabolism of homocysteine. We also need magnesium and zinc, but here we're looking at enzyme flaws. There is another enzyme, what we've referred to as the TMG enzyme, also known as BHMT (betaine: homocysteine methyl transferase). However, there is precious little data looking at this gene. So we'll focus on the vitamin dependent ones.

Folate

The gene in question here is the one that takes a version of folate and turns it into the active form. The enzyme is MTHFR, aka methyltetrahydrofolate reductase. Technically, there are several genetic flaws studied, but only one seems to have impact on homocysteine metabolism. So let's focus on MTHFR. This is the most studied of the three flaws.

One can have a heterozygous (single-parent) flaw, which means one of the chromosomes was not quite right. One can also have a homozygous (double-parent) flaw, in which case both parents contributed to the flaw, which makes it more severe. As a reference, one study looked at the activity in vitro and found that those with the single-parent flaw had about 71% of normal enzyme function, while those with the double-parent flaw had a mere 34% of enzyme function. (42) The good news is that taking folic acid as a supplement seems to alleviate serum homocysteine levels. A number of researchers have found that although this flaw plays a role, it's much more powerful if the patient is also low on

146

folate status. In one researcher's opinion, "A moderate average daily intake of folic acid appeared to counter the effect of the MTHFR variant on serum total homocysteine concentration." (43) Knowing how bad homocysteine is for your health, how can anyone claim that all supplements are useless?

In another study, to continue to confuse you, the researchers did not find a strong correlation between this flaw and homocysteine amongst 1,006 female twins. (44) They went on to state that "All our tested SNPs (gene flaws at a given location) were weaker predictors of plasma homocysteine than the strongest environmental factor, that of serum folate." This implies that studies to date have not yet examined the correct SNPs, or that other genes are involved. Two points here. These guys say that what's more important is the status of the vitamins in your blood. Their second point is: there may be other unidentified genes that are better predictors. In reviewing the literature, I think both statements have a lot of truth in them.

This MTHF flaw, as well as others, follows general patterns when comparing ethnic groups as well. For example, non-hispanic black subjects have been shown to have a higher frequency for the CBS flaw (B6) than do non-hispanic white and Mexican American subjects. (45) As the CBS enzyme is the only way to eventually shuttle out the homocysteine after it runs its course(s) through the cycle, a flaw in this enzyme may be the most important of all. This may in part explain why black Americans tend to die from heart disease at a younger age than do individuals of other races.

Methionine Synthase

The methionine synthase complex is a two-part enzymatic process, which requires a second enzyme, methionine synthase reductase, to keep synthase active. The MTRR A66G polymorphism is probably the most studied. At least two studies have shown that a double-parent flaw here results in higher homocysteine. (46) Frequency varies by populations. At the low end, the double-parent flaw for MTRR is 8-10% in Japanese in Hawaii and Hawaiians while at the high end it was 50% in Hispanics. (47)

An Italian study found no association between the MTRR A66G flaw and plasma homocysteine in 114 patients with vascular disease. (48)

Here's some more interesting information to ponder. The MTRR A66G flaw "seems to be a risk factor for neural tube defects, especially when the plasma B12 level is low, or when the MTHFR polymorphism (double-parent flaw) is present." (49) Remember that MTHFR activates folate, which contributes a methyl group to B12. What these researchers are saying is that in this virtual worst-case condition, flaws in folate and B12 metabolism, combined with a low B12 status, are, not surprisingly, linked to neural tube defects. Natural medicine may help you to conceive and it can also help determine your infant's risk for neural tube defects.

Two studies show that, "Women who have both the MTRR 66G and MTHFR 677T mutations appeared to have an increased risk of having a child with Down's syndrome." (50) This comes as no surprise either, as we're still within the realm of neurology. Why someone has a neural tube defect and another has Down's is likely linked to some other gene we have yet to uncover. It's probably similar to the events later in life where one person develops AD and another develops Parkinson's. From the data, it seems the causes may be almost identical, and so there may be another gene that pushes one way or the other.

Another set of researchers state that the MTRR flaw "seems to be correlated with an increased risk for the development of premature coronary artery disease." (51) The point is now clear. This MTRR flaw is CENTRAL in the methionine-homocysteine-methylation cycle. The primary consideration here is methylcobalamin, a relatively cheap and safe product when used in moderation.

CBS

Many alterations in this gene have been found to date, but there's very little data. The double-parent flaw here is not common. The highest reported frequency is in blacks from Brazil and Africa, where it was 3%. If you're in that 3%, then it makes a big difference. Single-parent occurrence for this flaw is much higher, averaging about 14% among whites of European descent. (52)

So what are we to learn from all of this genetic stuff? I think it's safe to say that we are in the beginning stages of our understanding and discovery of genetic information. It has enormous future potential to radically change the way we practice medicine, assuming we can get out of the way of our own policies. We can also begin to use it as a tool today for diagnostic and treatment needs. We know from dozens upon dozens of studies that elevated homocysteine is a bad thing, and we know how to reduce it. What we know today about these enzymes can help us to guide therapy more successfully.

Something missing from the studies I have reviewed is the connection to the brain. We know (at least we think we do) that there is a lesser capacity to metabolize homocysteine in the brain. So, it may be that someone with an MTHFR or MTRR/MTR flaw may do fine outside the CNS on low dose folic acid with no real overt signs, but the story in the CNS may be quite different. Remember that the important TMG pathway does not exist in the brain, and some research points to a less active P5P pathway there as compared to the rest of the body. This is likely why injectable methylcobalamin shows some success in a condition like Parkinson's.

We must also consider age in these trials and others down the road. If we are to examine subjects age 45 and under, we may not find as strong a connection than if we were to look at a significantly older crowd. We know that methylation declines as we age, and thus a genetic flaw would be less easily compensated for in the elderly than in someone with relative youth.

Nutrient deficiencies must also be considered. I know many doctors have stated that taking supplements only results in expensive urine. Yet even this contradictory and incomplete genetic research shows us repeatedly that if you do have one double-parent flaw and are deficient in that nutrient that lines up with that flaw, then expect poor outcomes. Should you have two flaws and be nutritionally deficient in both, you're definitely behind the 8-ball. Considering that B-vitamins are among the cheapest of supplements to take, they may be worth considering.

Chapter 6 Vascular Health

According to epidemiological calculations, making healthy food choices consistent with the Mediterranean diet, along with smoking cessation and physical activity, can prevent 80% of coronary-artery disease. (1) If true, why are we so hooked on taking so many drugs to supposedly reduce our risk of vascular disease? We'll first take a look at one class of drugs, the statins, the most prescribed drugs in the world.

Is there really any benefit in taking statins? It seems more and more people are being prescribed this class of drugs for preventative medicine. Is it just good marketing and sales on behalf of a corporation, or are these drugs just that valuable? How about cholesterol? We have all of these low cholesterol diets, and yet more and more people are on statins. I often get questions revolving around the side effects of statins, and what the other choices may be. So let's take a deep look into statins and cholesterol as they pertain to your vascular health.

Understand that the goal of this book is not to "bash" drugs and conventional medicine while putting all things "natural" up on a pedestal. There are a number of products, devices, practices, and practitioners in natural medicine that should be avoided. In addition, modern medicine provides a number of fantastic features for our health and longevity. There are drugs that can do things of which natural medicine can only dream. There are necessary life-saving procedures in acute care as well. Many highly trained, intelligent conventional practitioners bring a lot to the table for all of us.

With that said, there are places and times for everything. Many of our chronic degenerative diseases can be treated or avoided without drugs. There are uses for drugs, but they are also very often overused. A classic example would be antibiotics. If a mother brings in a child with a cold, which is caused by a virus, and she demands antibiotics, the doctor may cave in as she's the customer, even though the prescription will do no good. Antibiotics are in fact overused, resulting in more resistant strains for when they are actually needed. At least there's a push to reduce needless prescriptions in this area.

The opposite is true for statins. The market for statins keeps growing and growing, yet the clinical evidence behind their use is very limited. You may be shocked to learn some of this material, but then again, you probably won't find it too surprising. It was not an easy task to wade through some of the bullshit in the clinical data, as these trials are funded by the industry. One has to read all opinions, understand statistics and clinical trials, and throw in a little common sense to distill the truth. With that said, I'll offer up many statements and opinions from others, from which you can make your own informed decision.

Before today's statins hit the market, we had fibrate drugs from the 1960s to the 80s. After many years of use, a World Health Organization (WHO) study found that clofibrate increased the risk of overall death by 47%, and a Finnish study found that gemfibrozil caused a 21% increase in deaths. (2) <u>A blind man can see from a mile away that any drug that increases mortality, regardless of how it impacts certain parameters, is not a good drug</u>. Sadly, I'm not surprised these drugs were around as long as they were. *Thank goodness our government and the pharmaceutical industry have cleaned up their act?*

The statin came of age in 1987. In 2001, an expert panel as part of the National Cholesterol Education Program (NECP) updated guidelines from clinical trials to "assist" doctors in reducing their patients' risk of developing coronary heart disease. (3) These guidelines, or clinical practice guidelines, or standards of care, become VERY IMPORTANT in how we conduct medicine in this country. In theory, clinical practice guidelines (CPGs) are intended to present a synthesis of current evidence and recommendations performed by expert clinicians and may affect the practice of large numbers of physicians. (4) Ideally, you'd have a group of very intelligent, impartial, skilled practitioners establishing these guidelines for a whole nation to follow. Ideally.

The lead author, Dr. Scott M Grundy stated, "These statins are amazing drugs…" He and 13 others established these new guidelines. The bulk of these new recommendations address LDL cholesterol as the primary target of therapy. (5) If your primary care doctor tries to jam statins on you, you now know where that recommendation originated. There are a couple major problems with this whole scenario. Cholesterol is essentially not the cause of CVD, especially not alone. Second, 5 of the 14 experts who wrote the guidelines, including the chair, disclosed financial relationships with manufacturers of statin drugs. (6) Four of these five, including the chair, had relationships with all three manufacturers of the best-selling statins. (7) Hmmm.

In 2004, the NCEP met again to update the guidelines. The panel recommended even lower targets for "bad" cholesterol, which would effectively put more Americans on statins. (8) At long last, some responsible people began to step forward. A petition was sent to the NIH illustrating the weakness of the evidence, and that the panel members were biased, as 8 out of 9 of the "experts" on the panel had financial ties to the pharmaceutical industry. (9) In 2008, in a *BusinessWeek* cover story by John Carey, Dr. Rodney Hayward, professor of internal medicine at the University of Michigan Medical School, stated, "It's almost impossible to find someone who believes strongly in statins who does not get a lot of money from industry. Current evidence supports ignoring LDL cholesterol altogether."

The thing is, not all doctors are corrupt. The problem is that when you have centralization of decision making, which affects a great many people, like the centralizing of our federal government, then a lot of influence is placed in the hands of a few. So, if you have a business, and if you seek to influence the influencers, then it's much easier in a centralized scenario than otherwise. Doctors aren't required to follow these or any guidelines to the letter, but most do for several reasons: they want to practice what's perceived to be the best medicine, they want their medical decisions to be consistent with community standards, and most importantly they know that if they do not follow current guidelines, they have a greater risk of getting sued should something go wrong. (10) This is why it's so hard to find an M.D. who practices integrative medicine. These people put their livelihood on the line for something in which they believe.

In the *Journal of the Canadian Medical Association*, two authors penned a letter, which included the following statements:

"There are no statin trials with even the slightest hint of mortality benefit in women, and women should be told so. Likewise, evidence in patients over 70 years old shows no mortality benefit of statin therapy: in the PROSPER trial there were 28 fewer deaths from coronary artery disease in patients who received pravastatin versus placebo, offset by 24 more cancer deaths."

"The website of the ALLHAT study says it best: 'Trials primarily in middle-aged men demonstrating a reduction in coronary artery disease from cholesterol-lowering have not demonstrated a net reduction in all-cause mortality.' What is the point of decreasing the number of events without decreasing overall mortality, when the harm caused by the side effects of statin therapy is factored in?" (11)

So what are these trials anyhow? Drugs are brought to market through a series of clinical trials where efficacy (good clinical results) are supposed to be shown, and side effects (adverse events) are to be minimal. One of the problems with this scenario is that trials are relatively short in duration, and thus long enough to show benefit but usually short enough not to demonstrate bad or adverse effects. If you think this sounds like a conspiracy theory, consider the following.

The first generation of statins killed people, as already explained. They had been approved for use. Baycol from Bayer was pulled in 2001 for killing people; it had been approved. Vytorin, which is still on the market, is under review. A December 2008 posting from the law firm Parker-Waichman-Alonso LLP states that Vytorin is the subject of more than 140 class action lawsuits and the subject of a justice department investigation. The ENHANCE study showed the ineffectiveness of the drug, and Merck and Schering-Plough delayed releasing the results for more than a year. As the posting states further, such a delay is "something critics have likened to fraud." This delay prompted a congressional investigation, for whatever that's worth. This same posting notes that Vytorin is the subject of a Justice Department investigation, looking into the possibility of false claims. If this wasn't enough, the SEAS study showed no additional heart attack prevention, but did show higher rates of cancer for the drug. Congress expanded its investigation to include the handling of this trial.

At least Pfizer stopped the manufacturing of torcetrabip in 2006 when it was found in the ILLUMINATE trial that it increased the risk of death and cardiac events. The drug worked by increasing HDL, which it did very well, but at an obvious cost. <u>We need to look at the complete picture, not synthetically adjusted parameters.</u>

We mentioned the PROSPER trial, and the increased incidence of cancer. The IDEAL trial, which enrolled 8,888 patients with a median follow-up of 4.8 years, had an adverse (side-effect) event rate of a whopping 94%, with serious adverse events at 46%. (12) In this Pfizer-sponsored study, with four authors with connections to Pfizer, even they couldn't escape the obvious statements they made. "In this study of patients with previous MI (heart attack), intensive lowering of LDL cholesterol did not result in a significant reduction in the primary outcome of major coronary events. There were no differences in cardiovascular or all-cause mortality."

You have to understand that these big trials are carefully constructed in the hopes of yielding the best results possible. Subjects are carefully screened, and discharged if need be to make the numbers look better. For example, in an article entitled, "Should we lower cholesterol as much as possible?" from the *British Medical Journal* in 2006, the authors discuss how a significant increase in breast cancer was seen in the CARE trial, since then patients with a history of cancer have been excluded from statin trials. (13) Is this the real world? Highly unlikely, but this is one way to control the statistics.

Nowhere is this more evident than in the TNT trial where two doses of Lipitor were studied to see if intensive lipid-lowering at a higher dose provided any benefit. I have never seen so many patients excluded from a study before. They started with 18,469 patients, and then "started" the study with 10,003. (14) Subjects were excluded for a wide variety of reasons during the 8 week washout period, and then another 8 week pretreatment period to include, death, ischemic events, adverse events, and reasons not stated. I have to hand it to them, they did one hell of a job prescreening these subject for "success". They did lower LDL, and the higher dose arm had fewer major cardiovascular events, but over 4.9 years they showed no difference between the groups in overall mortality.

Of note, in this study funded by Pfizer, the lead author reports, "having received consulting fees from Pfizer, Merck, Bristol-Myers Squibb, and AstraZeneca and lecture fees from Pfizer." Remember Dr Grundy. He was a co-author in this study, and his disclosure states that he received, "lecture fees from Merck, Pfizer, Kos Pharmaceutical, Abbott, and AstraZeneca and grant support from Kos Pharmaceutical and Merck". The other disclosures from the remaining authors contain a long list of industry connections.

If we look at some very recent review articles on statins, articles that are supposed to impartially weigh all of the relevant data to come to a consensus on a topic, we quickly find two that support the use of statins. One from 2009 states, "Treatment with statins significantly reduced the risk of all-cause mortality" and "no evidence of an increased risk of cancer was observed." (15) Curiously, four of the authors had extensive competing interests. Seriously, under the heading "competing interests," it lists their numerous collaborations with industry. In a 2008 review, the authors emphasize the link between LDL cholesterol and CVD. (16) As stated in the paper, "This review was facilitated by Pfizer Canada, Inc., through honoraria (money) paid directly to each author."

I hope you understand that for the most part, you are not a person, not a father or mother, not a son or daughter, you are a dollar sign ($) to large corporations and a walking ballot box to a politician. The money and power at stake in healthcare and food is absolutely enormous, and these are but two aspects of our economy. According to IMS Health, statins revenue was over $17 billion in 2009. These are a lot of reasons to maintain the status quo. The smoke is out there, but you have to find the fire, as it doesn't often see the light of day, and when it does, it gets swamped in a sea of news. Three MDs went so far as to highlight this questionable interrelationship between doctors and the pharmaceutical industry in a paper published in *JAMA*. They were looking into the potential conflicts of interest for authors of the CPGs or standards of care we mentioned earlier. Remember, a few key "experts" have the ability to influence a nation full of providers. These three MDs found that 87% of the CPG authors had some form of interaction with the pharmaceutical industry, 58% had received financial support to perform research, and 38% had served as employees or consultants for a pharmaceutical company. (17) While only 7% admitted to believing that their own relationships influenced the treatment recommendation, curiously 19% believed their coauthor's recommendations were influenced by industry relationships. The authors went on to conclude that, "These specific interactions may influence the practice of a very large number of physicians."

So who should use statins? Some practitioners would argue that nobody should. I am in that camp, but others feel a segment of the population can benefit. As is argued in one review, statin use in patients without CVD does not reduce coronary heart disease or mortality. (18) Likewise, professor James Wright, director of a government funded initiative to review data on drugs says that, "Most people are taking something (statins) with no chance of benefit and risk of harm." (19) He does believe they can be life-saving in patients who have already suffered from a heart attack, but found no benefit in people over 65, no benefit in women of any age, and noted that even in middle-aged men there was no overall reduction in total deaths, despite big reductions in "bad" cholesterol." (20)

Similarly, Dr. Howard Brody, professor of medicine at the University of Texas Medical Branch, states that many drugs are effective in small groups, and with statins, that is with those who already have heart disease. (21) To support these two, John Abramson in his book, *Overdosed America*, discusses how the data supports most men taking statins who have established coronary heart disease, but questions its role for women. The crazy fact lost in all of this commentary is that although statins do reduce "bad" cholesterol, its impact on overall mortality is highly questionable. So should we even be looking at LDL and total cholesterol? Dr Steven Nissen, who does have extensive research support ties to the pharmaceutical industry at Cleveland Clinic, but who does donate consult fees and honoraria to charity, as of his 2009 article in Current Cardiology Reports, states, "Another major reason for skepticism relates to the almost religious belief on the part of many prevention experts that elevated LDL cholesterol is the dominant risk factor driving coronary heart disease. This perspective ignores the reality that approximately half of all patients developing coronary disease have normal lipid levels." (22)

So how do statins potentially help with these sick patients? Two trials point to a lowering of C-reactice protein (CRP) as the possible primary mechanism for their benefit. (23) CRP is a marker for inflammation. It is produced in the liver, and its presence in the blood closely correlates to CVD. So what we're talking about here is inflammation. Does this mean that statins are anti-inflammatory? Yes and no. Statins work by inhibiting a pathway in the liver that makes cholesterol. However, this pathway makes other things as well, like CoQ10. If you want a more in-depth analysis of side effects and supplements to consider, I highly recommend *The Cholestrol Hoax* by Sherry Rogers M.D. One of the things that is also hindered in this process is an enzyme called ROCK. ROCK plays a role in vascular tone, inflammation, oxidative stress, vascular immune regulation, vascular bone-link morphology, nitric oxide, and clotting. (24) This is cutting edge research of which almost no practitioner is aware. Because ROCK is involved in so many aspects of vascular health, the pharmaceutical industry has considerable interest in the development of drugs that modulate this enzyme. (25) I believe it will not only be the next generation of statins, but it will also be the next generation of almost everything, as it has such ubiquitous effects. The importance of the ROCK enzyme will now become obvious to you as we look at what science really shows to be the cause of vascular disease.

What Causes Atherosclerosis?

The human body requires cholesterol for its survival. Unfortunately, it has gotten a very bad wrap over the years. Among other things, cholesterol is needed for brain function and hormone synthesis. In fact, the data shows as we age, reducing cholesterol becomes more of a bad idea. (26) A report out of the Framingham study showed that deaths from diseases other than CVD were higher for those over 50 as cholesterol went lower. They stated that, "Physicians should be cautious about intiating cholesterol-lowering treatment in men and women above 65 to 70 years old." (27) We need cholesterol. Too low a value is associated with amnesia, memory loss, cancer, suicide, depression, Alzheimer's, other neurological diseases, accidents, CoQ10 deficiency, and more. (28)

You'd be surprised to know that your body makes a significant amount of your cholesterol. That's right, those high cholesterol foods like eggs, which are very good for you, have been avoided for no good reason. In fact, one study with adults who ate 12 eggs a week showed no difference in cholesterol when compared to those who didn't eat eggs. (29) You'd be further surprised to know that dietary cholesterol is not the real culprit here, but dietary sugar is. That's right, sucrose, table sugar.

When the body digests sucrose, it breaks it into glucose for energy, and fructose. Fructose (as in high fructose corn syrup) is a precursor to forming cholesterol in the liver. This was proven decades ago, but the truth seems hard to come by these days. In a study with 18 subjects confined without access to other foods, a fixed diet was initiated to determine the effect of sucrose on cholesterol. (30) At first they were given amino acids, a little fat, vitamins, minerals, and glucose. After 4 weeks on this diet their cholesterol dropped from 227 to 160. The diet was then changed, with only one quarter of the glucose replaced by sucrose. After three weeks their average cholesterol rose to 208. When the sucrose was replaced with glucose again, the cholesterol dropped to 150. It's simple biochemistry. The fructose is converted into acetate, which is the prescursor the body uses to make cholesterol, just as cholesterol is the precursor needed by the adrenal glands to make the many hormones originating from those glands.

However, there is such a thing as too much. The risk for CVD does increase with increasing levels of cholesterol, but not uniformly in all people. Even in those with genetic flaws from both mom and dad yielding cholesterol values upwards of 800 (which is through the roof) there is as much as a 30-year difference in when CVD is first clinically presented in these folks. (31) It is not so much the total level of cholesterol, but the amount of oxidized cholesterol in the body that counts. Likewise, the walls of the artery may become oxidized as well by such things as toxins and pathogens, and cholesterol will essentially serve as a spackle to cover up the compromise in the lining of the arteries. (32) We'll focus on oxidized cholesterol as the primary mechanism.

There are many facets to vascular health. CRP, insulin/glucose, HDL, triglycerides, Lp(a), hypertension, toxins, pathogens, fibrinogen, and low testosterone are all valuable topics, but as you address the points in this chapter, these others will fall into line as their roots are grown from the same oxidation and inflammation. The simple fact, as discussed by numerous researchers, is that atherosclerosis is a chronic inflammatory disease. (33-37) What causes this inflammation? Primarily oxidation. (33-39)

In the normal vascular wall, inflammation is regulated in response to injury or activation, and excessive inflammation is controlled. (40) However, in the presence of continual activation through oxidized cholesterol, the inflammatory pathways are up-regulated. Oxidized cholesterol is primarily the result of the intake of certain oils, which are oxidized or easily oxidized, and other pro-oxidative factors, such as smoking and high blood sugar. If you just consider smoking, we all know the increased CVD risk associated with it. However, smoking itself does not raise cholesterol levels. If cholesterol levels were the sole reason for CVD, then smoking would be irrelevant. But, smoking oxidizes cholesterol.

Once oxidized, cholesterol is toxic to the artery wall, which results in an extended immune response. This fairly well-defined immune and inflammation reaction evolves over time and results in terms like fatty streak, foam cells, and calcification. In essence, the initial response to the lesion results in much communication with the immune system calling on components to adhere, multiply, and calcify the "plaque". Calcification can occur in the middle layer of the artery as well, leading to rigidity. The end result is a scab of sorts in the lining of the artery. This scab is usually not the cause of death, even though it restricts blood flow, but it is a rupture of the scab, which travels through the circulation and stops blood flow at smaller arteries in the heart or brain.

On a positive note, diet and antioxidants have been repeatedly shown to reduce the risk for the initial oxidation. Ideally, you'd want to pursue preventative medicine, and not have oxidized LDL to begin with, which could in turn cause the initial lesion, which gets the CVD ball rolling. However, reversal of the plaque can be accomplished. As well, controlling the inflammation, much akin to stopping smoking, can reduce your risks, as 75-95% of men and women at autopsy have coronary calcification regardless of cause of death. (41) In other words, you may be able to prevent further deterioration of existing plaque by controlling it with diet.

Some quotes from a number of researchers may help to send home the message, as this may all seem to foreign to many.

A paper authored by 5 PhD's, an M.D., and an M.D/PhD states the following. "The clinical events resulting from atherosclerosis are directly related to the oxidation of lipids in LDLs. Research in the last two decades has shown that atherosclerosis is neither a degenerative disease, nor inevitable." (42)

A recent paper in the *American Journal of Clinical Nutrition* states the following:

"In today's society, in which sloth and gluttony are unfortunately prevalent, the initiation of the atherosclerotic process can occur early in life. Indeed, 1 in 6 American teenagers already has pathologic intimal (inside layer) thickening in their coronary arteries. Inflammation is central to cardiovascular disease." (43)

In a recent 2009 paper by two M.D.s and an M.D./PhD, the following statement is made: "Laboratory and clinical data suggest that oxidized or glycated LDL evokes an inflammatory response in the artery wall, unleashing many of the biological processes thought to participate in atherosclerotic initiation, progression, and complication." (44)

Another set of researchers out of the University of California state, "There is compelling evidence that oxidized lipoproteins are atherogenic and play a key role in the pathogenesis of coronary heart disease." (45) Some of their other comments cover many aspects, which include: dietary antioxidants reduce lesion formation, oxidized lipoproteins are found in the lesions, oxidized lipids in the diet may play a significant role in generating oxidized lipoproteins, oxidized fatty acids and oxidized cholesterol in the diet accelerates fatty streak formation, and it is well established that the typical western diet contains high concentrations of oxidized cholesterol products."

As you can see, conversely to what you've been told, it's not about cholesterol. A large part of your vascular health has to do with the pro-oxidative things you do, and the lack of antioxidants in your diet.

Oxidized LDL is not the whole answer, as you'll see in a moment, but it is a large part of the answer. As you take the steps necessary to protect your vasculature, which include whole foods, proper fats, vitamin A, D, E, and K, detoxification, homocysteine control, nitric oxide support, and more, other concerns you have, such as high blood pressure, will fall into place. High blood pressure and atherosclerosis are diseases of the vasculature. Control your vascular health from a holistic viewpoint, and you control the number one killer of Americans, while gaining other benefits, like eliminating erectile dysfunction.

ADMA

We can't begin a review of ADMA until we first understand nitric oxide (NO). NO, as the letters imply, is simply a molecule that contains one nitrogen atom and one oxygen atom. It may be simple in form, but its actions are immense, many of which are still being understood. When it comes to vascular health, NO plays a crucial role in dilation, or widening, of the arteries. This is a good thing, as a narrowing of the inside, or lumen, is associated with plaque accumulation and reduced blood flow. Beyond this, atherosclerosis causes rigid, or inflexible arteries, unable to adequately respond to demands by the body. NO also plays a role in the structure of the arteries, and in inhibition of platelet and immune adhesion and aggregation (blood clotting). Among many other places, NO is made by the cells within the vasculature. However, in many of the conditions associated with vascular disease, such as high cholesterol, high homocysteine, low antioxidants, high blood sugar, and high blood pressure, the ability to make NO is diminished. This leads to a chicken and egg scenario. Does low NO cause these other closely associated factors, or do they cause low NO, or some combination thereof?

According to the clinical data, it would appear as if all of these factors feed each other, in a downward spiral of disease progression. As you will see from the data, someone with a genetic flaw in metabolizing ADMA has a ridiculously high risk for CVD. However, the data also shows that the previous mentioned associated conditions adversely affect NO production. In essence, they all seem to work together. It's much like the pack mentality. Take one child, and you have little to no trouble. Add another five or six, and they feed off one another. Like all things, there is no one single solution, but a blend. Given lifestyle and genes, some things become more important than others.

I bring up NO and ADMA for three reasons. First, it has become a very strong marker for CVD. Second, like many things in this book, I hope to introduce you to information with which you are not familiar, instead of boring you with the same old talk of HDL, LDL, and triglycerides. Like a kid from a small town going to the city, there's a lot more out there than you know. Third, I mention them because they are for the most part a separate risk factor from cholesterol, which emphasizes the lack of vision when just looking at blood lipids.

The body is constantly building and breaking down proteins. One metabolite in this process is a byproduct called ADMA (asymmetric dimethylarginine). ADMA floating in the body is not a good thing. Some is excreted through the urine, but more seems to be broken down by a couple of enzymes we'll call DDAH. If too much ADMA accumulates in the body, it gobbles up much of the raw ingredient needed to make NO, which is an amino acid called arginine. Consequently, the body can't make enough NO to perform its many roles throughout the body, only a few of which we touched on pertaining to the vasculature.

Only recently has it been discovered that ADMA is increased in the plasma of humans with high cholesterol, atherosclerosis, hypertension, chronic renal failure, chronic heart failure, and other conditions. (46) Studies of the ADMA/NO connection began in the 1990s, and although there is much focus on it hidden in the clinical literature, it's not yet mainstream. You are now on the cutting edge of information. A direct quote from one paper published in the *Journal of Nephrology* may give an indication to its importance.

"During the last 20 years, substantial evidence has been accrued that all major cardiovascular risk factors individually and/or jointly may profoundly alter endothelial function by impairing NO synthesis or, in more general terms, by decreasing the bioavailability of this molecule at vascular level. Indeed, either reduced NO synthesis, or enhanced NO degradation triggered by oxidative stress, or blunted sensitivity to NO are all potentially conducive to altered endothelial function and, ultimately, to arterial damage and cardiovascular events." (47)

Several trials have been edgy enough to administer low doses of ADMA to healthy volunteers while measuring their cardiovascular response. (48) Following injection and lasting about an hour, ADMA reduced heart rate, reduced cardiac output, increased blood pressure, decreased forearm blood flow, increase systemic and pulmonary vascular resistance (the blood didn't flow as well through the whole body) and decreased blood flow to the kidneys. This was just temporary in healthy subjects. Imagine this all day long in an unhealthy person.

The AtheroGene study looked at ADMA levels in 1,908 subjects with stable coronary artery disease and found that those in the highest quarter had 2 ½ times the risk for a cardiovascular event. (49) They concluded that, "ADMA was revealed to be one of the strongest risk predictors of cardiovascular events among patients with stable coronary artery disease." In a trial investigating the association between serum ADMA concentration and the risk of an acute coronary event, researchers found that those in the highest quarter had 4 times the risk as compared to all others. (50) In yet another study in 153 men and women with stable coronary artery disease, those ADMA levels in the highest third had more than 5 times the risk of cardiovascular events. (51) To hammer the point home with one more trial, in 52 critically ill patients ADMA levels were the strongest independent risk factor for death, with those in the top quarter having over 17 times the risk. (52) Granted these people were quite ill, but the correlation is amazing.

If that risk didn't floor you, I have one that will. One of the themes in this book is the genetic variability between us. Genes regulate your height, eye color, and other easily visible features. What is less visible is what's on the inside, the biochemistry of the body. This is why some people gain weight faster, some people respond to mold poorly, and some people die from vascular disease at a younger age. Certainly there are many lifestyle factors that come into play, but genes are just as powerful. Like homocysteine, which we'll dive into in a moment, ADMA is no different. Researchers have found no fewer than 13 genetic flaws in the DDAH enzymes, the ones that degrade ADMA. (53) Although these flaws are rare, for those who carry one, the occurrence of coronary heart disease was over 50 times that compared to those who don't. (54) 50 times the risk! In my years of reviewing hundreds upon hundreds of clinical trials, I don't think I've ever seen such a strong correlation. If that's not a smoking gun, I don't know what is.

So if those who can't properly degrade ADMA like the rest of us are at such extreme risk, then it would be in our best interest to maintain our ability to metabolize this indirect toxin. To understand this, we must understand which factors affect our ability to make the DDAH enzymes that break down the ADMA. Antioxidants, taurine (which is an amino acid with antioxidant properties), vitamin A, estrogen, and inhibitors of the inflammatory agent NFkB (curcumin) all increase DDAH synthesis, a good thing. High glucose, like in diabetes, oxidized LDL as we've discussed, cholesterol, the inflammatory agent TNF-alpha, and homocysteine have all been shown to decrease DDAH output. (55) You'll notice that the good guys all have antioxidant properties. Yes, estrogen does, which may account in part for the differences between men and women for cardiovascular risk prior to menopause. The bad guys are pro-oxidants and pro-inflammatory.

At this time, the best way to quickly increase NO production is with arginine supplementation. If you recall, arginine is the substrate needed to produce NO. ADMA occupies arginine, in what's called competitive inhibition. So, large doses of arginine are administered to supply the body with the raw materials needed. It's like two birds in a nest. In hard times there's limited food, the larger chick will eat the food, and the smaller will die. In good times, there's enough for all.

In theory, you'd want to reduce inflammation, homocysteine, and pro-oxidative factors, such as oxidized LDL, to supplement your arginine. Of course this ADMA problem is not just limited to CVD. The lungs, for example, generate large sums of ADMA, and too much may trigger lung diseases such as idiopathic pulmonary fibrosis and asthma, to name just two. (56) In fact, children with pulmonary hypertension tend to have high ADMA, and abnormal DDAH metabolism. (57) The DDAH/ADMA/NO equation may also play a role in autoimmune diseases like RA and lupus. It's presence in the immune system at certain locations, and the fact that lupus patients with elevated ADMA levels have an increased risk for cardiovascular events, provides some initial evidence. (58) Your ADMA level can be measured through commercial labwork currently available.

One set of researchers stated that, "In reviewing prospective clinical studies, we find strong and convincing evidence of the role of ADMA in the development of cardiovascular disease." (59) Another researcher states, "ADMA is a novel marker of endothelial dysfunction." (60) Whatever you want to call it, ADMA is an influential part of vascular health, which may or may not be relevant to yours. It is but one piece in a puzzle of several, and emphasizes the connection of oxidation and inflammation as a root cause of disease progression.

Homocysteine

Dr. McCully of Harvard was the first to associate homocysteine with atherosclerosis back in 1969. To this day, the medical community has not bought into the concept. His observations came from working with young people with a condition known as homocystinuria. In plain terms, these people have genetic flaws so bad, that they have homocysteine values that are through the roof, resulting in half having a thromboembolic event by age 30, with a corresponding mortality rate of about 20%. (61) As is the case in many examples throughout this book, you can look to an extreme condition and correlate it to the general public. The vast majority of people are not in this risk group, but an elevated homocysteine level over the long haul is the consideration.

We won't address any debate about the correlation between homocysteine and vascular health, as the evidence is overwhelmingly in favor of the connection. Just as an example, a 1997 *New England Journal of Medicine* article showed that the risk of death was 4.5 times higher for those over a serum value of 20 as compared to those under 9. (62) In one more example, the odds of coronary artery disease was 4.8 times greater in subjects with a blood value over 14 as compared to those under 8. (63) There are literally dozens upon dozens of studies that show a relationship between serum homocysteine and coronary artery disease, peripheral artery disease, stroke, or venous thrombosis. (64) Homocysteine and methylation also have supportive data in conditions of brain health, such as Alzheimer's and depression, cancer, arthritis, eye health, and more. For our purposes here, we'll just focus on vascular health.

With the connection of homocysteine levels and vascular disease firmly in hand, one would think correcting it would be easy, and benefits would be seen. Unfortunately, much clinical data does not bear this out. For example, a study that lasted over 7 years using the three B vitamins associated with the methylation cycle--B12, folate, and B6--did not show any difference in cardiovascular events among 5,442 women. (65) Likewise in another trial, the same doses of the three B vitamins were used, and after an average of 5 years, there was no difference in the occurrence of death from cardiovascular events, but those on the B vitamins had 25% fewer strokes. (66)

Do we throw away this homocysteine connection in the absence of clear success? Absolutely not. We know that homocysteine induces physical changes on the vasculature and affects its immune component as well, likely oxidizes LDL in the body, and we now know its affects on NO production. On top of this, the correlation between homocysteine levels and CVD is amazing. In a quick review of the methylation cycle, we also know that this cycle becomes burdened as we age. Homocysteine and its precursor SAH are toxic to the crucial functioning of methylation, and by no chance homocysteine levels also correlate with age. This amazing cycle, which is flying along in our youth producing healthy bone, skin, hair, and every other component of the youthful body, slows down through the metabolic burdens of life. We need to get this cycle spinning faster again. So where is the research going wrong? There are several aspects to consider.

Diet will vary between patients. If one has more antioxidants, more vitamins, and so forth, the homocysteine levels or actions will be buffered.

There can be significant genetic variability causing higher or lower levels.

Many of these studies were done in patients with pre-existing CVD or risk factors, with advanced age. You can't undo years of arterial damage in a year or so while addressing only one aspect of vascular health.

As previously stated, homocysteine is but one aspect of vascular health. Other factors should be considered.

The "safe" levels for homocysteine are up for debate. Many researchers will argue that ideal levels to minimize CVD risk should be around 6-7. Much of the research only reduced homocysteine moderately, with eventual levels still much higher. For example, in the two trials previously mentioned, homocysteine was reduced to 9.8 and 9.7 respectively. This is a full 30-50% higher than recommended. In order to drive homocysteine values to where they need to be, I believe TMG is necessary, in addition to the B vitamins. In fact, the B vitamins can be lowered with TMG at the appropriate dose, 6 grams per day.

Lastly, not mentioned anywhere else, one must consider "on-board" mercury in the body.

Given our toxic environment, many undesirable compounds accumulate in our bodies over the years; mercury is but one. The reason I mention mercury is that it differs with respect to methylation. The EPA informs us that there are three different types of mercury, of which elemental mercury is one. This is the type in thermometers, light bulbs, and dental fillings. Mercury vapors are released from these fillings for many years after the procedure, and the rate of "off-gassing" is higher with such things as teeth grinding and brushing. This mercury finds its way into body storage. When you induce methylation, you can also methylate this elemental mercury into methylmercury, its more toxic cousin. Methylmercury is the form found in fish.

There is scant data to support my theory, but it would help explain why homocysteine reduction in older people isn't as remarkable as mercury accumulates with age. One study has shown that the administration of methylcobalamin, which is one of the two active forms of B12, causes inorganic mercury to be methylated. In the words of the researchers, "Methylation proceeded at a remarkably high rate when methylcobalamin and inorganic mercury were mixed." (67) The inorganic mercury they used is typically found in batteries, some disinfectants, and health creams.

Mercury

It must seem odd that mercury is a part of this chapter. However, the unfortunate effect of our toxic planet is that mercury content is just as much a risk factor as any other. Our primary exposure to mercury is through seafood. This is evidenced by governmental advice for pregnant women to reduce their exposure to mercury containing fish. The sad fact is that although fresh seafood is great for our health, it now has to be qualified as clean as well.

Just think for a moment about all of the synthetic materials that surround you in the course of a day. These include your car, house, furnishings, carpeting, plastic food containers, toys, your clothes, and much more. All of these are synthetic sources of toxins. In the end, they wind up in the environment somewhere. We have this notion that these things just magically disappear. Trash gets incinerated, de-icing fluid at airports works its way into the water supply, powerplants burn fossil fuels, and a multitude of other toxins work their way into our water. From there, it works its way up the food chain, most concentrated in the fish and mammals at the top of the food chain. We in turn eat the fish, and accumulate this highly toxic heavy metal.

Short of industrial exposure, the primary route we accumulate mercury is through seafood. The hotly debated secondary route is through your dental amalgam fillings. Yes, we put mercury into our heads! Those silver fillings are much more mercury than they are silver. At least 50% of the material is mercury. How insane is this country in which we live?

Mercury is extremely toxic, and can affect every organ system in the body. Some people have a better detoxification genetic profile and can clear more mercury than others. Those with compromises in detoxification pathways can't clear it as well, and serve as canaries in the coal mine, so to speak. The role of mercury in vascular health is multifactorial, with free radical production, inhibition of antioxidant status, and heart muscle dysfunction (both autonomic and physical) leading the list. We will only look at the increased level of risk in those with elevated mercury. Keep in mind that mercury is but one of several heavy metals, and heavy metals are but one class of the many other toxins we are exposed to, possibly leading the list of root causes to many of our ills.

The fact is that fish is supposed to be good for us, and that mercury concentrates in fish has not gone unnoticed by researchers. Quoting how several studies have failed to show a cardiovascular benefit from fish consumption, researchers postulated that mercury contamination may have something to do with it.

In the most striking of papers on the matter, Finnish researchers looked at 1,833 men aged 42-60, who were free of vascular disease. Those with the highest mercury levels had 3 times the risk of death as compared to those with the lowest levels. (68) They theorized that the mercury resulted in increased lipid oxidation, which in turn prompted vascular disease. Notice a theme here. Lipid oxidation.

A different study from 2005 found a significantly elevated risk in those men with the highest mercury content as compared to the lowest. (69) They also went on to say that the mercury negated the beneficial effects of the fish oil on cardiovascular health.

There are a number of other studies as well. One looked at cardiovascular risk parameters and concluded that, "The results support the notion that increased methylmercury exposure promotes the development of cardiovascular disease." (70) In a paper from the *New England Journal of Medicine*, those with the highest levels of mercury had more than twice the risk of heart attack as compared to those with the lowest levels. (71)

I'm not absolutely sure of many things, but I think you'd be hard pressed to find anyone who thinks mercury is good for you. Likewise, the unfortunate fact that our seafood is contaminated with mercury and other toxins is recognized by almost all. The sad truth is that it will only get worse. I'm not a negative person, just a realist. With that said, you may want to rethink fish as a part of your diet, considering location, amount, and type.

As for your own mercury levels, there are ways to look into this. There is much debate over whether we should be chelating these heavy metals out of the body, as some will invariably deposit in other soft tissue. On the flip side, you will have to "pay the piper" at some point, and if your mercury levels are the root cause of your health problems, it would seem to be in your best interest to chelate them out.

Chelation is the process of binding some other agent to the heavy metal, and once mobilized, it's theoretically ready for excretion. There are several ways to look at your heavy metal status. Red blood cell, hair, and urine are the three most common methods. You can work with a qualified practitioner in natural medicine to assess the need for such a test, and weigh your treatment options.

Aspirin

It seems as if almost everyone is taking aspirin for their vascular health. I think most people recognize that it is a "blood thinner", and as such helps to prevent the clotting associated with heart attacks and certain strokes, the ones caused by clots in the brain. However, this virtual universal recommendation is now being reconsidered. In essence, government agencies have told doctors to assess the risks and benefits between internal bleeding and clot prevention, and consider some general guidelines. Of course, doctors are usually behind the times, and yours may not be aware of this most recent data for years to come. In fact, this most recent data is behind the times, too, as the risk of bleeding from taking aspirin has been know for decades. In the end, it's your body, so you ought to be aware of the information, even if your doctor isn't.

Going back to 1980, a trial showed that aspirin was not recommended for routine use in patients who have survived a heart attack. (72) The overall death rate was higher in the aspirin group as compared to the placebo group, and internal bleeding was much higher. Granted the dose was a bit high, but it did not show reductions in coronary incidence.

More recently, studies are showing similar results. In the *Journal of the American Medical Association*, as conservative and conventional a journal as it gets, a 2010 study, which used a low dose aspirin among patients without clinical CVD, showed no difference in mortality, but a much higher incidence of internal bleeding, requiring admission to a hospital, which has both financial and other costs. (73)

The results from this trial and others feed the new recommendations to reconsider the use of aspirin. In essence, this trial says that it would be unwise to use aspirin for preventative medicine, in an otherwise healthy asymptomatic person. So who should be taking aspirin? It would seem that there is general agreement that low dose aspirin shows benefits in those who already have had a non-hemorragic stroke, angina, or heart attack. Other doctors may expand the scope further. The bottom line is that there is no consensus, which is not surprising. A 2010 article from the *Wall Street Journal* entitled, "The Danger of Daily Aspirin," discusses this lack of agreement in regards to gender, age, and other risk factors. Essentially, it comes down to a weighing of the risks. Do you want to risk internal bleeding as compared to a heart attack?

Before you answer the question, consider that internal bleeding can also result in a stroke. It's not just stomach ulcers we're discussing, but hemhorragic strokes. Hemorrhagic strokes are strokes where blood from the brain vasculature spills out into tissue where it does not belong, whereas a thromboembolic stroke is a cut-off in supply of the blood (with oxygen and nutrients) to the brain. Aspirin helps prevent one type, while increasing the risk for the other. This risk was made clear in a review of aspirin trials, finding that aspirin did cause an increased risk for hemorrhagic stroke. (74)

This same trial also found that there was a reduction in risks for both thromboembolic stroke and heart attacks. This all brings us back to the "new" guidelines. Essentially what you and your doctor are looking at here is a "roll of the dice". You're betting that your risks of a clot causing a heart attack or stroke outweigh the risks of internal bleeding in all its forms. This is why only those with strong risk factors for another event should be swayed into considering aspirin. I don't pretend to know all of the variables for all patients, at all times, but why not find an alternative, and stack the deck much more in your favor.

There are a number of natural products that accomplish the blood thinning of aspirin, without the risks. And these risks are real. If they weren't, Merck would not have tried to launch Vioxx. Vioxx was supposed to address pain, while not placing the patient at risk for internal bleeding from traditional NSAIDS, of which aspirin is one. The downside was that it quadrupled the risk of sudden death from clots, a risk that had been warned of for years prior to being pulled from the market. (75)

So what are these natural products? Vitamin E, garlic, and fish oil are the three predominant ones that come to my mind, all of which have good data in their support. It is beyond the scope of this chapter to dive into these options, but there are many excellent resources for you to consider as you plot your own healthcare. My only point here is to inform you that the assumingly benign and automatic aspirin recommendations are not benign, and should not be automatic. These authority figures in this troubled medical system are authorities on coding for maximal reimbursements, writing prescriptions, and shuffling through as many patients as possible. The average conventional practitioner is not keenly aware of the clinical data, and through the AMA and legal recourse, not in the best position to question it. But you can question authority.

Vitamin K

In the chapter on bone health, you realized how critical vitamin K is to the process. Vitamin K activates the Gla protein called osteocalcin in the bone matrix, and only then can it bring in calcium to build bone. The other most commonly referred to Gla protein is called MGP. MGP likewise requires vitamin K to activate it to do its thing, which we'll get to in a moment.

You may also recall that K1 is from vegetables, and predominates in the liver, presiding over coagulation of blood. However, K1 has little role in vascular health. Only one trial out of many shows K1 was of benefit in CVD. (76) Contrarily, vitamin K2 has been shown to have significant benefits in vascular health.

K2 is found at much higher concentrations in the vasculature as compared to the liver. Because of its longer serum activity, its higher potency, and higher activity outside of the liver, vitamin K2 is crucial in regulation of calcium in the most prevelant diseases known to man. This leads us to what's referred to as the "calcification paradox". This is the observed fact that as we age, the bones become less calcified, while the arteries become more calcified. It's a bit interesting once you give it some thought. Equally interesting is the fact that vitamin K plays a role in both ends of this equation. You already know its role in bone health. You also already know that our standard American diet is low in both K1 and K2. And now we'll review vitamin K's role in vascular health.

Although MGP was first discovered in bone, it is mainly produced by the vascular smooth muscles cells and the cells that make up your cartilage. (77) The cartilage connection is quite interesting as it pertains to calcification of that soft tissue, but we'll stick with the vasculature. This is important because MGP is required to keep your vasculature from calcifying. Calcification is not a good thing, as it contributes to a lack in flexibility of the arteries to increase blood flow on demand, and to the calcification of atherosclerotic plaque. These are the two aspects of calcification, one which occurs in the middle muscular layers of the arteries, and one which piles on top of the oxidized/immune regulated/inflamed lesion. In the end, you want neither.

The body makes MGP at both of these locations. It is a protective measure. Of course, normal healthy vascular smooth muscle cells make MGP, but at sites of calcification the levels of MGP are much higher. It's as if the emergency alarm went off and all the firemen are watching the firm burn, but have no water. You need vitamin K, preferably K2 to activate the MGP so it can do what it has been proven to do, be a potent inhibitor of vascular calcification. (78)

So what does MGP do exactly? Well, this is evolving science, but we now know enough to recognize the immense value of this highly under-rated vitamin. MGP not only directly inhibits calcium crystal formation, but it regulates several bone proteins within the vasculature. (79) That's correct, I said bone proteins. There can be a transformation of smooth muscle cells into bone-like cells under certain conditions, and this event is KNOWN to precede arterial calcification. (80) The process is kicked off by a growth factor called BMP-2. It's a bit like a starfish losing a "leg" and growing a new one. Under a set of conditions, certain cells can become other cells. This is also seen in some tumors.

MGP inhibits this BMP-2. In turn, you need vitamin K to activate MGP. As seen many times, the body responds to calcification the only way it knows how, to throw more and more MGP at it. It's up to you to ingest the vitamin K to help out your body's innate response. The problem is that we don't eat a diet that's in accordance with our evolution, and instead we try to out-think millions of years of cellular intelligence, and throw a drug at it. One class of drugs worth mentioning is the blood thinners like warfarin, which work by counteracting vitamin K.

Oral anticoagulants, blood thinners, such as warfarin, work by counteracting the metabolism of vitamin K. Its origin is that of a fungal mycotoxin, which caused uncontrolled bleeding and death. Initially marketed as a rat poison, its synthetic derivative is now used extensively in atrial fibrillation, stroke, and hypercoagulable disorders. (81) The problem is that in treating one condition you may be causing another. Warfarin is not just resigned to affecting vitamin K cycling as pertaining to clotting, but all vitamin K dependent proteins, to include osteocalcin in the bone and MGP in the vasculature. In animal studies, warfarin induces widespread vascular calcification in rats. (82) Of course, its affects are not limited to rats. Warfarin, through its inhibition of Gla proteins, has also been shown to increase coronary calcification in humans. (83) For example, in one study with 86 patients with calcific aortic valve disease (calcified heart valve), patients with long-term anticoagulation therapy were compared to those without it by CT scan. Patients who had been on the therapy had significantly higher cardiac calcification and in conclusion the researchers stated, "Oral anticoagulation may be associated with increased valvular and coronary calcium in patients with aortic valve disease, presumably due to decreased activation of the matrix Gla protein (GLA)." (84)

The potency of K2 as compared to K1 is also highlighted in regards to warfarin. In rats given warfarin plus K1, vascular calcification occurred in 4 weeks, whereas warfarin plus K2 yielded no calcification. (85) The fact that K2 is concentrated outside the liver, and K1 is concentrated inside the liver, may help dictate new guidelines in the use of warfarin. For those where warfarin is deemed necessary, the administration of K2 at the same time may allow for the benefits of warfarin while minimizing the side effect. If you are on one of these drugs, I'm not recommending you either discontinue warfarin or add K2 on your own. It would probably be best to consult an integrative doctor in this matter.

The connection of vascular calcification to MGP is made even stronger in two more examples. In mice that are bred to have no MGP, death occurs within 2 months due to arterial calcification, which leads to blood vessel rupture. (86) In addition, these mice had cartilage in the arteries, and calcium mixed in with cartilage. This has implications in arthritis.

In another strong connection between MGP and improper calcification, a very rare heridary disease known as Keutel syndrome causes extensive soft tissue, cartilage, and vascular calcification. This disease results from a genetic mutation of the MGP gene. (87,88) This is yet another example where genes play a role in one's health, and an extreme example can be extrapolated to the rest of us.

As the role of MGP has been proven, the role of calcification is also an issue. As calcification is almost invariably associated with atherosclerotic plaque formation (89), and important in heart function, it's worth noting the strong connection between uncontrolled calcification and disease. Likewise, I have some concerns over the crazes of high doses of calcium, and the new fad of potentially high doses of vitamin D in regards to calcification of soft tissue as well. Simply stated, excess vitamin D induces vascular calcification in both humans and animals. (90) High dose calcium supplementation can do the same. In one study, 1,471 postmenopausal women were given a placebo or 1 gram of calcium per day and monitored for five years. Those in the calcium group had more than twice the risk of a heart attack, which was more evident with higher compliance. (91) In fact these researchers concluded that these results weren't surprising, as calcium supplements acutely raise serum calcium levels, possibly accelerating vascular calcification. In fact, they also state that high calcium intakes have also been associated with brain lesions, other studies showing vascular calcifications, and mortality in patients receiving dialysis. (92) The brain lesion component is an interesting point, outside the scope of this chapter, but you may be well served to note that K2 is strongly represented in the brain.

The importance of coronary and vascular calcification is immense. Just consider that coronary calcifications are present in 95% of those who have a first-time heart attack. (93) Studies show that vascular calcifications carry a 7-12 fold increase in risk for coronary heart disease and death. (94,95) In fact, coronary artery calcification is so influential, one trial concludes that it's a better predictor of death than age. That's right. Your coronary calcium levels more strongly predict your longevity than your actual age. In this study, 10,377 people without symptoms were scanned for calcifications and followed for 5 years for all deaths. Those with the highest degree of calcification essentially had 30 years tacked on to their actual age. (96)

Conversely, vitamin K has been shown to be protective. In two studies looking at serum osteocalcin markers (an indication of vitamin K status) the authors found that lower vitamin K status correlated with more bone loss, and more risk of vascular calcification. (97,98) Vascular calcification, and the loss of bone calcium intertwine with many of the most costly medical conditions in our country. Many times over, vascular calcification has been shown to be a strong predictor of morbidity and mortality, a fact which lends it an amazing amount of weight. Coronary calcium content has literally been shown to be the strongest predictor of future cardiac events, with those in the highest level having more than 20 times the risk. (99) Vitamin K sits in the crossroads of these two conditions. On the one hand, it plays a key role in activating osteocalcin in bone, and on the other hand it activates MGP to keep blood vessels from becoming bone-like. Our current diet is for the most part low in both K1 and K2, although the distinction being that vitamin K2 prevents arterial calcification, while K1 does not. (100) This has led researchers to comment that, "Over the past decade it has become evident that vitamin K plays a far greater role in human health than previously thought." (101)

We have had this obsession about cholesterol and cholesterol drugs literally shoved down our throats, and yet sudden death from a heart attack is more highly correlated with vasculature calcification than with cholesterol. (102) You aren't aware of the uses of vitamin K because it is not in commercials, because it can't be patented. Simply consider that most everything revolves around money and power, and with that said, the truth can be hard to find.

Diet

I find it baffling and disappointing that there is an abundance of clinical data pointing to the almost certain causes of most vascular disease, which also point to ways in which to avoid it. Instead, we find ourselves in different hyped modes over the decades pursuing the wrong avenues. We are getting a little better as time passes. Margarine was once hailed as a better alternative to butter, but with the recent dissemination of information on trans-fats, we are changing our habits. Polyunsaturated oils, such as the typical vegetable and corn oils bought at the grocery store, have also been in vogue, but the word is getting out on those oils as well. What's still in vogue, and becoming more so as each year passes, is the use of prescription drugs for the treatment of what's essentially a nutritional disease. You have been browbeaten with ads based on fear, and doctors have been swayed through various questionable practices to force medications down your throat. Now that you are armed with more data than most, to include your practitioner, you can make the call.

So if vascular health has its origins in nutrition for the most part, as something like smoking is a lifestyle factor, then how does one do their best to avoid the costly drugs with a laundry list of side effects and to avoid our number one killer at the same time? Believe it or not, there is a wealth of clinical data going back decades, data which is hidden in the clinical literature, that explains everything to the best of our knowledge. If you so choose, you can hop onto **Pubmed.com** and read the clinical data yourself. It takes a while, and can be very dense, but you'll get the hang of it. It is here from which data is pulled and health and medicine books are written. This is the initial research, most of which does not make it to the nightly news. Why? It may have something to do with the dollars from advertising that some companies spend on the networks, as compared to the lack of money spent by others. How often do you see commercials for drugs? How often do you see a commercial for extra virgin olive oil?

So what does this research say? In the beginning of this chapter you read about the most likely scenario for the development of vascular disease. This connection of oxidation-immune response-inflammation is at the core of your vascular health. This is why half of all heart attacks occur in people with normal or low cholesterol levels. This is why some people with genetically very high levels of cholesterol will die at wildly varying timepoints. This is why smoking is such a risk factor - oxidation. If you have higher levels of cholesterol but have a diet high in fresh whole foods, then the research tells us that your risk for vascular disease is much less as you'll have adequate antioxidants on board, while not insulting your body with oxidized oils. If, on the other hand, you have relatively low cholesterol, but consume oxidized oils through cooking, and eat processed/dead food, then your risk for vascular disease is higher.

The cholesterol hypothesis is not a totally wrong hypothesis; it's just not the whole story. What is primarily missing is the word "oxidized" from the equation. If you can control the level of oxidized cholesterol, then you can in theory control the consequent immune response and inflammation. Other measures of vascular health, such as Crp, fibrinogen, blood clotting, calcification, and more, are usually downstream factors from the initial insult to the walls of your arteries from oxidation. Sure there are other aspects, such as mercury, homocysteine, pathogens, and smoking, but guess what, they all have roles in oxidation as well. I can't package up "a cure" for all vascular disease in one pretty little package, especially in one chapter. What I can do is provide you with evidence, which we should all try to follow, and which would apply to the majority of cases. The scope of this chapter is to show you the flaws in the system as it is, the most probable underlying cause of vascular disease, a few extra considerations addressed best through natural medicine, and what I perceive as your best course of action to protect your arteries. It's up to you to make a decision. So what does the data have to say?

A couple of dietary trials highlight the power of dietary and lifestyle changes over what's conventionally done. For example, Dean Ornish ran a trial for five years to test just that. He took patients with moderate to severe coronary heart disease and divided them into two groups. In the control group, the patients followed their conventional doctor's advice, and took drugs like statins, if prescribed. In the experimental group, the patients were given no drugs, and put on a regimen that included a low fat vegetarian diet, moderate exercise, and stress management. After one year, the experimental group reduced their LDL by 37%, while the group that followed their conventional doctor's advice only dropped their LDL by 6%. The experimental group had a 91% reduction in episodes of angina, while the other group had a 165% increase in angina episodes. As for cardiac events, the conventional group had 247% more of them than the experimental group. (103) This study was published in the *Journal of the American Medical Association.*

If a vegetarian diet is not to your liking, consider the Lyon Diet Heart Study. The premise of this study was the finding that diets focusing on low cholesterol, low saturated fat, and high polyunsaturated fats weren't yielding good results. Instead of focusing on reducing blood cholesterol, their diet followed in accordance with other successful ones that focused on low intakes of total and saturated fats, higher omega-3 fats, and higher intakes of whole foods, which are higher in overall nutritional value. (104)

This is essentially a Mediterranean type of diet, of which you may have heard. Following a first-time heart attack, patients were asked to follow this Mediterranean type of diet, or a diet dictated by their attending conventional physicians. With an average of almost 4 years of follow-up, the results were quite striking. A number of cardiovascular outcomes were measured, and every way the data was cut, the results were impressive. For example, in probably the most important outcome, that of cardiac deaths, there were 3 times more in the conventional group. One of the interesting findings was that a high white blood cell count was a significant risk factor in developing a cardiovascular event. This brings to light the connection between the immune system and the cardiovascular system. They cite the fact that high white blood cell counts have been shown to be a marker for increased risk of coronary heart disease in many trials. They postulated several mechanisms behind the relationship from a number of studies. The simple fact here is that there are many ways to measure your CVD risk other than cholesterol.

There are many reasons why one diet is better than another for vascular health. The two primary ones we'll consider here have to do with the concept of the Mediterranean diet. Fresh foods provide nutrients, and

180

among these are antioxidants. The diet also provides more omega-3 fatty acids both by plant and animal, and more oleic fatty acids, the primary source being olive oil. Let's first take a brief look at the antioxidant connection.

Within natural medicine there are plenty of antioxidant products you can buy. Some are better than others, but they are worth consideration. Ideally, you'd be eating fresh foods from a chemical-free garden, clean animals, all grown and harvested locally. As we do not live in such a world, we rely on supplements. However, others around the globe do live in this manner, and the ones with the most recent attention surround the Mediterranean and live in Japan, more specifically Okinawa. It all only makes sense. Fresh grains, fruits, vegetables, olive oil, and seafood are better for you than pizza, cheeseburgers, milkshakes, and cookies. We live in a society on-the-run, and one in which we've lost connection to the farm and food. We rely on others with corporate interests in mind to tell us that dairy or drugs are good for us. When you boil it all down, it becomes simple common sense.

There is a ton of data in support of antioxidants, most notably vitamins E and C in the pursuit of vascular health. These two work together to "quench" free radicals. Vitamin E has probably the best data, and studies which you may have seen using the synthetic d,l-alpha tocopherol version are not the way to go. We want to replicate vitamin E in its naturally occurring state as much as possible, but cheap vitamin E products in your grocery store or in a pharmacy probably won't cut the mustard.

For example, in one study, the blood levels of vitamin E, blood pressure, and cholesterol were compared to the incidence of heart disease. These researchers found that low vitamin E status was a much stronger predictor of heart disease than blood pressure or cholesterol. (105) They quote numerous human, animal, and in vitro studies supporting the link between antioxidants and oxidation of cholesterol as a causation of atherosclerosis. They cite interesting data, such as finding oxidized LDL in freshly harvested artery plaques from humans. They discuss many mechanisms supporting vitamins A, E and C, and state that essential antioxidants, mainly vitamin E, are important underrated factors in heart disease, which may substantially counteract the previously known classical risk factors such as cholesterol and hypertension.

Similarly, a Scottish study showed that low plasma vitamin E status "predisposes to angina" and that smoking may increase the risk of angina by lowering plasma vitamin C levels. (106) There are many more books and studies that attest to the role of antioxidants for vascular health. With that said, we'll address a second major component of a healthy diet, that of fat intake.

Our low-fat diets have been a failure for weight loss just as our low-calorie diets have been. Have you ever noticed someone who weighs much more than they should drinking one of those low calorie sodas? I'm pretty sure it's not working. Likewise, low fat diets aren't working great either, and in fact aren't very healthy. The body needs fats and cholesterol. These are crucial components to our health. Saturated fat is required by the body. Cholesterol is a precursor for a number of hormones, the brain, and, in the case of the vasculature, actually serves as a band-aid to prevent a hemorrhage. As the lining of the artery can be oxidized like the cholesterol floating around in the blood, a patch is needed to prevent internal bleeding.

Fats behave in different ways inside the body. Although some saturated fat is good, too much is not. Likewise, some omega-3 fatty acids are good, but again, too much has been shown to be detrimental. It's not only the type of fat, but also the level of oxidation. For example, the oils used to fry your french fries at high temperatures are exposed to air and light for days on end. It contains a soup of identified and unidentified oxidized fatty acids of a variety of forms, not intended for use in the body. Even those vegetable oils on the grocery store shelf have been highly processed, and when at home likely cooked at temperatures that are too high. They also sit in your kitchen exposed to heat, air, and light, which further oxidize the product. Make no mistake about it, the oils you expose yourself to are one of the most crucial aspects of your nutritional status.

This is why oils like extra virgin olive oil and extra virgin coconut oil have been gaining more use. The downside is their cost. It's much cheaper to buy vegetable oil than the labor-intensive healthier oils. Saturated fat is pro-inflammatory and has been shown to reduce HDL levels. (107) However, they are the most stable to oxidation. As they have no double bonds, the fatty acids don't react as readily. On the flip side, fish oils are highly oxidizable. This is why a little is good, but too much is not. In the middle we have the omega-6 polyunsaturated fatty acids, such as corn oil. They oxidize more readily than saturated fats, but not as quickly as fatty acids from fish oils. Unfortunately, given our diets and exposures, these oils oxidize in the body and can lead to vascular damage. If only there was something that offered up the best of all worlds.

Olive oil is primarily comprised of oleic acid, which is a monounsaturated fatty acid. It has only one double bond, and thus doesn't oxidize as readily as the polyunsaturated oils. So why does any of this techno-babble matter? Well, fatty acids comprise the cell membranes in your body, and are also a constituent of your LDL. Limiting our focus to LDL, we can have particles that are high in one fat or another. These changes in composition lead to an LDL that will oxidize easily, or not. This is crucial for the health of your arteries.

One set of researchers states, "Significant amounts of data have been accumulated to show that linoleic acid (omega-6, ie vegetable oil) can induce marked injury to endothelial cells (the cells that line your arteries). For example, it was reported that this fatty acid can disrupt endothelial cell integrity, alter functions of gap-junctional proteins, increase concentrations of intracellular calcium, and induce cellular oxidative stress." (108) In another study, researchers showed that monounsaturated fats like those found in olive oil were more resistant to oxidative damage in the body, and the authors suggested that they be used in place of omega-6 fats. (109)

I mention extra virgin olive oil as it has not been processed like the others. For a book on oils and processing read, *Fats That Heal, Fats That Kill*, by Udo Erasmus. Vascular health largely boils down to oxidation. Yes, there are other factors such as infection, toxins, and genetic flaws that predispose one to vascular disease, but oxidation is applicable to all of us. Dietary fats and antioxidants are but one aspect of how eating impacts your health. I realize that in our fast-paced lifestyle, some people don't want to change their diets, and would rather take a drug instead, which theoretically allows them to have the best of both worlds. They think they can literally have their cake and eat it too. From a cost and overall health viewpoint, you may want to consider natural options that have been shown in trials to have more efficacy, little to no side effects, other health benefits, and may even cost less. As for the diet, if this hasn't swayed you, then a broader look at nutrition may help.

Chapter 7   Dietary Choices

How the time flies. When you're a kid home for summer vacation, by August you're almost looking forward to going back to school because you've run out of things to do. As you get older, and especially after having kids, time goes by entirely too fast. Life is short, and the amount of time you're vital and vibrant is even shorter. As people, we've been looking for the fountain of youth for thousands of years. It's man's ability to be cognizant of his mortality that drives this phenomenon. Animals don't give it any thought, as they are, for the most part, a living bunch of electrical and chemical impulses. We do think about it and look for ways to extend the length and quality of our lives as best we can.

With that quest in mind, there have been in years past, and still exist today, many snake-oil salesmen who are more than happy to part you from your money. Also of concern are the many practitioners within the mainstream medical establishment who buy into a corrupt medical system where service to the patient is dead, and drug slinging doctors who are brainwashed by biased information from big-business lead the charge. Don't expect our government to do much, as our politicians are bought and paid for on both sides of the aisle. It is up to you to seek out and distill the information, and do with it the best you can in this system, which prides itself on one thing, the almighty dollar.

We have a good concept of how long life has existed on this little rock in the universe. We're aware that dinosaurs once roamed this planet. We know of the black plague. We watch movies about the American Revolution and wonder what it must have been like to live back then. We know these events happened, even though we weren't there. Billions of people have come before us for hundreds of thousands of years. Those of us alive today share in this amazing time of knowledge. When we go, that's it. We won't be able to experience whatever is to come. People in the future will read about us in some book, just as we read about those who have come before us. It's a shame not to know what the future holds.

As you can gather, as I am a person of science, I do not have religious tendencies. I truly wish there was something considered an after-life--that would be fantastic--but it is highly unlikely. Some of you reading this book are religious, and therefore have your own beliefs. So you have your beliefs, and I have mine, and in the end they are both beliefs. I will concede that it is possible for some type of after-life to exist, if you will concede that it's possible that there is none. That being the case, wouldn't you want to make the most of your time on earth, both in duration and quality? I know I do. You may only get one chance at it, you know.

Our modern standard of living is better, more comfortable, more secure, and more enjoyable than any of our predecessors ever knew. We have access on a year-round basis to a wide variety of foods, even though the quality may be questionable at times. We have come to learn a great deal about the human body as well. Although we have much to learn, we understand many basic principles of health. It is unfortunate that some of this valuable knowledge gets twisted by those with power, at the expense of your health. I hope that I will have given you enough examples to point you in the right direction.

Conversely, all we know about health isn't buried in science journals. Much is common sense. We know we need to exercise, to eat fruits and vegetables, to avoid unhealthy habits like smoking, and we know that the highly processed foods we eat are not good for our health either. Yet I'm amazed at what people buy in the grocery store. I'm amazed at what people feed their children. I'm amazed that 1/3 of Americans are overweight, and another third are obese! I can't figure out how the average American watches 5 hours of television a day. These things should concern all of us. There is a nationwide financial impact on us all, whether it's in taxes, the cost of our health insurance, or other expenses.

I am not alone in my opinion. Obama stated during the election campaign, "This nation is facing a true epidemic of chronic disease. An increasing number of Americans are suffering and dying needlessly from diseases such as obesity, diabetes, heart disease, asthma, and HIV/AIDS, all of which can be delayed in onset if not prevented entirely." (1) I don't agree with his socialist views, but in this case, I couldn't agree more. In 2008, $2.1 *trillion* was spent in the U.S. on medical care. At least 75% of these costs were spent on treating chronic diseases, such as heart disease and diabetes, which are preventable and even reversible. (2) Those involved in natural medicine know that the human body has an amazing ability to heal itself. You need to know that too. However, you also need some good guidance on how best to do it, and how to try to avoid an illness in the first place. Heart disease, diabetes, prostate cancer, breast cancer, and obesity account for 75% of health-care costs, and yet these are largely preventable and even reversible by changing diet and lifestyle. (3) I have addressed these diseases and others at various points in this book, when applicable.

We have some obstacles preventing us from moving forward on healthcare as a nation. Some of these obstacles are outside our control, and some within it. Of those we can control, there are five, in my opinion, that prevent progress.

- Some Americans are simply lazy, and want quick, cheap solutions.
- Americans are so busy they don't have the time to eat right and exercise.
- Americans are confused about proper food choices.
- People are resistant to change.
- Components of processed foods lend themselves to ill health unknown to you.

Before I tackle this list, let's understand a thing or two. This is not a diet book. This is not intended for you to lose weight quickly for a wedding, the beach, or because you're looking to land a date. The goal of this book is to present you with data, much of which you've probably never seen before. This data is intended to help direct you to making choices in preventative care, or considerations for existing conditions. In the end, the goal is to save you money, pain, and suffering.

Morbidity is the condition of ill-health. Ideally, we want to minimize morbidity, and maximize our life span. What if, instead of taking fifteen different medications, buying an electric mobility scooter, keeping the nursing profession gainfully employed, and tripping over numerous other ancillary medical supplies, you were to live a long healthy life. That would be nice. But, it requires us to face some truths about ourselves. Be honest with yourself.

- Some Americans are simply lazy, and want quick, cheap solutions.

In general, humans can be lazy. It boils down to conservation of energy. Why expend energy when you don't have to? I don't mention this to be offensive and insulting; I mention it because it's true. It may not be true for you, but I guarantee it is for someone you know. Have you taken notice of people at the beach, or in the general public? Seeing people in good shape is a rare thing. Staying in shape over the years is hard work. It's much easier not to exercise and eat right.

When at the grocery store, I'll look in the carriage (cart) of the person behind me while waiting. I'll see soda, cookies, candy, beer, ice cream, and all of the other usual suspects. Then I'll look at them. They look exactly as you'd expect given the contents of the cart. We all know that those contents aren't good for us, but we buy them by the boatload anyhow. Years ago, an economics professor of mine posed the following question: "In which aisle of the grocery store have studies shown that consumers spend the most time?" I figured I had the answer and said, "The produce aisle." According to their data, I was wrong. It's the cereal aisle. I guess there are so many cereal choices, people can't make up their minds. If you're eating healthy, the answer should be the produce aisle.

I see parents buying their kids candy and soda all the time. I see children under the age of 10 who are obese. In November of 2008 a report came out on 70 youngsters enrolled in the Children's Mercy Hospital study. The researchers performed ultrasound imaging on the arteries in their necks. They found that more than half had a "vascular age" of about 30 years older than their actual age with the detection of fatty deposits in the carotid arteries of children as young as 10. This doesn't mean that they'll be having a heart attack or stroke in the coming weeks, but it does put them at risk at a much earlier age.

About 16% of American kids are considered obese, and we talk of their blood lipids as if they were in their 50s or 60s. To make matters worse, if not disgusting, the American Academy of Pediatrics recently recommended cholesterol-lowering drugs for kids as young as eight. How is it that we are a nation so addicted to the nonfactual notion that drugs will save us from our behaviors, that we are now recommending them more and more for our children? This is borderline criminal, and at best poor medicine and poor parenting. Do you think we could instead consider a dietary change? I mention these things not to be an arrogant ass. I mention them because they are fact. People don't typically like to hear the truth about many things, but in order for us to get anywhere with this we can't continue to bury our heads in the sand.

Why is it that new and improved diet fads and those Saturday morning abdominal machines continue to sell? Is America in any better shape now than it was 20 or 30 years ago when these things started to hit the mainstream? No, we're worse as a nation. We're sicker on so many levels, but we want our instant gratification here in America. We want to look like a movie star in three 15-minute sessions a week on some device for three installments of $19.99. We think reducing calories alone will do the trick, regardless of the quality of those calories. We have the classic American drive-through mentality. I want it, I want it now, and I don't want to pay a lot for it, whatever it happens to be.

Today, we watch more television than ever. Instead of a handful of stations that come in poorly, as was the case 30 years ago, we have potentially hundreds. We now have video games too. Our kids spend more time playing inside than running around outside actually playing a sport with their body instead of on a screen. We eat more, and we eat more crap. Mostly gone are the days when you'd all come home nightly to a meal that mom cooked. Today, it's all about picking up something on the run. The Institute of Food Technologies informs us that, "We never get out of the car for 24% of our meals." That was in 2006. I'll bet it's a bit higher now. I'm not saying that mom always cooked a healthy meal, but on average it was much better for you than the fast food of today. In that fast food you're throwing down the hatch, there are a number of agents that aid you in your weight gain as well. Sure we live a bit longer now than then, mostly from massive reductions in smoking and mild reductions in saturated fats. We also live sicker now, we're on a host of drugs starting at a young age, we spend insanely more on health care, and at least 2/3 of us are carrying too much weight.

It very simply boils down to poor choices for the vast majority of us. Yes, there are cases where bad genes or circumstances have dealt someone an unfair hand. It could be cancer at a young age, or something less sinister. I truly feel for those people, especially for the children. And yes, some of us have tougher hills to climb than others, and those hills will vary. My weakness may not be yours, but we all have them, and thus we all have our challenges to surmount. What choices do you make?

I think some people to some degree like to be lied to. Think of the wife who asks her husband if she looks fat in her dress. We all know his answer is supposed to be "no". What if he said, "Well, honey, you could stand to lose a few pounds." He'd be ridiculed in the media. Our useless gossip-queen modern "journalists" would be parked in his front yard. He'd have to go on some daytime talk show where a bunch of women brow-beat him into submission demanding an apology. Then 2 months later he'd have his own reality show.

Why did she even ask the question at all? She knows the answer. She just wants an empty approval. The same is true when we buy into all of these gimmicks. The truth is a bit more complex, and requires more effort. There are many patients who seek out a provider in natural medicine for many good reasons, but expect to trade out an Rx bottle for an OTC one, and be better instantly, with little effort on their behalf. The road to recovery may be longer and harder than you had hoped. You may have been sick for years, and your recovery, even when in the hands of a talented provider, may take time and effort. Be honest with yourself.

- Americans are so busy they don't have the time to eat right and exercise.

I'd be surprised if you don't fall into this category. How many of us have the time to prepare our foods? Aren't we all running around like chickens with our heads cut off? Not to make blanket statements, but the answer is mostly "yes". I'm not naïve. I know many of you have demanding jobs and lifestyles. Some of you are killing yourselves to just make ends meet. Still we make choices. Even if you're busy, changes can be made. These changes include not just diet and exercise, but lifestyle choices as well. In my 40 years, I have been witness to some interesting social and economic changes in America. If you're my age, or older, this may sound familiar.

Not too long ago, Dad went off to work each morning while we went to school. Dad worked a reasonable number of hours. His commute wasn't an insane multi-hour traffic jam, over long distances. We lived in a reasonably sized, affordable home. We didn't get a new car every three years. Mom didn't even have a car until I was about five. Mom stayed at home and took care of the household. There really wasn't daycare, or at least as it exists today. Taxes were low. The cost of things was low. We didn't fly to some resort every year for vacation. We had one television, which had poor reception, and no remote. At most, we did one activity at a time, such as sport, a musical instrument, or a language. We had only enough basic toys to keep us busy. Somehow, we survived, and may have even been happy.

Contrast that to today. The dynamics of time, stress, and energy have changed substantially over the years. Both parents may have to work to pay the bills. If you consider today's cost of living, while the average family income is about $50,000 per year, then yes, both do have to work. This in turn ensures further costs, mostly related to daycare. However, we also do make choices. Why do we need three televisions, two computers, three cars, and pricey annual vacations? Why is it our children get mountains of plastic toys, which you have to trash or donate on an annual basis? Why do we enroll our kids in every possible activity under the sun? Don't we realize someone has to drive them? Multiply that craziness times the number of kids you have. Why do we have to have a 3,000 square foot home, which has to be heated, insured, and taxed? I won't get into the political-economic-social reasons why the costs for taxes, goods, and services are high, but suffice it to say, they are.

Some of the issues that contribute to our lifestyle are mostly out of our control. But, guess what. Many are within our control. It's human nature to want to keep up with the Joneses. We want to sing the praises of our children. We want to live life to its fullest, however you happen to interpret that. This is human nature, but consider this point. Although these may seem like basic needs, it is a higher thought process that is able to overcome that, and put it in perspective. Isn't the end goal peace of

191

mind and happiness? Do you have peace of mind? Are you content with your life? If not, make the changes. We live only once. Your children are young only once. Have no regrets.

Sleep problems are one of the biggest reasons patients seek medical attention. Many of us can't sleep, which is as basic as it gets. If you're so stressed out that you can't sleep, then consider why. If you look and feel like garbage, isn't it time for a change? I'm not saying, "get rid of everything." I'm saying, it's not the end of the world if you cut back on things. Do you need the new cars, the huge house, and the material things that in the long run really don't matter? This isn't just fluff talk here. One of the key aspects to natural medicine is peace of mind. When stressed, it's hard to sleep. If you can't sleep, you can't heal.

I see people racing around every day. When you are able to put things into perspective, and place fewer demands on yourself, you free up time and energy. That's the point of this section. *Find more time for you.* Make time for yourself and your loved ones. Learn to say "no". Do you currently say, "I don't have time to exercise"? "I don't have time to put together a good meal." Make the time. Do it. Unhook the cable TV. I did. You'll be amazed at how much it sucks you in, and when gone, at how productive you can be. Do you know the average American watches five hours of television a day? FIVE HOURS! There's some time. Make the time for your health.

Take time to exercise. Get up and play soccer with your kids in the back yard. You'll tire fast and realize that you used to be able to play all day. Being winded, you could sit down and resign yourself to aging, or you could use it as motivation to get in better shape.

Realize this whole process is a slow one. Here in America, we want instant gratification. We want a drive through meal, and we want it now. We want the house, the BMW, the boat, and we want it now. In general, we lack patience. One healthy meal, one healthy day, isn't going to make you healthy. It is a long process. If you're ill, it took you a while to get there, so it may take a while to get out. You know this is true. You know deep inside that to lose weight properly will take time. You know it, but you don't like it. That's why the gimmick weight loss diets and "exercise" products are a multi-billion dollar industry. Save your money. Spend it instead on a gym membership, good food, and proper supplementation.

Speaking of gym memberships, did you know that the average gym may have 3,000 members, but only about 400 to 500 are regulars? That's it. The gym couldn't survive financially off the regulars; it needs the majority. It needs those with good intentions, but who lack the follow-through. Did you join a gym you didn't use?

I readily admit that changing habits and routines takes time and effort. There's the time at the grocery store, the time at the gym, the time preparing your food, and the time to clean-up after a meal. It's time consuming. That's why fast food is so popular. Fast food is quick, cheap, easy, and instant. I realize that everyone can't live a totally healthy lifestyle for whatever reason. Do what you can. Take selective bits and pieces from this book to improve upon your health status.

- Americans are confused about proper food choices.

Have you ever talked to a nutritionist or doctor, and while they were telling you what to eat, you couldn't help but wonder why they're 30 pounds overweight and look like hell? Seriously, I see it more often than I should. There are many "experts" who preach proper diet, but who are grossly overweight, have poor complexions, dry hair, poor energy, lousy personalities, and other undesirable traits. The question begs itself: "Do they know what they're talking about"? The same is true for personal trainers, right? Have you been at the gym, and seen some trainer "teaching" a new member how to exercise, and the trainer is in horrible shape? I've seen it too. I would think if you're going to pay your hard earned money on a trainer, then hire someone who looks the way you'd like to look. Your odds of getting a decent trainer under those conditions is higher than if you opt for something less. Shouldn't you expect the same of a practitioner who lectures you on food choices? They may think they know, and they may sound like they know, but many don't. Again, use common sense and reasoning. If your practitioner is bald and is selling you on products to grow your hair, think twice.

Practitioners who are partially educated, partially immersed, and less than passionate about what they do, will often lend inaccurate information. Conflicting data in the media will also confuse and frustrate you. Unfortunately, some of this comes in the form of marketing. It seems that many companies will say anything to separate you from your money. The food group with the most amount of confusion surrounding it has to be dairy products. This is why I have written an entire chapter dedicated to it.

You think dairy is a proper food choice because it's been hammered into your head since you were a child. Dairy is a part of the food pyramid. Dairy is a source of calcium. What could be better than wholesome dairy? Dairy foods, in the forms of cheese and yogurt especially, are quick and easy. Just throw some in with your child's lunch. Not much effort required there. Misinformation has you thinking milk is nature's perfect food. Dairy has been a part of our culture for thousands of years, and thus ingrained into our habits.

Dairy can produce an extreme amount of mucus in the body. For example, I had someone ask me about his son's runny nose. Every time I saw the kid he literally had non-stop goo running out of both nostrils. I asked if he gave him dairy, to which he said yes. He ate milk, yogurt, and cheese, the usual suspects. I told him to take him off of dairy products for a while and see what happens. I knew what was coming next before he asked the question, because I get it all the time. "What about calcium?" I went through high calcium foods, which we resist feeding to our children because they'd rather eat garbage. It's part of conditioning the child for his own benefit.

So what happened? The mucus was gone in a few days, never to return. We'll never know how much I saved him in doctor's visits and drugs for ear infections and the like, and then the downstream problems that antibiotics can cause. This is but one example of food confusion. It's not your fault. We've been trained, and it's time to un-train, which is a nice segue into change.

- People are resistant to change

Habits formed over a lifetime are hard to change, and I realize that. The way we do things is a part of who we are, and how we were raised. If cooking has never been your thing, you hate to exercise, or you've been seeing dr. so-and-so for a lifetime, it will be hard for you to fully adapt.

The best example I can give here is in choosing your practitioner. Most of us are programmed to see our practitioner of modern medicine whenever something isn't quite right. We plan on walking in with symptoms, and getting that "magic in a bottle" to cure us. We don't often know what the consequences are of either short or long-term use of a given prescription, but we go for it anyhow. We don't know why we got sick, when someone else didn't. We're told repeatedly that we have the best healthcare in the world, but chapter one may dispel that gospel. In any event, we still go, and in droves like never before.

Another example is that of milk. People become very defensive and visceral about certain things. Politics, parenting, and even milk are topics where we feel we're right. If I told you that you've been doing something wrong your whole life, you'd get defensive, like the nurse who tried to tell me that chocolate milk was good for my son. When people become defensive, they can also become irrational. This book isn't meant to insult you, just provide you with information to refine your thoughts. For some people, even with mountains of evidence, rational thought still eludes them. How else could O.J. Simpson have been freed?

There are numerous points in this book. Pick as many as you think you're capable of doing. These changes aren't the big stressful ones like moving or starting a new job. These are reasonably simple ones, like eating differently, spending money wisely on supplements, and considering alternative medicine. Most people are resistant to change. I know that. Hopefully I will be able to provide you with enough evidence to muster the drive from within to make the changes, and stick to them.

- Components of processed foods lend themselves to ill health unknown to you.

Beyond the obvious issues with dietary choices, there are the hidden ones with which you are only vaguely familiar. You may know that preservatives aren't particularly good for you, but you may not know the difference between a preservative and a food ingredient. You are also likely unaware of how significant your reaction can be to seemingly innocuous chemicals added to your foods. If we refer back to the chapter on IBD, we already have an excellent example of how chemicals can cause one set problems, which lead to more downstream. The whole root of your illness could be related to a chemical. It could be that simple.

The offender doesn't have to be a chemical either. Did you know that there is an enormous amount of evidence linking dairy consumption to a whole host of diseases, including type 1 diabetes? The list of diseases potentially and likely caused by dairy is enormous. Do you get headaches frequently? That could be an allergy to dairy, or to some other allergenic food. These labs can be run for you, or elimination diets can be undertaken to find the culprit.

We have a tendency to explain away these problems, and attribute symptoms to some general untreatable complication. Oh, my mother always had headaches, and I have them too. Maybe your mother and you have the same food allergy. Maybe since you were raised by her, and quite possibly cook the same way, maybe you're ingesting the same offender. Whenever a naturopathic provider, or at least one worth their salt, looks at a condition, the number one thought should be, "What is causing the condition?" This is at the heart of natural medicine, to find the root cause. In the end, this is a much better form of medicine than taking drugs to treat a symptom.

We all know that our modern medical community writes prescriptions by the boat-load to alleviate your symptoms. We discussed this in "Our Current Healthcare Model". I mention this because those drugs also have hidden components that can result in ill-health via an array of side effects. We all know this to be true, as people move to natural medicine in droves, hoping to avoid the side effects from drugs. Wouldn't you rather try something more natural that has been proven to have fewer side effects, while trying to address the underlying cause?

Take soy as another example. It's billed as our modern miracle food. You might be surprised to know that the marketing information you've been exposed to isn't entirely accurate. Soy can cause problems ranging from thyroid issues to hormonal imbalances and worse. These components of soy, these "side effects," are unknown to you. Unless you go looking for this information, it's likely you won't find it. The truth on soy is out there; it just gets trampled by the incessant marketing that serves to separate you from your money.

Understand that natural/integrative medicine has just as much to do with what you eat, as it does with supplements, labs, exercise, and a good mental state. I can't underestimate the value of a good diet. This is followed closely by proper exercise. These two combine to form the best thing you can do for your health. The other stuff exists to get you out of the hole you're in, or tries to keep you from getting into one to begin with.

We all have heard that it's not healthy to be overweight or obese. We know it's linked to cardiovascular disease, type 2 diabetes, and even cancer. With all the hype behind health and losing weight, as a nation we still continue to get heavier. It seems to me that you can tell someone to do something, and they may or may not do it. Or, you can explain in detail WHY something is good for them. So that's what I'll attempt to do for the rest of this chapter.

I address obesity not only because it is so prevalent, but also because it is a risk factor in a broad array of diseases. Conversely, the benefits of exercise have broad support as a model to health. From a monetary viewpoint, heart disease, prostate cancer, breast cancer, diabetes, and obesity account for 75% of healthcare costs. Obesity is a central factor in all of these disease states, as well as numerous others. To address obesity, is to address the healthcare cost crisis of this country head on.

What's involved in the process of weight gain? Fat is just fat, right? As you eat more, and exercise little, this stuff called fat accumulates in the body. Technically speaking, the process of weight gain reflects the accumulation of triglycerides in fat tissue, which leads to an increase in size of the fat cells (adipocytes) and the generation of new ones. Once you've generated a new fat cell, it's yours to keep. You can shrink it along with the others, but it won't go away, unless of course you have liposuction performed. This plays a significant role in the quick regaining of weight after a diet. Each time you fall off the wagon, your body is able to regain weight quickly, in part from the extra fat cells that you did not have in your youth. Obesity is also caused in part by a defect in signals telling the body when to eat and when to stop. There is also manipulation of our food with man-made chemicals, MSG for example, which alters your eating habits. Additionally, there's hormonal system dysregulation through genetic variability, flaws, if you will, that will make it easier for some to gain weight as compared to others. However, obesity is only rarely attributable to mutations in genes that encode for hormones or receptors. (4) Researchers conclude that genetic effects alone could not account for the doubling of obesity in one generation alone. (5) Both of these statements make perfect sense to me. As common sense tells us, two obese parents are more likely to produce a child prone to obesity than two non-obese parents. However, overweight and obese people in the U.S. are now the norm, which is an epidemic not of genetic origin.

So, you've been told to lose some weight, or maybe you're telling someone to do the same. But why should you lose weight, other than that "it's good for you"? As research has progressed, we understand more about how the body works. The amount of information at your fingertips is overwhelming. In the example of adipose tissue, there have been excellent advances in our understanding. Adipose tissue is composed of fat cells embedded in loose connective tissue that contain precursor cells for new adipocytes, immune cells, and others. Our traditional view of fat as a form of energy reserve, cushioning, and an insulator has been changed. Fat tissue is now regarded as an active endocrine (hormonal) organ, which releases a large number of mediators, perhaps in the hundreds, which affect blood pressure, lipid and sugar metabolism, inflammation, and food intake, to name a few. (6) I won't burden you with some of these agents that have been identified, especially since we are in the beginning stages of understanding their roles and interactivity. I will mention two of the more studied as a case in point.

The most abundant protein produced by fat cells is called adiponectin. It is a "good guy". It sensitizes cells to insulin, making them better able to respond to insulin, which is a good thing for someone with insulin resistance. It also plays a protective role in atherosclerosis. It has been shown that more adipose tissue is associated with less adiponectin, and more insulin resistance and ultimately type 2 diabetes. Another "good guy" you may have heard of is leptin. Leptin represses food intake, promotes energy expenditure, improves peripheral insulin sensitivity, and helps beta cell function. In fact, the administration of leptin has been shown to reverse insulin resistance.

Now that insulin resistance has been brought up twice, let's review insulin and some physiology to better understand this discussion. Insulin is secreted by the beta cells located at the pancreas in response to increased blood levels of glucose (sugar) and amino acids (protein) after a meal. The regulation of blood glucose by insulin is done by suppressing liver glucose production and promoting liver and muscle glucose storage (glycogen). It also increases triglyceride storage in adipose tissue, and amino acid storage in muscle. Insulin is therefore a powerful growth stimulator, as well as regulator of these basic units in our body. Our capacity to produce insulin is determined by the total number of beta cells and their functional activity at the pancreas. We are capable of increasing the number of beta cells, but that can be offset by other factors that cause them to die.

To take this one step further, insulin resistance is a pre-diabetic condition where peripheral tissues, to include muscle, liver, and adipose tissues, do not respond as well to normal insulin levels. Insulin resistance also occurs in obesity, as you would imagine, but it's also present in hypertension, autoimmune diseases, cancer, and more. For example, in the case of cardiovascular disease (CVD), insulin resistance is considered to be a pivotal event in the increased risk of plaque instability through different pathways. (7) In one such pathway, it has been shown that high concentrations of insulin directly increase inflammation at the site of atherosclerosis, causing the plaque to become unstable. (8) Insulin also induces production of an enzyme that makes plaque unstable. (9) Whether through these mechanisms or others, a state of hyperinsulinemia and insulin resistance poses an increased threat of plaque instability, possibly contributing to a cardiovascular event. Since high insulin is so closely related to obesity, this is one of several biochemically proven dangers of obesity for your consideration.

Here's another. As fat cells increase in size and number, certain good-fat derived hormones are decreased, while unhealthy ones are increased. You probably didn't know this, but fat tissue promotes inflammation. Inflammation can be a good thing for fighting off an infection; however, it's not so good chronically as it has unwanted effects on blood vessels, mutates DNA (carcinogenic), constricts airways (asthma), attacks cartilage (rheumatoid arthritis), or causes GI distress (all causes of IBD). Amazingly, the inflammatory agents produced by adipose tissue have their effects throughout the entire body. As one researcher states, "The products arising from inflamed adipose tissue contribute to an inflamed state in distant cells, such as endothelial, arterial and bronchial smooth muscle, and pancreatic islets, which help drive conditions that progress to hypertension, diabetes, atherosclerosis, asthma, and certain cancers." (10) So excess fat tissue produced these pro-inflammatory agents that have negative affects throughout the body, which should come as no surprise since we already know that increased risks for all of the listed diseases are associated with obesity. Inflammation is not just relegated to fat tissue, it is a normal part of our immune response, without which we'd die. However, it is the up-regulated rate of inflammation by excess adipose tissue that plays such an important role. A very interesting feature of the inflammation response that emerges in the presence of obesity is that it appears to be a trigger, and to reside predominantly in adipose tissue. (11) In other words, systemic inflammation seems to be controlled to a degree by the fat tissue.

In addition to the fat cells that produce inflammatory agents, there are immune cells within the fat tissue. Of course, we want properly controlled immune cells; that's a part of their job. But for some reason not completely understood, these specific immune cells (macrophages) infiltrate the fat tissue in significant numbers. Between the two, they kick off appreciable quantities of pro-inflammatory agents. So what are these agents? TNF-alpha and IL-6 are the most widely studied cytokines produced by adipose tissue. You remember TNF-alpha. We discussed this very important player in the role of IBD. TNF-alpha causes inflammation everywhere, not just in the GI tract. TNF-alpha is directly proportional to fat mass. (12) *Weight loss decreases TNF-alpha.* IL6 has been shown to decrease adiponectin, that "good guy" protein. Together with other inflammatory agents, they play a key role in ensuring their success, and your failure. How do they do this? Their increased expression in adipose tissue has a proven link to insulin resistance.

The idea that inflammation is associated with insulin resistance has been known for a long time and is consistent with the finding that stress induced cytokines like TNF-alpha cause insulin resistance. (13) These elevated pro-inflammatory cytokines are positively correlated with, and can predict, insulin resistance in metabolic syndrome patients. (14,15) Many researchers have shown the link between the two. There is some debate on exactly what's going on, and to what degree they play a role, but there is a mountain of evidence correlating these inflammatory agents with diabetes and the conditions that precede it. For example, not all researchers find that IL-6 is elevated, but overall levels are increased in the obese and in those with insulin resistance. (16) It is thought that TNF-alpha and IL-6 modulate insulin resistance through several different mechanisms. (17) Others lend more weight to TNF-alpha and state that, "TNF-alpha may be causal in the insulin resistance of the metabolic syndrome of aging." (18) It has also been shown that TNF-alpha and free fatty acids (fats) from both plasma and stored triglycerides (fat cells) impair insulin signaling. Yes, I mentioned free fatty acids. What does this mean and why is it important? Free fatty acids are basically fat in its smallest form that you're able to absorb from the GI tract into circulation. If you eat a high fat diet, you have more circulating free fatty acids. I will next present one reason why a high-fat diet is not particularly good for anyone concerned about their blood sugar.

You thought you just had to keep your blood sugar under control, right? There are two parts to the blood sugar equation. Briefly, elevated blood sugar helps to drive insulin resistance in peripheral cells, and to compromise its own production at the source, the beta cells of the pancreas. As we know, when beta cells are exposed to elevated levels of glucose for a prolonged period of time, the glucose becomes toxic to insulin secreting gene expression and beta cell survival. This phenomenon is referred to as glucotoxicity. The other part of the equation is that high blood sugar causes extensive damage throughout the body, which is why diabetics have issues with CVD, the eyes, and their feet, to name a few. So, controlling for blood sugar is a great thing from preventative and reversal of insulin perspectives. This is still only half of the story. The

201

other half, which you have not heard, regards lipids. It has been known for 40 years that free fatty acids (FFAs) are able to induce insulin secretion. (19) Great, that's good for science geeks, but what does that mean for the general public?

Again, as the years have gone on, our knowledge has grown. We went on to learn that FFA-induced insulin secretion in beta cells is dependent on glucose as well. (20) In other words, in a fasting condition, the amount of insulin in response to FFAs is minimal. However, as higher levels of glucose are introduced, the insulin response is maximized by the FFAs. (21) Further translation is as follows. If you eat a fat on an empty stomach, or with a protein, in the case of a steak, then your insulin won't shoot up markedly. If you were to instead eat a carton of ice cream, the fats would have a synergistic effect with the sugar on your insulin secretion, sending it up higher than if you had eaten the sugar alone.

As research progressed, we came to a clearer understanding of how FFAs induce insulin resistance through a cascade of events. As we already know, excess fat ingestion increases triglycerides and FFAs in the blood, which in turn induces insulin resistance, which further increases glucose. (22) The increase in blood sugar further increases glucose-stimulated beta cells to make more insulin, which further increases triglycerides. In the end, defective insulin secretion is the result of chronic exposure to elevated levels of fatty acids, which inhibit insulin gene expression by functioning as beta toxic agents. (23) The knowledge that chronic exposure of beta cells to high levels of both blood sugar and blood FFAs results in impaired insulin production, led to the old "which came first" question. Are the FFAs the initial agent, or is it the high blood sugar? This led to the term "lipotoxicity" among researchers, as they have more recently struggled to find the smoking gun. In my review, it seems to me that it is the high blood glucose levels that provide the initial insult, where once damage has begun, the FFAs pour gasoline on the fire. My conclusion is backed by other researchers who make similar claims. The argument is basically as follows. It seems that high FFAs have a detrimental affect on beta cell survival, but only for those pre-diabetic, insulin sensitive, or diabetic. (24,25) They may in fact be so crucial that they are the straw that breaks the camel's back in many instances.

So we're left with the following understanding of the cascade of events as they are related to blood sugar and FFAs. Bear in mind this is based on the findings of many researchers, who are not all in complete agreement, but of the information to which I am exposed, most seem to go with this general progression, which seems to be well supported by data.

- Poor dietary habits cause high spikes in insulin chronically.
- In time, peripheral cells become less sensitive to the effects of insulin.
- More insulin is produced to compensate for higher blood sugar levels.
- Peripheral cells respond less to insulin.
- High blood sugar and/or sugar consumption combined with fats accelerate damage and death of the beta cells where the toxicity of both share targets. (26)
- Insulin production may be significantly reduced by damage, making high blood sugar a systemic problem.

This doesn't take into account the inflammation induced by the fat cells we discussed earlier, which also plays a role in insulin sensitivity and beta cell death. There is a silver lining in the fat-ingestion equation. Recent research has backed up a fact we have known for a long time. You should aim to cut down on saturated fats. Researchers used longer chain saturated fatty acids, usually palmitic acid, and also used monounsaturated fatty acids, ones you'd associate with olive oil, to discern effects on beta cells. So what did they find?

They found that the <u>monounsaturated fatty acids improved beta cell secretion and not only had no effect on causing beta cell death, but promoted beta cell proliferation</u>. (27,28) They also showed that only the long chain saturated fatty acids synergized with high glucose to kill beta cells, and reduce their proliferation. The differences caused one researcher to state, "The distinct effects of the saturated fatty acid and the monounsaturated fatty acid on beta cell turnover and function are striking." (29) That's a lot coming from a researcher. I think we can be comfortable with this data. The fact that FFAs longer than 15 carbons may be harmful to various cell types has been reported in numerous studies. (30) This does not include saturated fatty acids from butter or unadulterated coconut oil, but mostly from animal fats.

There are a number of possible theories behind how the differences in these two fatty acids can have such different impacts on our insulin production. It is likely that their toxicity is exerted through the metabolites, but the exact mechanism is not completely understood at this time. Does it really matter? We have now proven that longer chain saturated fatty acids, when combined with high blood sugar, can kill and/or dampen the insulin response from the pancreas. This high FFA impact is not seen in everyone. Although not all patients show high FFAs in the prediabetic state, circulating FFAs and triglycerides are commonly elevated, particularly within overweight subjects. (31)

Now let's take this fatty acid thing one step further. Fatty acids are an obvious fuel source, not just for making components that require fat cells. The powerhouse of the cell is called the mitochondria, and one of its main functions, in addition to producing energy for every cell, is to remove fatty acids through a process called beta oxidation. (32) If the process of beta oxidation and its associated clearance rate of fatty acids is overwhelmed, then they can reach toxic levels in the cell. These fatty acids are then dumped from adipocytes and distributed into the periphery. These released triglyceride deposits are associated with the development of insulin resistance in muscle and liver, and are also lipotoxic in pancreatic beta cells. (33)

Excessive FFAs are also implicated in endothelial dysfunction, death of vascular smooth muscle cells, induction of adhesion molecules, and others. (34) Translated this means that there are severe consequences to your vasculature directly posed by high serum FFAs. Atherosclerosis is itself a disease of inflammation. It can be characterized by the accumulation of leukocytes (white blood cells), proliferation of smooth muscle, and neoangiogenesis within the vascular wall. (35) All of this contributes to formation of the aforementioned arterial plaque.

A small insult to the vasculature may begin things. It could be from a stimulus such as something mechanical or maybe chronic oxidized lipids from a deep-fried diet. The body must act to respond to these insults. It's a choice between the body's perceived instant survival, and dealing with this imperfection in the vasculature down the road. Under normal circumstances there would be a normal response, or hopefully none needed at all. In the case of chronic inflammation, you have a heightened number of adhesion molecules called chemokines and the inflammatory molecules called cytokines, of which TNF-alpha is one. They make the white blood cells stick when they normally wouldn't. A less-than-ideal pattern ensues where inflammation and adhesion stimulate cell proliferation with plaque formation as the end result. The stability of the plaque itself is dependent on how you care for yourself. So as you can see, the role of high serum fatty acids is not simply pathogenic in regards to the pancreas and insulin receptors, but they have systemic effects.

In review, we can try to lump the previous pages around the beta cells of the pancreas, and the vasculature. We know that high serum insulin levels have negative consequences for both. We know that high serum saturated fatty acids do the same, whether dumped from adipocytes, or from the diet. We know that the inflammatory agents, cytokines and chemokines, which are produced from adipose tissue, negatively impact both the beta cells and the vasculature. We also know that a poor diet combined with a sedentary lifestyle sets the stage for obesity, insulin resistance, and inflammation, which all keep this cycle going.

So when someone says "eat right and exercise" they're saying a whole lot more than they know. Of course, even among experts, there are disagreements as to what "eating right" actually means. Some things are fairly universal, like eat your fruits and vegetables, while others are in dispute, such as dairy and protein intake.

In an attempt to clarify this for you, the next three chapters will address key aspects of diet. The little known consequences of dairy and iron will be reviewed extensively in the next two chapters, while I will try to roll up a dietary conclusion within our ideal diet.

Chapter 8   Dairy

How is it that cheese, yogurt, and milk could be bad for us <u>humans</u>? I must be lying. I must have some agenda to bash the dairy industry. I must have something to gain by scaring you away from dairy, and towards other foods. Well, if you can uncover my master plan and my angle, please fill me in. However, I'm pretty sure I have nothing to gain in this process. As I have stated before, this is merely information. It is up to you to determine what is best for you and your loved ones. You can choose to ignore it, or you can implement changes to varying degrees. If you are interested in improving your health for the short and long term, then at least give this information fair consideration.

You are beaten over the head repeatedly with marketing from a wide variety of companies eager to separate you from your money. One of the best marketing programs has been the "got milk?" slogan. You see famous people with the milk moustache enticing you to drink milk to be healthy. Everyone else tells you to drink your milk to get calcium. Yes, I know, you were already thinking about your calcium. "If I don't get it from dairy, then where will I get it"? We are all told how important calcium is to our health, and we are told to get 1,000 mg per day as an adult, or 1,200 mg perday when we're over 50. Think about this. If dairy products were so good at preventing osteoporosis, and here in America we are one of the top global dairy consumers per capita, then shouldn't we have the lowest rates of osteoporosis? Wouldn't you be surprised to find out that's not the case? In fact, the highest dairy consuming nations also have the highest rates of osteoporosis, such as Great Britain, Scandinavia, and the United States.

I'm going to attempt two approaches here in my case against dairy. I'm going to appeal to your logic, and show you technical information as well. I will be able to quote numerous researchers who feel the same as I about dairy. You will see that I am not alone in my wacky free-range, tree-hugging, dolphin-safe, off-the-grid, organic mindset. Actually, I'm just as regular as any of you, illustrating that you don't have to be "out there" to live a healthy, happy, lifestyle living amongst the masses.

You may find that there are some things in this book with which you decide to comply 100%, and others you choose not to comply with at all. I realize we are all different, have different challenges, have varying degrees of discipline, and have different outlooks on life. I don't want anyone to become neurotic about the topics in this book. We don't want to detract from any dietary improvements with the detriments from neurosis. To have the few things you crave the most on rare occasion is not the end of the world. Life is to be enjoyed, as much as cherished. I get it. You will find your own levels of moderation over time, and they themselves may change as time passes. Again, consider the facts, and make your own call. I know I'm bashing an old stand-by here, but it's still the truth no matter how little or how much you may disagree. We are on average resistant to change. Probably nowhere else in this book does that apply more than it does with dairy. So, what's wrong with dairy anyhow?

First, let's establish what dairy is, and what it is not. Dairy products are derived from a milk source. Milk, ice cream, yogurt, and cheese are dairy products. Butter comes from dairy, and is a fat, consequently not containing some of the problematic proteins. I'm sure few of you will try to argue the benefits of ice cream, and so we'll spend our time on milk, yogurt, and cheese, which in effect we can lump together under the category dairy. Let's apply some common sense to kick things off.

As a baby, our perfect food for the first year or so of life is milk from our mother. Milk from a human is different than the milk from a cow. Our own FDA states, "The best first food for babies is (human) breast milk. More than two decades of research have established that breast milk is perfectly suited to nourish infants and protect them from illness. Breastfed infants have lower rates of hospital admissions, ear infections, diarrhea, rashes, allergies, and other medical problems than bottle-fed babies. A baby should drink breast milk, not cow's milk, for a full year. We've known for years that the death rates in third world countries are lower among breast-fed babies. Breast-fed babies are healthier and have fewer infections than formula-fed babies. Human milk contains just the right amount of fatty acids, lactose, water, and amino acids for human digestion, brain development, and growth."

You see, we're raising a human infant, not a calf. Human breast milk is designed for us. For example, breast milk contains much higher levels of the amino acid taurine, which is important for brain development. Last I checked, cows weren't particularly bright animals, and don't need nutrients valuable for brain development like taurine, linoleic acid and DHA. You know DHA; it's the main reason you're taking fish oil. Breast milk has more DHA. Cow's milk also has five to seven times the mineral content. This includes calcium. If we don't need that much calcium as a rapidly growing infant, then what makes you think we need that much calcium as an adult? Cow's milk is geared to develop an animal from about one hundred pounds at birth to several hundred pounds when ready to wean. They require big bones to support those big bodies. They have four stomachs, while we have only one, although I wonder about some people. Breast milk is loaded with immune enhancing components geared for us. Cow's milk has immune components for a cow, but not after pasteurization. Pasteurization also kills off many to most of the beneficial enzymes that aid in digestion. Cow's milk is also loaded with casein. Casein is the protein component of milk. Human breast milk is mostly whey, which is much easier to digest. Cow's milk contains about 3 times the amount of protein as does human milk, and upwards of 20 times more casein, depending on who's referenced. Like lactase, as we age we lose the ability to make another enzyme, rennin, which breaks down casein.

Whether you were breast-fed or not, at some point you and your mom were genetically programmed to end the feeding process. You were weaned. You grew some things in your mouth called teeth. Your immune system was up and running, as was your digestive tract. You went on to eat solid foods. Animals do the very same thing. As a cow ages, it goes on to eat grass. Here in America, however, where we have radically screwed with nature, we also have cows eating grains, other cow parts, and more.

So, why is it that when another mammal is weaned from its mother, it only goes on to eat the foods of that adult mammal? If you're a fan of nature shows on television, you'll actually watch a mother mammal turn away her young at the time she feels it's ready to feed on its own. This has been part of our evolution over millions of years. Why is it that we as humans decided to throw biology out the window and go on to consume milk for our entire adult lives? Not only do we eat it, we also heat it, add sugar to it, and a whole host of other wonderful add-ons. Is it that we are so smart, that we have decided to out-think our genes? In fact, we are so smart that we are not only consuming milk in our adult years, but we're also consuming it from another animal. This makes no sense to me.

Do you go running for the bathroom 20-30 minutes after consuming milk? If so, you probably have lactose intolerance. A whole industry geared to making an enzyme, lactase, has sprung up so that we can consume more dairy. An intolerance to lactose is not a milk allergy. It is a compromise in the ability to digest the sugar in milk, lactose. At birth, we have the enzyme that splits lactose into smaller digestible sugars. That enzyme is lactase. Here's something to consider. As we age, most of us lose the ability to produce this enzyme in quantities that make it plausible to consume milk to any significant degree. This major drop usually occurs before adulthood. Why would our body reduce its ability to digest milk at a youthful age if it was something crucial to our survival? If you really think about it, and discount the fact that people tell you to drink milk for your bones, would you drink it at all, considering how unnatural it seems to your logic?

Consider our ancestors. They evolved over hundreds of thousands of years, hunting, scavenging, and gathering food to survive. Our genetic make-up comes from them. How long has the cow been domesticated? Scientists think that around 8,000 years ago the ancestors to our "cow" were initially domesticated. How many thousands of years after that did it take for that domestication to spread to your ancestors? Perhaps many of you don't have ancestors that loved the cow. If you're ancestors came from the far east, or were American Indians, or a host of other peoples, then your ancestors never got on the bandwagon, pulled by a cow, by the way. Today billions of people do not consume cow's milk and they suffer much less from bone demineralization. No, our ancestors, all of our ancestors, came long before the domestication of the cow. The few thousand years of dairy production pale in comparison to hundreds of thousands, if not over a million years of evolution our genes have adapted to. The records show that our Paleolithic ancestors had solid bones, no osteoporosis there. How could that be? They didn't consume any dairy products. What were they eating?

Is this starting to sink in yet? There's more. Have you noticed, as I have, that girls seem to be maturing earlier these days? I've seen heavy-set second graders developing breasts. When I pose this question to people, I get the same response every single time. They say, "It's the hormones and stuff in the food." Would you be curious to know which foods? Sure, it's not all due to dairy, but dairy certainly shares the blame. Hormones and chemicals that mimic hormones are lipophillic. They like fat. They bond with fat. So, the more animal products you consume, the more you ingest concentrated hormones and chemicals that have adverse effects on your health, to include earlier puberty. Here's an interesting study to illustrate the connection.

This data comes from Japan, published in *Preventative Medicine* by Yasuo Kagawa in 1978. As part of an annual survey, detailed statistics are taken from tens of thousands of citizens. This offers an interesting model in that prior to their defeat, the Japanese lived one way. After the conclusion of the war, the occupation of Japan by the Americans brought change. Among the many changes, food was also subject to influence. 21,707 Japanese were analyzed in 1975 and compared to the 1950 numbers. Remember that the war ended in 1945. So, in 1950, 5 years after the end of the war, the average annual dairy consumption was 5.5 pounds. That's it. Twenty-five years later, in 1975, the average annual dairy consumption was 117.4 pounds. That's an increase of 2,127%. Would you like to know what else increased? Heart disease was up 35%. Breast cancer and colon cancer were up 77%. Their weight also increased. In 1950 the average 12-year-old Japanese girl was 4'6" and weighed 71 pounds. By 1975 her height was up 4.5 inches, and she weighed 19 pounds more. The only thing to go down was the onset of the first menstrual cycle. In 1950 the average Japanese girl began her period at 15.2, while in 1975 it had dropped to 12.2 years old. The quality of milk has gotten much worse since then, but we'll get to that later. In fairness, their consumption of protein went up during that time, which would contribute to growth as well. That amount went up by 759%, significant, but not nearly as much as the dairy.

"Expert" opinions on dairy are not uniform. The data is very strong against dairy, and those who continue to push it are ignorant of the science and are falling in line with the big industry machinery, of which the government is included. Perhaps nutritionists, practitioners, and other "experts" in this field are innocent in their lack of knowledge on the subject, because any one of us only has so much time in a day. We all can't sift through books and research articles endlessly looking for the hidden truths. You will now be armed with more information than most professionals, and you can then choose your own direction.

Let's look at much of the science. Research has shown that dairy products are frequently contaminated with cow's blood and pus, pesticides, hormones, and antibiotics. They are also linked to a number of diseases, which include but are not limited to allergies, diabetes, heart disease, and numerous cancers. Allergies are first up.

Allergies

Allergies to food are the cause of an enormous number of medical visits, and consequently are of considerable cost to you, and to our healthcare system. The only problem is that you may not know your condition has any connection at all to a food allergy. The symptoms of food allergies and the offending food or foods can both be difficult to grasp. If you go to see your practitioner due to eczema, diarrhea, GI distress, asthma, or an ear infection, it is quite possible that your visit is related to ingesting a food to which you are allergic. This is not to say that all of these conditions have causes based in foods. Clearly there are other connections such as chemicals, stress, and more that play a role. The food allergy may exacerbate the symptoms of another allergy. To make matters even more confusing, you may have more than one food allergy.

Let's begin with defining the term "food allergy". We come to the splitting of hairs again to separate an allergy, from a sensitivity, from an intolerance. The term allergy implies that there is an immune-mediated reaction, while we could classify the non-immune-mediated reactions as an intolerance. The hypersensitivity reactions would be a subset of the immune-mediated ones, but apply only to an IgE response. Although the IgE reaction can be accurately connected with a food to a large degree, there are difficulties in separating an intolerance from an allergy. As you will see in this section, there is much confusion over this, and since we have no reliable tool with which to define the two, and since it really doesn't make a difference to someone who's suffering from a symptom, then at the expense of making the nit-pickers unhappy, we'll refer to all adverse events from food as a food allergy for the purposes of this book.

Approximately 20% of today's U.S. population has been reported to experience adverse reactions to food. (1) While over 140 different foods have been shown to produce allergic reactions in humans, the most often documented offenders are cow's milk, wheat, citrus, eggs, peanuts, soy, shrimp and other seafood, tomato, chocolate, nuts, and seeds. (2,3) Our focus here is on cow's milk, but we need to have a broader understanding of food allergies in order to better grasp control of one based in milk, and to be fair in our implications.

Cow's milk contains more than 25 proteins capable of inducing an antibody response in humans. (4) Although the connection of symptoms, particularly hives and gastric upset, can be traced back over 2,000 years to Hippocrates, it was a much rarer event until recently. The most likely suspect of this phenomenon is the movement away from breast-feeding, and the move to cow's milk and milk-based formulas in western countries. As usual, the incidence is significantly lower in less developed nations. Cow's milk allergy is primarily a disease of infancy and early childhood, although well documented cases have also been described in teenagers and adults. (5) Infants and young children who have been properly diagnosed with milk allergies have shown remission rates in three clinical trials, but suffice it to say that by age 5-7 most do not show an active allergy. (6) Although this statement is true, it also leaves many allergic adults undiagnosed. The provider may very well be operating under the incorrect notion that these allergies should have been outgrown. To further complicate things, the original symptoms may disappear, and new ones may take their place for the same allergy. It's very hard to estimate exactly the percentage of cases that are caused by a food allergy, since it is hard to test for conclusively, it is often missed, and it is often labeled as another disease, implying some other origin.

To make matters even more complicated, allergic symptoms can present themselves as different symptoms to the same food between people. The most common symptoms of milk allergy are gastrointestinal, skin, or respiratory. Gastrointestinal symptoms can range from diarrhea to constipation, can manifest themselves in the stomach, small intestine, and/or large intestine. Whether the label is gastroesophageal reflux, enteropathy, or colitis, you want the symptoms gone. The most common dermatologic symptom is hives (urticaria), while eczema and atopic dermatitis are also symptoms. Respiratory manifestations include wheezing, asthma, or ear infection. Basically think mucus. Since respiratory mucus is a consequence of milk allergy, then mucus, and a possible subsequent infection of the mucus within the sinuses and beyond, can be problematic. Other possible links are irritability, hyperactivity, and insomnia. In the case of insomnia, for example, in a study of eight infants with insomnia, researchers eliminated cow's milk exposure, and "cured" all of the patients. To prove this wasn't a fluke, upon rechallenge with milk proteins, four regained their sleeping problems. (7) As further proof of the connection, all of the infants had high IgE antibodies to milk. We do know from clinical trials that the majority (75-92%) of infants with a cow's milk protein allergy have more than one symptom, and the majority (over 70%) have symptoms from more than one organ system. (8)

To further complicate things, one could present with one of three different reactions based on time, immediate, delayed, and late. An immediate reaction would occur within about 60 minutes or so from the time of ingestion. This is an IgE mediated (hypersensitivity) allergy. These are the easiest to identify since you're able to link symptoms with ingestion in a reasonable time frame. The second reason why this is easy to identify is that tests such as the skin prick test measure for an IgE reaction to a food, and this test has relative reliablility. Those with the IgE reactions tend to develop reactions more to other foods, such as nuts and fish. Also, since an IgE reaction can be more systemic, these patients tend to have more inhalant allergies as well. Inhalant allergens have been reported in about 50% of IgE mediated children by age three, and in about 80% before the age of puberty. (9)

The second type of reaction possible is the delayed version. This is where the symptoms occur at over one hour from ingestion, up to a day or so later. As time rolls on this kind takes on the complications of the next type of reaction. Slight delays over an hour or so may depend on the meal, the individual, or the quantity of allergen. Both the delayed and the late response have been linked with an increase in inflammatory cytokines, particularly TNF-alpha. (10)

The third type, and probably the most confusing is the late reaction. This is where the symptoms don't develop for a day or more. As you can imagine, it's hard to isolate an offender under these conditions. Diagnosis via the IgE test is probably a waste of money. It's also possible that tests for IgG and IgA antibodies are a waste as well, since trials have yielded conflicting results. (11) Allergy panels in natural medicine also have a level of inaccuracy. A false positive is possible since carrying the antibodies to milk protein is natural. The formation of IgG, IgA, IgM, and low levels of IgE antibodies to cow's milk is a normal physiological response, which has been demonstrated in normal children. (12) It is also more difficult to test for this reaction by food avoidance, given that it can take significant time for inflammation to resolve itself. You may not have the patience for this process, especially if you're on a hypoallergenic diet trying to gradually add back offenders while looking for possible multiple allergies.

The confusion in symptoms and allergen exposure are exemplified well in the following trial. 47 children aged 4-66 months with clinically proven cow's milk allergy were challenged with milk proteins, and their antibody response was measured. The variability in the responses had them placed into one of the three groups I just previously illustrated. Those in the immediate reaction group had mostly dermatological symptoms, which were associated with a high IgE level. Delayed reactions, defined as within 1-20 hours, were mainly vomiting and diarrhea, with no IgE response. Late reactions, defined as over 20 hours, were dermatologic and gastrointestinal. In these, the dermatologic reactions had an elevated IgE, while the GI did not. (13) As you can see, the "immediate hypersensitivity" of an IgE response can be quite delayed. Also, if you have an IgE response, it doesn't mean you'll just have a dermatologic problem only, as you might infer from this trial. Delayed reactions following an immediate IgE response occur in some, and are accompanied by inflammation and subsequent tissue damage, which may play a role in gastrointestinal symptoms from foods such as dairy, soy, and gluten. (14)

Another factor that can cause confusion is that one could have multiple food allergies and not know it. If you went to see your doctor with symptoms, and she was able to link them to a food by suspicion or otherwise, if your elimination proved fruitless, you may revert back to consuming the offender. The fact that a second offender is present could easily be missed by all.

For all these reasons, your first action should be that of a hypoallergenic diet. Technically, there is no diet that's hypoallergenic for everyone, but there is one for the masses. We just have to hope that you are helped by this, and statistics show us that you will be. It's easier for me to tell you what's not in a hypoallergenic diet, than what's in it. A hypoallergenic diet excludes dairy, wheat, soy, egg, seafood, corn, nuts, and citrus. That's your hypoallergenic diet for food, which differs from the steps necessary to rule out a chemical sensitivity, as per our IBD discussion. Keep in mind the likely big offenders for the general population are dairy, wheat, corn, and soy. In the event you do not want to consider a hypoallergenic diet because it will be inconvenient for you given the prevalence of these foods in the average American diet, I will now illustrate proof of its use.

27 infants with chronic constipation were investigated for the connection to a cow's milk allergy. When put on a milk-free diet for one month, 21 patients had resolution of symptoms. When rechallenged with milk, constipation reappeared within 48-72 hours. In 15 of the 21 "cured" patients, lab tests indicated an immune connection. (15) This tells us a few things. One, all constipation does not have its origin in milk, or milk only. Two, for those cases where milk is the agent behind the symptom, removal yields resolution in a reasonable period of time. Three, all patients with a proven milk allergy will not show a "testable" immunologic response.

In another study, 104 children aged 1.5 to 9 years old with recurrent ear infections were evaluated for food allergies by skin prick (IgE) and food elimination/challenge. Those found to be allergic by IgE response were taken off the offending food for 16 weeks. The elimination diet led to a significant reduction in symptoms in 86% of the patients. A rechallenge of the offending food provoked a recurrent ear infection in

94% of the children. (16) How often do our dairy-raised children develop ear infections resulting in medical visits, prescriptions, time, and money?

In yet another trial, 52 patients with chronic constipation were enrolled in a milk protein-free diet. During the first two weeks, bowel movement normalized in 24 subjects. The remaining patients were then placed on a more restrictive hypoallergenic diet. Bowel movements normalized in another six subjects. Upon rechallenge with the offending foods, constipation was reproducible showing that all 30 patients who had resolution had a milk allergy, and six of them had multiple food allergies. (17) This shows us that eliminating just dairy may lead you to believe that dairy is not the culprit, assuming you have multiple food allergies. A comprehensive hypoallergenic diet where allergenic foods are gradually added back 1-2 weeks at a time is the best way to detect food allergies. Longer periods may be warranted for cases of extreme inflammation. Re-challenging with the suspected offender can further confirm suspicion, and labwork from a provider of natural medicine will also be helpful.

In more support of the allergenicity of dairy, researchers took 51 children whose dermatitis was thought to be caused by milk protein allergies. They performed a skin challenge (IgE) test on these children. 35 of the children reacted in minutes with hives at the site of administration. (18) This shows that milk clearly plays a significant role in their dermatitis. It could be that for those who did not respond, they may have also had milk allergies, but as we've learned, all do not present with an IgE mediated response, and thus they would have been missed.

In another trial, 42 infants with a known IgE mediated allergy to milk were followed for at least two years to evaluate for remission of the allergy, or the occurrence of additional ones. Prevalence of symptoms in the children were as follows; eczema 57%, asthma 69%, egg allergy 67%, peanut allergy 55%, and 83% demonstrated allergies to three or more allergens. At the end, cow milk allergy naturally remitted in 13 patients, while the allergy persisted in the remaining 29. The incidence of allergy to inhalants, egg, and peanut was greater in those whose milk allergy persisted. (19). In other words, the children with milk allergies started the study with very high rates of other allergies and symptoms of allergies. For those kids who "outgrew" their milk allergies, they had a slightly less allergic profile than for those who didn't. This study shows us that the longer you expose your allergic child to the offender, the longer you dysregulate the immune system of your child, and the more likely it is that your child will go on to develop other allergies.

For those of us beyond childhood, 20 adults identified as milk-sensitive or controls were subjected to a milk challenge test. Only two out of nine milk-sensitive subjects had a detectable serum IgE response. This was not a lactose intolerance test, but an immune marker test. Basically, they were determining if the administration of milk affected one or more of several immune responses. Given the immunological responses, the researchers concluded, "Milk hypersensitivity in adults, occurring as gastrointestinal reactions, may be more common than previously thought." (20) This study illustrates that relying on an IgE based test for milk allergy will miss a great many people who are allergic, particularly in the case of GI symptomology.

This next study was published in the *Journal of Pediatrics* in 1995. The researchers had previously noticed that infants with milk allergies, who were suffering from diarrhea, dermatitis, and bronchospam in their first year of life, went on to suffer from chronic constipation later at ages 2-3. With that premise in mind, they prospectively analyzed 27 infants with chronic constipation, and showed that 21 of the 27 had resolution of symptoms as they responded to a one-month milk free diet. In 15 of the 21 who improved, immune-reactive tests confirmed hypersensitivity. Upon re-feeding with cow's milk, constipation reappeared within 48-72 hours. The serum IgE did not differ between responders and non-responders. (21) This trial illustrates several previous points. The symptoms of milk allergy are variable, IgE tests are highly unreliable when GI symptoms are the primary complaint, constipation in infants may well have an allergic pathogenesis, and a hypoallergenic diet with re-challenge is fairly accurate in assessing hypersensitivity.

In one last allergy study, the subjects were 65 children with constipation, defined as one bowel movement every 3-15 days (ouch). They had been treated with laxatives without success. The children were placed on diets with soy or cow's milk for two weeks, then had one week free of milks, and then switched for two more weeks. Constipation resolved on the soymilk in 44 children, while <u>all</u> on cow's milk had constipation. To prove that it wasn't a fluke, the responders were all re-challenged with cow's milk and the connection to constipation was confirmed. (22) Take into consideration two things here. One, all children didn't respond to the milk-free regimen, possibly due to other food allergies, soy included. Second, soy demonstrated a better symptom profile than milk, not only because milk is more allergenic, but also because it has a slightly unfair advantage. Milk is usually the first complex protein ingested in a young immature GI tract, setting the stage for early hypersensitivity. It is possible that had these children been raised on soy milk, the numbers would be somewhat reversed.

It seems everyone is constipated, and they're looking for something to move things along. Products that make people poop are very popular. If you love the concept of cleanses, I suggest you start by eliminating dairy. I get questions very often about which cleansing protocol is best. My comments are always the same. There are a million cleanses out there; some sound almost reasonable, and some sound risky. I believe that your diet should serve as its own cleanser, and you should pollute yourself as little as possible in the course of the non-cleansing days. If your diet has fiber, nutrients, and few toxins and allergens, then you are on track. If you want to do a "cleanse" then just eat less food for a period, since digestion places a burden on the body to a certain degree. However, you must keep in mind that you need to ingest those nutrients for your detoxification process. If you look at the longest-lived healthiest peoples on earth, cleanses are not mentioned in the literature. You can start by just eating less, and taking out those food allergens.

For the best overall health, which includes the possible elimination of allergies from cow's milk, the best step is that of avoidance. For the infant, human breast milk is the best thing for your baby. In the legitimate instances where breast-feeding is not possible, you should be aware of the downside of your other options. This is where providers usually recommend a soy-based formula. I don't recommend it. Along with a host of other issues, it also has its own allergenicity. Adverse reactions to soy have been reported to occur in about 17-47% of children sensitive to cow's protein. (23) Soy-induced lower GI issues are mostly of the non-IgE type, and thus these sensitive infants are usually equally sensitive to the soy proteins. (24) In fact, the American Academy of Pediatrics recommends that in patients with GI symptoms caused by non-IgE mediated cow's milk allergies, soy formula should be avoided. Although raw goat's milk is most likely a better option than cow or soy, it may not be ideal for your child since it shares some cross-reactivity among its proteins and the proteins of cow's milk. (25)

Clinical trials have shown that hydrolyzed formulas are best suited for an infant in regards to allergenicity. The term hydrolyzed refers to the fact that the proteins have been "chopped up" and denatured to the point that they aren't whole and thus have almost no reactivity. You may find that some formulas have been hydrolyzed more than others, and even in the best products the success rate isn't 100%. In that event, an amino acid based formula might be your best consideration. We're talking about a very rare person here, once the breast milk, goat's milk, and hydrolyzed formula regimens have all failed.

Speaking of infants and formula, this brings us to gastroesophageal reflux (GER). GER is considered normal when the child is healthy, and is resolved in 98% of the time by age two. (26) However, when GER is caused by a food allergy, it becomes GERD (D=disease), which can be difficult to separate from the normal vomiting of most infants. You're familiar with GERD. You see those commercials all the time on T.V. Our diets are so bad, that sales of heartburn and GERD (chronic heartburn) medications top $14 billion a year. Isn't it concerning to you that in February of 2008 two forms of Nexium, which is a proton pump inhibitor (PPI), were approved for use in children aged one to eleven? Once again, we have been saved by the FDA and the drug companies. Never mind the fact that reduced gastric acid has been shown to increase your chances of a food borne infection. Never mind the fact that an increased sensitization to food antigens has been shown in humans treated with PPIs, and never mind the fact that we need adequate HCL in our stomachs to activate certain nutrients such as calcium. We should note that in a Canadian study in people over fifty, 7 years or more of PPI use has been shown to increase the risk for a hip fracture by 4.5 times. I only mention this because 30% of seniors who break a hip die within a year. I mention all of these things because I think it is completely irresponsible of the government, parents, and pharmaceutical companies to be "drugging up" our children in the same way we treat ourselves as adults. At least we have a choice.

Your child has a choice as well. In one study of 10 children with unremitting diagnosed gastroesophageal reflux, including biopsy abnormalities of the esophagus, with symptoms on average for 34 months, all were placed on an amino-acid based formula for a minimum of six weeks. Two children had improvement and eight had resolution. All patients redeveloped their symptom on an open food challenge. Prior to this treatment, all children were unresponsive to standard GERD treatment. (27) This shows a connection to a food allergen; however, in this case the allergen was not identified. As previously stated, as bad as milk may be, it is not the only cause of allergy symptoms.

In another formula study, 18 infants with an average age of 7½ months had reported hypersensitivity to hypoallergenic formulas (no whole milk proteins). These infants were given an amino acid formula for two months. Following this two-month reprieve, the infants were then rechallenged with the formula that had reportedly been best tolerated previously. In 12 of the infants, irritability, vomiting, diarrhea, and/or eczema flares developed during the re-challenge. Allergies were to soy and hydrolyzed milk protein products. (28)

In summary, for dairy allergies, if you can't breast feed your infant, evaluate your other options while realizing that milk may not be the only offender. In children over one year old, the best practice would be to avoid dairy altogether. The introduction of other allergenic foods should be done one at a time for upwards of 2-4 weeks until status can be verified. As an adult, consider dairy as a cause or contributor to a disease for which it seems there is no link.

Diabetes Type 1

Numerous studies show a strong correlation between the consumption of dairy products and the incidence of diabetes. I'm not talking about diabetes from the weight gain that one would expect by eating tons of dairy products. That is relatively easily reversible with a good diet and exercise. I'm talking about type 1 diabetes, expressed through damage to the cells of your pancreas that produce the insulin itself. One of the most striking studies comes to you from Finland and Canada, and was published in the *New England Journal of Medicine* in 1992. The researchers make significant statements to support the connection between dairy proteins and the development of type 1 diabetes. They looked at bovine (cow) serum albumin antibodies in the serum of 142 newly diagnosed children with insulin-dependent diabetes mellitus (IDDM) as compared to healthy controls. The researchers found high levels of antibodies to a specific cow's milk protein in 100% of the 142 children with diabetes. That strikes me as more than coincidental. They went on to state that these antibodies are capable of reacting with "beta cell specific surface proteins" and that these antibodies could participate in the development of islet dysfunction. (29) Those beta cell surface proteins are components of the cells that produce insulin.

Finland is the source of yet another study that found diabetic children had higher levels of serum antibodies to cow's milk. (30) Yet another 1998 study from Finland found that children with insulin-dependent diabetes mellitus (IDDM) had higher levels of cow's milk protein antibodies than the matched controls, and these high levels of antibodies are an independent risk marker for IDDM. (31) This was after controlling for factors such as age, duration of breast-feeding, age at introduction of dairy, and recent consumption of dairy. A more recent analysis of dairy consumption and diabetes was published in 2006. The researchers looked at two factors in children from Iceland as compared to children from Scandinavia, which includes Norway, Denmark, Sweden, and Finland. Iceland is not considered a part of Scandinavia; however, the roots of its people can be traced mostly to Scandinavians. I think this is even more evidence dispelling the concept that there is genetic risk factor, since the diabetes rate in Iceland is significantly less than for Scandinavia. It was found that the lower consumption of dairy products in Iceland might be related to the lower incidence of type 1 diabetes in Iceland as compared to the other nations. The consumption of dairy proteins is likely more important in younger childhood since correlations between dairy proteins and IDDM were found for the two year olds, but not for the 11-14 year olds. (32)

Finland should be researching this connection. As one of, if not the highest dairy consuming nation on the planet, their rates of type 1 diabetes are also the highest. If you look at other high consumers of dairy, such as people in the U.S., you will also find a correlation between dairy and type 1 diabetes. If you look at nations with little to no dairy consumption, you'll find their levels of type 1 diabetes are a fraction of the others.

The next study comes to us from the University of Rome, published in 1996. These researchers looked at the immune response to a certain protein from cow's milk, from 47 patients with a recent onset of IDDM, as compared to 36 healthy controls. They found antibodies to the protein were present in over a third of IDDM patients and relatively non-existent in healthy individuals. (33) Another Canadian study reported in the *American Journal of Clinical Nutrition*, in March 1990, found "a significant positive correlation between consumption of unfermented milk protein and incidence of insulin dependent diabetes mellitus in data from various countries."

Although I didn't include any U.S. studies, be certain they exist. I'm trying to illustrate a couple of points here. One point is that this research, much like other research, is global. There are many others who recognize that there is very likely a connection between the consumption of dairy products and the development of IDDM via the destruction of the cells in the pancreas that produce insulin. The other point is clearly that there is an abundance of current research that seems to show support for these findings. Is this to say that dairy causes all cases of type 1 diabetes? No. Is it a very significant contributor? It would seem that way.

Let's get a little deeper into our understanding of what's going on here. The very premise of this milk-diabetes connection is based on the contention that there is destruction of cells called beta-cells, which produce insulin at the pancreas. Insulin places blood sugar where it needs to go, and removes from the blood. As far as I can gather, there is no real debate here. It is known that this destruction does occur, and as a result, insulin production suffers. It has been estimated that at the time of diagnosis, only 10-20% of the insulin-producing beta-cells are still functioning. (34) Whether or not these cells can be regenerated, is a bit of a debate. There is some evidence that fish oil, for example, as well as other natural products may be able to play a role in this regard.

There is clearly an autoimmune issue going on here. In other words, the body of an IDDM patient is making antibodies that destroy these cells. There are seemingly four related antibodies, and their presence is the first warning sign. The number of detectable antibodies is unequivocally related to the risk of progression to overt type one diabetes (35). Should you develop one of these antibodies, the risk is in most cases not terribly high. Should you go on to develop two or more of these four antibodies, then your risk goes up significantly. It has been shown that your chances of developing clinical type 1 diabetes are 60-100% over the next 5-10 years if you test positive for three or four of these antibodies. These antibodies can develop at a very young age. So how are these antibodies formed?

There are three main concepts that drive this debate: genes, conferred protection, and triggers. The theory behind the trigger is that it gets the ball rolling, and keeps it rolling until progression has resulted in disease. There is seemingly not a lot of argument over these concepts, from a macro standpoint. The debates lie in the specifics about which gene confers protection, and what is the trigger? So let's first look at genetic variables.

We first have to recognize that there must be a genetic issue at play. If there were not, then you'd see a much higher prevalence of IDDM given the fact that so many Americans are fed off a milk-based product as infants. You'd see just about everyone fed a milk formula go on to develop IDDM, which is clearly not the case. Only about 1% of us progress to IDDM. There are many of us, who were fed a milk-based formula, and milk for many years later, who never went on to develop IDDM. So there is some type of genetic risk that compromises those unfortunate few.

I think this marker is still yet to be identified. There has been a lot of attention given to a class of genes referred to as HLA. However, fewer than 5% of these HLA "high-risk" individuals go on to develop IDDM. (36) To further refute this argument, in yet another Finnish study, 16% of

HLA susceptible children had a rotavirus infection within 6 months of beta cell antibody detection, as compared to 15% for non-HLA susceptible children. In other words, the rates of the risk for diabetes were the same in all the gene pools analyzed when a suspected autoimmune initiator (rotavirus) was present. In addition, there is also a lack of supporting evidence when looking at celiac disease. The HLA connection is similar here as well, yet many do not go on to develop celiac disease. While about 20% of Caucasians have the HLA susceptibility, only about 1.3% go on to develop celiac, even considering that most of us are exposed to gluten on a daily basis.

Beyond this HLA conversation, you also have to consider my earlier comments in regards to the Iceland-Scandinavia trial. Why is it that these nations of peoples with the same origins go on to have such differences in a given disease? We do know that the Scandinavian countries have some of the highest rates of dairy consumption in the world, while Iceland has significantly less. We also know that the incidence of IDDM has occurred in many groups who have moved from an area of low risk to an area of high risk. In yet another point, we know that in Puerto Rico the incidence of IDDM is about 10 times that of Cuba. Again, we have arguably peoples of similar backgrounds, in a similar range of geography, with wildly varying rates of disease. It is of note that fewer than 5% of mothers breast-feed in Puerto Rico while breastfeeding is the norm in Cuba. This last point, given in an area of warmth and sunlight brings us to our next point, the possible protective role of vitamin D.

It could be that vitamin D, or more specifically a lack thereof, plays a role in the progression of IDDM. When you consider that the nations with the highest rates of IDDM are also in colder climates, then the connection seems to have plausibility. There has also been shown to be a seasonality with the initial antibodies presenting in the fall and winter months. Vitamin D has been shown to be protective of the beta cells, as shown in an amazing Finnish study with over 10,000 infants born in 1966. These subjects were monitored for vitamin D intake as infants, and then years later for type 1 diabetes development through to 1997. It was found that those infants *in their first year of life* who consumed vitamin D supplementation, had almost a 78% lower chance of developing type 1 diabetes when taking 2,000 IU/day or more when compared to those who did not supplement. Additionally, those suspected of rickets in the first year of life, (those with a vitamin D deficiency), showed three times the risk of developing type 1 diabetes. (37)

Vitamin D certainly plays a role. Whether it is that of an anti-inflammatory agent, an immune-modulator, or something else, we don't know for sure. In another similar disease, vitamin D was administered to see if it could alleviate the intentional multiple sclerosis-like damage to mice. There is good evidence to support low vitamin D and the prevalence of MS. I did not tackle MS in the vitamin D chapter, since there is potentially an enormous array of diseases where it can help. In this mouse model, it was shown that vitamin D drove down the inflammatory pathways by essentially telling the immune components that were causing the sustained inflammation to die. (38) This is not the first time that the uncontrolled genetic-immune-inflammation model has been discussed in this book.

With that said, vitamin D is not the whole answer either. As you have seen, the data in Puerto Rico as compared to Cuba does not support the connection entirely. Additionally, we know that there are locations in northern Europe having an incidence of IDDM far less than in Finland. Russian Karelia and Iceland are two that come to mind. Consider that their diets may be different, but the sun exposure is similar. The vitamin D connection is without a doubt an important protector, but not the whole answer.

The other highly likely protective measure is breast-feeding. There are a number of studies that show breast-fed children develop IDDM significantly less than those who weren't. Breast milk contains a host of growth factors and cytokines, mostly species specific, many of which appear to have a role in the maturation of the intestinal tissues. (39) Hopefully the mother is passing on healthy breast milk to the infant, which helps to confer immune protection against pathogens, improve the integrity of the GI tract, and help develop a less-sensitive hyper-inflammatory response. It only makes sense that the properties in mother's milk need time to build this whole new defense system to foreign particles ingested for many years to come. Remember from earlier chapters, the GI tract is this amazing intricate balance within the body. It is a tube running through in which foreign matter bumps up against the inner workings of your body in an attempt to gain nourishment while keeping out the bad guys who'd love to feed off of you. Expose an infant slowly to complex proteins, especially allergenic ones.

There is data to support this slow introduction. A large review was performed on all studies deemed valuable as to whether early feeding practices had any influence on the risk of the development of IDDM. The researchers showed that patients with IDDM were more likely to have been breast-fed for less than three months, and to have been exposed to cow's milk before the age of four months. (40) Given this, as a parent you'd likely want to consider breast-feeding for as much of that first recommended year as possible. When food is introduced, avoid highly allergenic ones such as wheat, dairy, soy, egg, corn, and nuts.

So what's the offender? What is it that kicks off this process of inflammation and self-destruction? It is likely a combination of the above. The early introduction of a highly allergenic food, with subsequent insult to the GI tract, a possible background of genetic susceptibility, and a lack of protection, which limit the inflammation response, all likely contribute. Given that dairy is the most allergenic food we have, and that in industrialized nations it is the first allergenic protein introduced, and it is in these industrialized nations where the predominance of IDDM occurs, then we must place dairy at the top of the list of suspects. There are five principle proteins in milk, caseins (70-80%), beta-lactoglobulin (10%), alpha-lactalbumin (5%), gamma-globulin (2%), and bovine serum albumin (1%). (41) We must include the protein bovine insulin in this equation as well.

The studies support allergenicity predominantly to the caseins, bovine serum albumin, beta-lactoglobulin and bovine insulin. Although the data is amazingly consistent in matching dairy consumption with the development of IDDM, the data is not in agreement on which protein is the culprit. Those in favor of casein can make a strong argument over the fact that there is so much of it in cow's milk as compared to human milk, and it is by far the predominant protein in milk. Those who support the bovine insulin case can make a good argument that bovine insulin differs from human insulin by only three amino acids, and that an allergenicity to this foreign protein can kick off an immune response that could mistake its own insulin as an enemy. Those who support the bovine serum albumin or beta-lactoglobulin case, like the other two have many trials on which to hang their hats. *We do know that antibodies to cow's milk are present in virtually all infants exposed to it, and it is thus considered a normal response.* (42) Additionally, we also know that antibodies to the proteins in cow's milk decrease over time with exposure.

I should add that other allergenic foods seemingly aren't even close to being as highly problematic. Many researchers make the argument that dairy proteins receive too much blame due to the fact that they are usually the first allergenic protein introduced. However, studies show that in patients newly diagnosed with IDDM, there is not the corresponding increase in antibodies to other introduced proteins, such as the gliadin protein responsible for celiac disease. (43) Milk proteins certainly seem to own the stage on this one. Diabetes develops to a much lesser degree in countries that do not make a habit of consuming cow's milk. So milk is not the whole answer, but it is a seemingly significant portion.

From the standpoint of exposure to dairy proteins, consider these points. There are several proteins within milk, all of which have data to support their proven allergenicity and connection to IDDM. All likely play a role. Milk is the first protein usually introduced, but is also the most allergenic, and others don't have the same impact. Finally, we'll probably all produce antibodies to these foreign proteins, but due to several factors, most of us will pass through and essentially become inoculated, if you will, while others won't be able to control the inflammatory response.

This brings us to the agent (trigger) that kicks off the inflammatory process. Viruses, particularly enterovirus and rotavirus, get a great deal of attention here. The Illinois Department of Public Health tells us that enterovirus-caused infections are second only to those caused by the common cold. There have been over 60 different kinds identified, and the primary ones in the U.S. include coxsackieviruses and echoviruses. Lining up with the development of IDDM, children are less likely to be immune than adults.

Finnish researchers claim that enterovirus infections appear to be the most probable trigger of beta cell antibodies based on the data from three clinical trials. (44) As you might guess, all studies don't support this theory, and of course testing models vary between research labs. We do know that enterovirus RNA has been detected in the blood of about one third of patients with IDDM, but only in 5% of healthy controls. (45) A number of other studies prove the toxicity of enteroviruses, and the respective claims. In vitro studies show that the enterovirsus infect beta cells easily, and induce impairment and cell death. (46) Other researchers state that variants of the coxsackie B virus are present in the general population and that they are able to induce beta cell damage in susceptible individuals. (47) In addition, recent studies show that the enterovirus itself can be detected in the beta cells of IDDM patients. (48)

The rotavirus has been analyzed as well, but perhaps not to the same degree as the enterovirus. In any event, one study showed that the appearance of diabetes antibodies was associated with a significant rise in rotavirus antibodies. (49) This shows that a recent or current rotavirus infection may initiate the inflammation response in conjunction with already ramped up antibodies to dairy proteins necessary to destroy beta cells. In our previously mentioned study when we discussed the proposed HLA link, it was shown that about 15% of children and infants experienced a rotavirus infection in the 6 months preceding the first detection of antibodies.

This all sounds eerily like IBD, doesn't it? We have many of the same components. Here, we have a compromised intestinal tract that never reached maturity prior to the introduction of allergens. We introduce this highly allergic food, which even in a mature healthy gut will produce antibodies. We can also assume that this infant is deficient in some vitamins, notably A and D, further setting the stage. Consequently the infant, or child for that matter, is chronically exposed to the host of allergenic dairy proteins that ramp up the immune response, causing GI permeability and a host of other issues. The introduction of a pathogen tips the scale. Since the child has not either been breast-fed for long enough, or not at all, the immunity transferred from the mother is lacking, to include but not limited to probiotics. The infection ramps up the inflammation, and the antibodies to these foreign proteins now become overpowering. We know through gut permeability and serum studies that this gut associated event moves out systemically. The proteins on and in the cells of the pancreas look a lot like the proteins we're trying to kill in a different downstream location. Given the likelihood of low levels of vitamins A and D and omega-3 fatty acids to keep the inflammation in check, the beta cells are killed by the body's own immune system.

It's quite possible that you don't need either of the two aforementioned viruses to set off the inflammatory response. Just as in IBD, it could also be a bacterium. We see the same uncontrolled inflammation in IBD, the only difference is that it's the cells of the intestine that are bearing the brunt of things. Again, we could use the example of MS provided earlier, where the initiator and autoimmune component has yet to be agreed upon, but here the inflammation has a neurological manifestation. So back to the bug. As we know in IBD, bacteria can kick off the course of events. Given that milk has been shown to be loaded with bacteria, and even shown to carry viruses, don't you think it is more than possible that the milk could not only be the source of the allergen, but also the source of the pathogen initiating the cascade of events responsible for type 1 diabetes?

So what are you to take from all of this? Realize that there is no known genetic marker that has yet been identified to test a newborn's risk reliably. Also realize that your race probably has little impact on your potential, or more importantly the potential of your child, to develop IDDM. From the genetic component, there is really nothing you can do. Therefore, your action lies in the ability to prevent exposure to triggers and other complimentary considerations. A first line consideration is to take fish oil and vitamins A and D at the very least. Take it as an adult, take it as an expecting mother, a breast-feeding mother, and give it to your children. These supplements can play a significant role in regulating an autoimmune response that may save the beta cells of your child's pancreas. Breast feed your child for as long as possible, and introduce complex foods slowly over time. Build up the immunity and maturity of your child's GI tract. You can't live in a bubble, so the exposure to pathogens may be difficult. However, you can avoid them to a certain degree by ensuring clean eating habits. Last, but certainly not least, do not give your child dairy products of any kind. The health of your child depends on your informed choices.

Osteoporosis/Calcium Myth

To reiterate my important point from earlier, if dairy products were so good for our bones, then why is it that the nations that consume the highest amounts of dairy have the highest incidence of osteoporosis? Sure, bone is primarily made of calcium, and dairy products contain substantial amounts of it. Why is it that nations which consume less dairy and protein have much less osteoporosis? For how many years have you been hearing about osteoporosis, calcium, and dairy? As a nation, do you think we are any closer to the answer today than we were 10 or 20 years ago? Why is it that our Paleolithic ancestors seemingly had no problems with bone mineralization in their dairy-free lifestyle? Could it actually be that dairy products contribute to osteoporosis? It sure seems that way. The high protein content of dairy products has been shown to cause a leaching of calcium from the bone. This was evidenced in the Harvard study, which looked at 78,000 women and found that those who got the most calcium from dairy products actually broke more bones than those who rarely drank milk. (50) In an earlier study on the other side of the globe, Australian researchers showed that a higher dairy consumption among elderly men and women was associated with an increased fracture risk. When those in the highest consumption group were compared to those in the lowest, there was an almost doubling of the risk of hip fracture. (51) Additional studies have produced the same results.

An extensive review done in 2005 of the existing literature on bone mineralization and children yielded some interesting results. The researchers looked at 58 studies in regards to the relationship between dairy and/or calcium intake, and bone mineralization and/or fracture risk. This extensive review showed that "neither increased consumption of dairy products nor total dietary calcium consumption have shown even a modestly consistent benefit to child or young adult bone health." This doesn't seem like such a stretch when you consider the low amount of calcium consumed in other less affluent nations during those same years, and how as adults, osteoporosis is virtually non-existent in those non-dairy consuming nations. The bone mineralization will come with a healthy and dairy-free diet as a child develops. As an adult, it is more important to reduce bone loss. Doing away with excessive animal protein, which certainly includes dairy, is a good start. A significant portion of the absorbed calcium is excreted by the body to compensate for the protein in the milk. When you consider that people absorb only about 25% of the calcium in milk, then excreting a significant portion of that 25% to compensate for the acid-base balance from the protein isn't ideal. For cheese it's even worse. Most of the calcium is excreted, since cheese doesn't have all the water of milk, but is a concentrated protein source.

How can we increase our bone formation, and more importantly as the years roll on, reduce our bone loss? We need to reduce those things that cause calcium to be purged from the bone and sent into the blood. We have covered a high protein diet. Other recommendations include exercising, reducing your salt intake, cessation of smoking, and eating more fruits and vegetables. Those fruits and vegetables seem to keep coming up when people talk of a healthy diet. This does not include cooked ones. Applesauce, cherry pie, overcooked broccoli, and other dead fruits and vegetables don't count. We're talking about fresh fruits and vegetables, and partially cooked vegetables. Those green leafy vegetables are great for your bones. They have magnesium to help absorb the calcium, they have vitamin K to help build bone, they have potassium to conserve calcium loss from acids, and they are low in protein. It should be mentioned that bone requires more than just a few minerals, and fruits and vegetable are loaded with these other nutrients as well.

How is it that cows, elephants, and other large herbivore mammals build such large bones? They consume greens. While the animals may eat grass, we can digest leafy greens, and other vegetables, beans, nuts, and seeds. Researchers at Yale reviewed 34 published studies, which encompassed 16 different countries. Some of our usual suspects were included, such as Sweden, Finland, and the U.S. They found that those countries that consumed the most animal food, which obviously included dairy, had the highest rates of osteoporosis. They also showed that African-Americans, who consume much more calcium on a daily basis than South African blacks, were 9 times more likely to suffer from a hip fracture.

Looking at one of these groups specifically, we see that the Bantu women in Africa consume no dairy products at all, and take in only about 250-400mg of calcium a day from vegetable sources. This 250-400mg is a fraction of the RDA set for us here in America. After having multiple children, and breast-feeding all of them for months even with no dairy intake, osteoporosis is virtually unknown among these women. (52)

If the calcium intake in undeveloped countries ranges from around 300-500mg/day, and they don't experience osteoporosis nearly to the extent we do, then why do we recommend 1,000-1,200mg/day for adults? Why is it that the World Health Organization (WHO) recommends 400-500mg/day? I think our intake of milk and other dairy products is a habit, a remnant of our past, much like our school summer vacation. Many years ago children had to help raise and harvest the crops to keep the family fed throughout the winter. Obviously today, we walk into a grocery store at our convenience. Why couldn't we convert to the metric system? Why do we still swear in our new president in January, even though the election results came in November? My point is that habits are hard to break.

Our consumption of dairy is similar, but goes back even further. It is a remnant from Europe. If you were to have lived in a colder climate, your growing season would have been shorter, and you'd need more food to hold you over through the rest of the year. For those of you who have a garden, think about the few days of the year when you can actually go out there and pick something fresh to eat. Now think, if you had to support your family for an entire year, how would you go about doing that? First you'd need a much larger garden. Second, you'd have to find a way to preserve the harvest. In some years your garden does better than other years, right? How about the weeds and grass? That seems to grow well every year. So if you could harness the spare land, the greens that grow every year, and if your day-to-day survival during the long cold winter depended on it, you'd do it. This, of course, brings us to dairy. Cheese keeps very well. Butter doesn't do too poorly either since all of the water has been extracted. Milk you can get by feeding stored dry grass to the cows. So here you have a supplement, or even an emergency reserve of food for day-to-day survival.

Thankfully, we no longer live in that world. We have a spoiled, comfortable, safe world where we can get "fresh" produce harvested from around the world a couple miles down the road. We don't need that emergency dairy. Get rid of it. It's not a part of your gene pool.

IGF-1

In my research, the best resource for this chapter is Robert Cohen's book, *MILK-The Deadly Poison*. This section reviews his book with added updates and commentary. Should you like to know more about this topic, as well as the scope of corruption and greed between Monsanto and our federal government, I suggest you read it.

The scientific community had known for many years that isolated bovine growth hormone injected into another cow would increase milk yield. It does this through a variety of effects on the mammary glands in the udder mediated by insulin-like growth factors since the mammary tissue of cows does not contain binding sites to BGH. However, extracting the BGH was not economically feasible until biotechnology companies came up with the economies of scale processes through recombinant technology.

In the spring of 1994 the FDA approved the use of a genetically engineered hormone called "recombinant bovine growth hormone" (rBGH). That little "r" comes when a naturally occurring hormone in one species is recombined with genetic material from another species. In this case, Monsanto merged the genetic material from the bacteria E. coli with the naturally occurring bovine growth hormone to yield a marketable product that would increase milk production in cows, which it does. Sounds yummy, and I'm sure it's good for us. Monsanto says so. Of course, the FDA's assumption that rBGH is safe for humans is based upon short-term rat experiments done by Monsanto-sponsored scientists. Other independent investigators question the Monsanto data.

Not relenting to pressure, Japan, the European Union, Australia, New Zealand, and Canada all ban the use of rBGH because of concerns over the health and welfare of cows, as well as humans. In fact, in 1998 reviews by Health Canada determined the use of rBGH increases the risk of mastitis by 25 percent, affects reproductive functions, increases the risk of clinical lameness by 50 percent, and shortens the lives of cows. Monsanto then lobbied the Canadian government for rBGH approval. Dr. Margaret Hayden, a Health Canada researcher, reported to the Canadian Senate that officials from Monsanto had offered between $1 million to $2 million to Health Canada scientists, offers she said, could only be understood as an attempted bribe. (53)

Of course Monsanto, and now Eli Lilly which paid $300 million for the drug in August 2008, want their product to succeed. Monsanto spent about a half billion dollars developing the product, called Posilac. They are also intertwined with the FDA. Why else would the FDA force dairies that opt not to treat their cows with rBGH to state on their labels that "no significant difference has been shown between milk from treated and untreated cows"? What use could possibly come of this policy other than to serve financial interests? Unfortunately, state politicians aren't much better than those at the federal level. Pennsylvania, Ohio, and Indiana have had less than desirable results supporting the rBGH-free labels. In 2003, Monsanto asked the state of Maine to stop issuing an official quality seal, which the state only grants to dairies that do not use rBGH. Maine refused. Later that year, Monsanto sued Oakhurst Dairy, Maine's largest dairy operation, over its rBGH-free labels. Ultimately, Oakhurst changed its labels, adding the statement, "FDA States: No significant difference in milk from cows treated with artificial growth hormone." (54)

The states can't seem to get their act together, but some businesses that survive off of consumer decisions are in the lead. In 2007, Kroger and Safeway banned the use of rBGH-treated milk in their store-branded dairy products. In January 2008, Starbucks stopped using rBGH-treated milk, and in March 2008, WalMart banned rBGH use in their store-brand milk products. I recommend you check with your town to see if rBGH is used in the milk supply at school. Or you can pack a lunch like I do, and avoid the fiasco altogether.

If this hormone is such a good thing according to those with money and power, then why do numerous dairy farmers report extensive problems with it, and many others proudly advertise that their product is rBGH-free, or at least attempt to do so. What is it that other nations, farmers, and consumer action groups know that you don't? What is so wrong with rBGH?

Even Monsanto states in its package insert that the drug increases the risk for mastitis. Mastitis is an infection of the udder, which produces a white blood cell response, better known as pus. This infection is an indication of the health of the animal, and requires antibiotics to resolve. The journal *Nature* reported that Posilac increases somatic cells (pus) in the milk by a whopping 19 percent! Researchers estimate that an ordinary glass of milk contains between one and seven drops of pus. You get to drink pus, antibiotics, and more.

Beyond the issues rBGH causes to cows, there is no valid concern that rBGH will be passed down to the human consumer. rBGH is not directly the issue. rBGH causes cows to increase their production of a growth factor, in particular insulin-like growth factor-1. As humans, we have no receptors that can effectively recognize this rBGH protein, so it cannot do to us what it can do to a cow. IGF-1 is another story. In an amazing coincidence of nature, both the bovine IGF-1 and human IGF-1 are identical.

Pasteurization does not adequately destroy the IGF-1 protein. The acidic environment of our stomach doesn't either, since the calcium in milk decreases acidity. This is similar to the logic of drinking milk when you have an active ulcer since there is temporary relief in the acid effect. In essence, the buffering capacity of milk, the casein, and even homogenization are all incriminated in allowing these proteins to escape degradation, and move downstream into your intestines for absorption.

There are those who would argue that IGF-1 is destroyed during pasteurization and digestion, but studies have disproved this. Dr. Samuel Epstein is professor emeritus of Environmental and Occupational Medicine at the University of Illinois School of Public Health, and Chairman of the Cancer Prevention Coalition. He has published some 260 peer reviewed articles, and authored or co-authored 11 books. He has stated that rBGH injections cause substantial and sustained increases of IGF-1 levels in milk. He further states, "IGF-1 is not destroyed by pasteurization, survives digestion, and produces potent growth promoting effects." In fact, it is against the law to sell milk from a cow in the beginning of lactation due to the increase in hormones present. Why would the government impose this law, if they thought these orally ingested hormones had no impact?

Even if the milk you drink is not tainted with rBGH, it still contains levels of IGF-1 you may want to avoid. Consider the Japanese study referenced earlier, or the following data. Monsanto conducted a survey of 100 bulk tank milk samples to ascertain the naturally occurring range of IGF-1 in untreated milk. These samples would have been drawn from millions of pounds of milk in total, collected from numerous cows at various points in time, providing a reasonable number for what you might expect in milk you'd buy. They found that the average concentration was 4.32mg/ml. (55) Robert Cohen was kind enough to run some calculations for us to shed some light on what these numbers mean to the average American. When looking at milk not treated with rBGH, the amount of IGF-1 in a 12 ounce glass of milk is roughly equivalent to the amount of free (unbound) naturally occurring IGF-1 in an adult human. In other words, one glass of milk doubles the amount of IGF-1 floating around your body looking for a receptor.

The ranges seen for increases in IGF-1 in rBGH-treated cow's milk vary significantly depending on who's referenced. We'll go with one Cohen referenced, which is on the low end of quotes, at an average increase of **78%**. So, if you drink a glass of rBGH treated milk, that's another 78% above the doubling of free IGF-1 you're already receiving from untreated milk, if you're an adult. What if you're a child?

You're familiar with human growth hormone therapy. It's touted as an anti-aging remedy, and is quite pricey as well. I won't be elaborating on the pros and cons of HGH, but I will say that the effects of HGH are mediated by insulin like growth factors. There are several types of IGFs, but IGF-1 is the most potent. In fact, it's the most powerful growth hormone in the human body. As we've stated, IGF-1 from bovines is exactly the same molecule as it is in humans, containing the identical 70 amino acids in the same sequence in both species. It is the BGH induced increase in IGF-1 that has its effects on the mammary glands of the cow. So if it's identical in humans, and can be absorbed into our blood stream intact, then don't you think it can have an impact on human breast tissue?

IGF-1 receptors surely aren't limited to breast tissue; they are ubiquitous in the body.

IGF-1 on its own does not cause cancer. Cancer, as we best understand it, is the unregulated growth of tissue resulting from some insult. IGF-1 is a growth promoter. It doesn't care which tissue holds its receptor. It will plug into the receptor and initiate its cascade of growth results. Simplistically, this is seemingly all well and good if you're a competitive athlete and have no aberrant cells. However, should you have some cells replicating as they should not, then it's a bad thing.

IGF-1 has been implicated in the growth promotion of numerous cancers. The scientific community has come to learn over recent years that many of us have "cancers", just not in the way we picture them. According to the national cancer institute, more than half of all American men have some cancer in their prostate gland by the age of 80, yet only 3% will die from the disease. Most do not progress to the point of endangerment. In 1994, an article written in the *New York Times* referenced data showing that although 1 percent of women between the ages of 40 and 50 are diagnosed with breast cancer, autopsy studies within that same age group show that 39% of these women had a breast cancer. Our bodies seemingly keep in check the progression of these aberrant cells in most cases. Do you want to feed these cells with fertilizer, and chance losing that control? Pancreatic, colorectal, central nervous system, lymphomas, and other cancers have much evidence to support the IGF-1 connection. Let's take a look at some quotes from researchers.

In a research article published in 2001, researchers looked at IGF-1 status and Tamoxifen. As you may know, Tamoxifen is the most commonly used agent in the treatment of hormone responsive breast cancer. In addition to its action on the estrogen receptors, the drug also acts on IGF-1 in a positive manner, mostly by increasing the binding proteins that eat up the free hormone. (56) This researcher states in a pathology journal that, "IGF-1 is a potent growth promoter for breast cancer, increased IGF-1 concentrations have been found in breast cancer patients when compared to controls, and that it is now accepted that high concentrations of IGF-1 are a risk factor for premenopausal breast cancer." This rationale is probably partly based on the findings from the

Harvard Nurses Health Study, where in 1998 it was published that, "Premenopausal women with high IGF-1 levels in their blood had almost five times the risk of developing breast cancer than those with low IGF-1 concentrations." It is also of interest to note that the author states, "Healthy subjects with high IGF-1 concentrations when controlled for binding proteins, have been shown to have an increased risk for breast cancer." In other words, when you consider the free/unbound IGF-1 in the blood as opposed to the IGF-1 that is bound up by proteins, the risk increases. It is the unbound IGF-1, or any other hormone that is able to carry out its mission. This refers back to Robert Cohen's calculations earlier on doubling the free IGF-1 from a glass of milk in an adult.

In a review on IGF-1 and how it may promote cancer published in 2003, the author states, "Multiple large case-controlled studies in the past five years have reported positive associations between high circulating levels of IGF-1 and the risk for different types of cancer. Circulating IGF-1 may facilitate cancer development, though it likely does not cause cancer to form." (57)

In another review on IGF-1 and cancer from 2003, the authors state, "The IGF-1 receptor is commonly over-expressed in many cancers, and many recent studies have identified new signaling pathways emanating from the IGF-1 receptor that affect cancer cell proliferation, adhesion, migration, and cell death; functions that are critical for cancer cell survival and metastases (spread)." (58)

An in vitro study from 1994 on ovarian cancer suggested that their data, ". . . support a role for IGF-1 in the proliferation of ovarian cancer and suggest that IGF-1 and estradiol interact in regulating this malignancy." (59) Remember that milk contains estradiol as well.

In a 2008 trial looking at IGF-1 and its binding protein on colorectal cancer, results mimic others previously stated. The researchers measured the plasma levels of IGF-1, IGF-1 binding protein, and other parameters in 527 patients participating in a randomized trial of first-line chemotherapy for metastatic colorectal cancer. They found that higher binding proteins were associated with a significantly better chemo response rate. Remember it is the binding proteins that tie up the free

IGF-1, preventing it from freely promoting cancer growth to a large degree. (60)

Our next example comes from Canada. Testicular cancer is the most common cancer among Canadian men aged 20-45. The researchers analyzed data from 601 cases of testicular cancer and 744 healthy controls between 1994-1997 for dietary correlations. Their results suggested that a high dairy product intake, in particular a high intake of cheese, was associated with an elevated risk. (61) Depending on the cheese, it can take up to 10 pounds of milk to make one pound. All of those hormones, pesticides, and IGF-1 have been concentrated into a smaller source for your ingestion. The connection to cheese here is not unique. There are many other researchers who link the high IGF-1 in cheese to cancer.

A review article that commented on several cancers had an interesting point for your consideration. They stated that epidemiological studies consistently show a positive association with high consumption of milk, dairy products, and meats. They went on to state that these factors tend to decrease the active form of vitamin D in the body, which at low levels may enhance prostate carcinogenesis (62). Said another way, the more vitamin D you have in your body, the more likely you are to not get cancer. More support for vitamin D.

I hope you've come to understand the connection between milk, whether treated with rBGH or not, IGF-1, and the prospect of cancer promotion. Of course, the rBGH not only increases your IGF-1, but also increases the amounts of pus and bacteria you'd consume above and beyond that of an untreated cow. So far we've covered milk's impact on allergies, bone health, type 1 diabetes, and now IGF-1. I have skipped a number of other diseases linked to dairy, as we can't cover them all. We still have one more lesser known unpalatable section to cover, that of contamination.

Contamination

The number of pus cells in milk is an indicator of the health of the cow. Considering cramped quarters, artificially extended lighting, abnormal food, poor air quality, drugs to induce more milk, and a host of other conditions that render a cow useless in about 3 years, I'd say you're asking for unhealthy cows. The USDA does not allow milk containing 750 million or more white blood cells (pus) per liter to be shipped across state borders. The average number of pus cells per liter of milk in America seems to hover around 300 million+, depending on whom you reference. In an analysis of milk quality from five of the largest milk plants operating in the state of New York published in 2002, the researchers found on average 363 million cells per liter. It is interesting to note that they also found over 24 million bacteria per liter. (63) The white blood cells were present in the milk as part of the immune response to the bacteria. We won't even mention the antibiotic residue violations. Speaking of bacteria, in 2000 it was reported that dairy products were the foods most often recalled by the U.S. Food and Drug Administration (FDA) from October 1, 1993 through September 30, 1998, because of contamination with infectious agents, mostly bacteria. (64) Don't bet the farm on the pasteurization process.

Researchers at the National Mastitis Council define normal and abnormal milk based on the number of pus cells. The concentration of pus cells in normal milk is almost always less than 100 million per liter. I'm not so sure I want any. In another New York study, Consumer's Union tested milk samples in the NY metro area in 1992 and found the presence of 52 different antibiotics. Published in the *Wall Street Journal* in 1989 was more news on the contamination of our milk supply. Milk samples were taken in 10 cities, and it was found that 38% were contaminated with sulfa drugs or other antibiotics. A similar study published in the Nutrition Action Letter in 1990 found a 20% contamination rate for samples from Washington D.C.

Hormones found in cow's milk include: Estradiol (estrogen), Estriol (estrogen), progesterone, testosterone, 17-ketosteroids, corticosterone, IGF-1, growth hormone, and oxytocin, to name a few. (65) Dairy cows aren't necessarily taken "off line" when they are pregnant. So any extra hormones racing through their blood and milk may wind up in your blood.

Dioxin is a toxic deadly substance created mostly from industrial chlorination, incineration of municipal waste, and the production of certain herbicides. In fact, in 1983 the United Press International reported, "Dioxins are the most deadly substances ever assembled by man…170,000 times as deadly as cyanide…" It fits on a receptor similar to the estrogen receptor on our cells. This known carcinogen changes the metabolism of estrogen, disrupts insulin, IGF-1, and TNF, as well as activates cancer genes and deactivates tumor suppressor genes. The lipophilic (fat loving) nature of these toxins results in deposition and concentration in the fats of animals, and us. Animal sources are the number one source of dioxins for human consumption. Many of you demand certificates of analysis on your fish oils, demanding to know if it is free of toxins such as PCB and Dioxin. Are you as passionate about the meats you eat, or the milk you drink? If you're worried about the Dioxin content in a glass of milk, you should consider other milk-derived products. If it takes 21.2 pounds of milk to make one pound of butter, wouldn't you think twice about throwing it on your food? It also takes 10 pounds of milk to make one pound of hard cheese or 12 pounds of milk to make one pound of ice cream. Speaking of ice cream, a man by the name of Steve Milloy spent his own money to test for the amount of dioxins in a single serving of Ben and Jerry's World's Best Vanilla. It was found that the ice cream contained **almost 200 times more Dioxin** than the "virtually safe daily dose" determined by the EPA. The findings were reported in the *Detroit Free Press* in November of 1999. If you consider all of the hormones, drugs, and toxins in just one glass of milk, then what is the equivalent number of glasses of milk you're consuming in a day accounting for milk, cheese, butter, yogurt, and ice cream? How much is your child consuming? Pizza and milkshakes anyone?

You're familiar with Mad Cow Disease, aka (BSE). You may recall that prions are the little guys responsible for the transmission of the disease. The latest technology is now detecting these proteins in milk, whether the milk is organic or not. Pasteurization doesn't seem to solve the problem either. (66) I'd reconsider the dairy.

The Bovine leukemia virus was found in cow's milk in 1969, but since the technology of the time couldn't detect antibodies in humans, its importance was shelved. More recent technology in 2003 detected evidence of infection with bovine leukemia viruses in 74% of the people tested. It's amazing that this isn't more well known. Stunningly, it is estimated that 9 out of 10 cattle herds in the U.S. are infected, and that ¾ of people who consume dairy may show immunologic signs of infection. (67).

Let's now look at yet another impactful contaminant found in milk. Milk is involved in a controversial, yet probable connection to Crohn's disease. Cattle and other ruminants, such as sheep, goats, and deer, may contract a deadly disease called Mycobacterium avium paratuberculosis (MAP). MAP is akin to what we refer to as human tuberculosis. In animals the disease is called Johne's disease, in reference to its discoverer. The primary site of Johne's disease is the distal ileum, which is strangely the primary site for Crohn's. This invader is able to resist defenses in some way, and in fact reproduces within the GI tract, causing severe damage. As a part of the inflammation response the intestines become thickened, which prevents nutrient absorption. Explosive diarrhea and weight loss progress to an eventual death. Not only is MAP transmitted in the feces of the infected cow to its milk and other uninfected cows, but MAP is also transmitted in white blood cells. It colonizes and multiplies inside these white blood cells. Remember the National Mastitis Council defines normal milk on the number of pus (white blood) cells, and that the concentration of pus cells in normal milk is almost always less than 100 million per liter. Remember that rBGH increases mastitis, and mastitis increases white blood cells (pus) in the milk.

MAP causes Johne's disease, and the consequences of Johne's disease on animals (in this case cows) is not in dispute. The big question is: If a dairy cow is infected, can it be spread to humans and cause disease within the human GI tract? Many researchers believe it can, and I'll shed some evidence on the topic.

Let's first look at its prevalence within our dairy and beef herds. Our most recent evidence from Johnesdisease.org informs us that:

- One out of ten animals moving through a livestock auction has Johne's disease.
- The National Animal Health Monitoring Systems Study in 2007 reported that 68% of U.S. dairy operations are infected with MAP.

It also suggested that at least a quarter of U.S. dairy operations have a relatively high percentage of infected cows.

- It is estimated that 8% of beef herds are infected. (note that about half of U.S. ground meat comes from dairy cattle)

I would say that represents significant exposure to MAP for you and your children. The dairy industry doesn't seem to disagree. In fact, in 2000 they asked Congress for $1.3 billion to pay dairy farmers to cull infected cows with MAP. A spokesman for the milk producers said the program's aim is to reduce the levels of infection of the "mysterious" (my quotes) bacterium called MAP. MAP at the time had been found in one or more cows involving 22% of the U.S. dairy herd. This information comes to us courtesy of Lance Gay from the Scripps Howard News Service.

Now go back and look at the numbers in the last two paragraphs. In 2000, an estimated 22% of U.S. dairy herds were infected. The most recent data from Johnesdisease.org suggests that 68% of U.S. dairy herds are now infected. That is in line with other predictions. In 1996 the USDA estimated between 20-40% of dairy herds were infected with MAP, and the folks at crohn's.org expected significantly higher numbers in the years to come. I'd say that's significant growth. Do you think the dairy farmers and the U.S. government have a good handle on the situation?

This same dairy spokesperson, Christopher Galen states, "This is an animal health issue." He's the one who also stated that MAP is a "mysterious" bacteria. It was first discovered in 1905 by the german bacteriologist and veterinarian, Heinrich Johne (pronounced "Yo-nee"). I'm pretty sure I'm not willing to believe a spokesperson for the dairy industry. I'm pretty sure he's downplaying the dangers to you and your family because he doesn't want the country to stop consuming dairy.

We pasteurize our milk, so shouldn't that kill it? Pasteurization is what the dairy industry is hanging its hat on. The merits, or lack thereof, of pasteurization will not be a part of this book. We do pasteurize our milk, and we are told that MAP does not survive this process. This is where the debate lies. Of course there are numerous analyses that show MAP does survive the process.

The first evidence that MAP may survive pasteurization came in 1993. Then, in 1998, the University of Wisconsin found that MAP was able to survive the process. Since then a slew of research has shown the same. Some of the research uses varying methodology, and that's where those who have a vested interest in you buying milk make their stand. I won't get into the details of variations of techniques used by the labs. For the sake of argument, we'll agree there was variation in methodology. Also for the sake of argument, we'll say that if it's possible to find live MAP bacteria in pasteurized milk for sale to the public, then it's reasonable to agree with the researchers that MAP can and does survive pasteurization.

In 2002, British researchers published their works on exactly that. Over a 17 month period, they took 814 milk samples from 241 approved dairy processing establishments throughout the United Kingdom. They tested for MAP, and to see if they could culture living MAP as well. They were able to culture living MAP from 3.3% of the dairy processors in pasteurized milk. (68) They (the British) use the same commercial pasteurization processes as we use here in the states. It's simply a well known fact among these researchers that MAP is far more resistant to heat than are the bacteria that pasteurization is designed to kill.

How about an example closer to home? The following comes to us from a press release generated by the Paratuberculosis Awareness and Research Association, Inc. (PARA). In August 2004, Dr. Jay Ellingson of Marshfield Clinic Laboratories presented his findings at the International Association for Food Protection meeting in Phoenix. His team had tested 702 samples of milk from retail grocery stores in California, Minnesota, and Wisconsin. They found that 2.8% of the samples contained MAP that was alive and capable of multiplying. This number is eerily similar to the 3.3% from the U.K. The consensus seems to be that pasteurization does significantly reduce the quantity of living MAP, but does not eliminate it completely. If you're calculating your risk at only 3%, then consider how many separate milk products you buy in the course of a year. If it's 33 or more, then your odds are effectively 100%.

Whether or not MAP will survive and thrive in your body is another issue, as all people who drink milk do not have Crohn's. Now that we know MAP survives pasteurization, the question begs, "Can it successfully inhabit the human body and cause disease?" In research conducted at St. George's Hospital medical school in London, professor John Herman-Taylor found that over 90% of the Crohn's patients taking part in the study were infected with MAP. The professor went on the say, "Careful research in our own laboratories and others in the U.S. and elsewhere shows unequivocally that when the tests are done correctly almost everyone with Crohn's disease is found to be infected with MAP."

In a comprehensive review of 49 studies, researchers looked at the detection of MAP in patients with Crohn's, and in control subjects who were uninfected. As this was published in 2008, the latest understandings of MAP detection were utilized to consider the data. The researchers found sufficient evidence for the presence of MAP in the gut of patients with Crohn's. This remained consistent across many sites, many investigators, and when controlling for a number of variables. (69)

A review published about a year earlier came to the same conclusion. They analyzed 28 case-controlled studies comparing MAP in patients with Crohn's to those free of Crohn's. They showed that positive tests for MAP are substantially more common in Crohn's disease as compared to others. (70)

The piece not completely proven is whether MAP is directly responsible for Crohn's disease. In my opinion, there are a number of factors that can result in the disease we call Crohn's. Given that MAP is found in these patients with so much more frequency than in controls, and given that drugs specifically geared to kill this very specific pathogen can have such marked results, it is certainly reasonable to make the claim that MAP is either directly or indirectly the cause of Crohn's or Crohn's-like symptoms in a significant percent of the population diagnosed with Crohn's.

If it were not a concern, then why would the Food Safety Authority in Ireland adopt the following measures in 1998 to remove MAP from the food chain?

- Animals diagnosed with Johne's disease must be removed from the food chain.
- From the time an animal is diagnosed with Johne's disease until it is culled, milk will not be used (pasteurized or raw) for humans or calves.

If MAP were not the issue that the dairy people want us to think, then why is it that in April of 2007 the FDA approved the investigational new drug application (IND) for the development of a product called Myoconda to treat patients with Crohn's disease infected by MAP. The drug is a combination of three previously registered anti-mycobacterial drugs, which have shown promise by visionary practitioners. The company, Giaconda Ltd goes on to state that MAP is considered the most likely infectious cause of Crohn's disease, and that current research indicates that between 40-50% of Crohn's patients are MAP positive. If MAP couldn't survive pasteurization, and if it couldn't colonize the human GI tract and cause disease, then do you think a pharmaceutical company would spend millions on bringing a FDA-approved investigational drug to market that kills a pathogen that doesn't exist? Do you really believe the dairy people?

What the Experts Have to Say

If you don't want to trust me, or the many researchers I have quoted, then maybe you'll recognize some of the following names. Perhaps you may even heed their advice. Educate yourself. The evidence against milk is overwhelming. Don't listen to the lemmings in the medical community who tell you to drink milk for calcium. These people are not "in the know". They are regurgitating information from biased sources. Have they done their own independent research? Do they look healthy to you?

Dr. Benjamin Spock – He spoke out against feeding cow's milk to children, saying that "it could cause anemia, allergies, and insulin-dependent diabetes, and in the long term will set kids up for obesity and heart disease. Do you remember the study looking at the carotid and coronary arteries of children in the chapter on food choices, and how it was shown that more than half had clogged arteries, as much as someone about 30 years older? Do you think all this dairy we shove down their throats has anything to do with it?

The American Academy of Pediatrics – They recommend that infants under one year of age do not receive whole cows milk. Certainly they could have improved upon these weak guidelines, but it's something. Data shows that these poor infants are at the greatest risk for milk induced deficiencies in iron, fatty acids, and vitamin E. Milk has been shown to cause blood loss from the intestinal tract, which over time can cause a reduction in overall iron. One set of researchers from the University of Iowa stated in the *Journal of Pediatrics* that "in a large proportion of infants, the feeding of cow's milk causes a substantial increase in hemoglobin loss. This blood loss is likely the result of the allergic reaction to the casein protein."

Walter Willet, PhD – Dr. Willet is the chair of the Harvard School of Public Health's nutrition department. Based on the latest research, he states that Americans are getting more calcium than they need. It is his opinion that 600mg of calcium a day is probably enough for most people to keep their fracture risk low. He also states that there may be real drawbacks to overdoing calcium, especially if dairy foods are the source. He points out studies linking dairy products to ovarian and prostate cancer.

Dr. Neal Barnard – Dr. Barnard is the author of *Food for Life* and was director of the Physicians Committee for Responsible Medicine. He states that the consumption of cow's milk is totally inappropriate for humans, and that the scientific literature is filled with evidence of the inadequacy of cow's milk for human nutrition, which it is. He states in a 1995 news release, "There is no nutritional requirement for dairy products, and there are serious problems that can result from the proteins, sugar, fat, and contaminants in milk."

Dr. Frank Oski – Author of *Don't Drink Your Milk,* the former physician-in-chief of John Hopkins Children's Center, and Professor and Chairman of the Department of Pediatrics at John Hopkins University School of Medicine had this to say about milk: "Why give it at all–then (referring to infant use) – or ever? In the face of uncertainty about many of the potential dangers of whole bovine milk, it would seem prudent to recommend that whole milk not be started until the answers are available. Isn't it time for these uncontrolled experiments on human nutrition to come to an end?"

Dr. Christiane Northurp – Author of *Women's Bodies Women's Wisdom* quotes other health problems associated with the consumption of dairy foods to include conditions of the breast, recurrent vaginitis, acne, menstrual cramps, fibroids, chronic intestinal upset, and increased pain from endometriosis.

Harvey Diamond – Author of the *Fit For Life* series of books, Harvey spends a great deal of time trying to convince you not to consume milk, assuming you have an interest in good health. Some of his quotes are as follows. "There is 300 percent more casein in cow's milk than human milk. The by-products of the bacterial decomposition of casein end up in thick, rope-like mucus that sticks to mucus membranes and clogs our bodies." "Dairy products are the leading cause of allergies." "The list of ailments that can be linked to dairy products is so extensive there is hardly a problem it at least doesn't contribute to."

Dr. John McDougall – Dr. McDougall has authored several books on health and nutrition, and has an informative website at **drmcdougall.com**. He states in his February 2007 newsletter, "Even in the face of solid scientific evidence to the contrary, because in part of the annual $206.5 million advertising campaign of the dairy industry, mothers, doctors, and government officials have bought the dairy industry's propaganda about calcium. Misleading marketing might be forgiven if the only consequences were wasted money and efforts; but the costs deepen. The result of selling dairy foods to correct a problem that does not exist – calcium deficiency- is that consumers buy foods that actually make them sick."

Dr. Robert Kradjian – The former chief of breast surgery at Seton Medical Center states, "So don't drink milk for health. I am convinced on the weight of scientific evidence that it does not 'do a body good.' Inclusion of milk will only reduce your diet's nutritional value and safety."

Dr. John Postley – Author of *The Allergy Discovery Diet* calls milk "one of the most common causes of food sensitivities." He recommends avoiding milk products.

Hippocrates – The 'father of medicine' and the man who brought us the Hippocratic oath of ethics still in use today, suspected that the white stuff is the commonest cause of childhood allergies.

If you *must* drink milk, then get it locally, and raw from a clean goat, and consume it in moderation. A local animal given no extra drugs, given land to roam, fresh air, the appropriate food, humane care, and no pasteurization will produce much healthier milk than you can find in any store. This is compared to the unfortunate commercial dairy cows, which are drugged up and burnt out so badly that they produce about 10 times what they would naturally, and are culled in about three years, a fraction of their milking life. Guess where the meat from those sick cows winds up? Fast food burgers anyone? However, ensuring that your animal is clean is not done easily. I had called around to government agencies and labs, and couldn't even find someone to send a sample to. Since this process is impractical for most, just avoid dairy altogether.

Chapter 9   Iron

You're probably thinking I'm going to rave about the benefits of iron, and express concern in regards to anemia. I will grant you the obvious importance that iron plays in our health, but it can come at a cost. Let's understand iron in its many facets to better enable you to make the best decisions for you and your loved ones. Like most other things, moderation and proper usage are key.

When you think iron, most associate it with anemia. Anemia is a condition whereby the blood is low in red blood cells or low in the iron containing hemoglobin portion of the red blood cells. There are three types of anemia. One can become anemic from excessive blood loss. Trauma is obvious, but conditions that perpetuate internal bleeding such as IBD or NSAID use can make one anemic. Anemia can arise from excessive red blood cell destruction, as you would associate with sickle-cell anemia. The third and most common mechanism for anemia is deficient red blood cell production. The most common cause of this type is a nutritional deficiency.

There are three possible nutrient deficiencies that can cause anemia; folic acid, vitamin B12, and iron deficiency can all lead to anemia. Folate and vitamin B12 create what's called a macrocytic anemia since the red blood cells become quite large, while an iron deficient anemia is microcytic in nature. Vitamin B12 is derived from animal sources although some foods are fortified. Those at risk are vegans, those with low gastric acid, patients with IBD, and those genetically lacking intrinsic factor. If unresolved, a vitamin B12 deficiency can result in serious disturbances within the nervous system.

Folic acid deficiency is the most common vitamin deficiency in the world. The amount of folic acid stored in the body is sufficient to sustain itself for only one or two months (1). Those at higher risk of suffering from a folate deficiency are alcoholics, IBD patients, and pregnant women and the fetus. You will sometimes see highly dosed supplements with just vitamin B12 and folic acid, so both possible deficiencies may be addressed, while also not having the folate mask a B12 deficiency. In other words, supplementation with just folic acid will correct the anemia of a vitamin B12 deficiency, but it will not resolve the B12 deficiency itself, which can result in nervous system damage (2). In essence, it can mask the need for B12.

We last come to iron deficiency anemia, which is the most common type. Iron not only plays a role in the transport of extracellular and intracellular oxygen, but is also critical in other aspects of growth, enzyme function, and cell differentiation. The fatigue associated with iron deficiency anemia (IDA) is a recognizable symptom of an ongoing deficiency.

Almost two-thirds of the body's iron is found in the hemoglobin, with smaller amounts found in the myoglobin (muscle oxygen transport), and enzymes. Iron is primarily stored as ferritin, and is transported in the blood by the protein transferrin. Levels of ferritin may rise or fall depending on your state of health. Iron that is not bound in some way, shape, or form is referred to as free iron. As with calcium, the body regulates iron absorption based on need. There are two types of iron that can be derived from the diet, heme and non-heme. Non-heme iron comes from plants. Heme iron comes from animal sources, and is much easier to absorb. Depending on whom you reference, heme iron ranges anywhere from 2-35 times more absorbable with many estimates in the 3-10 times range. The best sources of heme iron are chicken liver, oysters, beef liver, beef, other mollusks, and sardines. The capacity and efficiency of iron absorption depends on your iron stores, the rate of blood cell production, and dietary components, such as amount and type of iron, inhibitors, and enhancers.

Those at highest risk for IDA are infants, those with low stomach hydrochloric acid (HCL), vegetarians, teenage girls, and pregnant women. Infants and pregnant women need adequate iron for the intense growth processes in place. Teenage girls are also growing quickly, with a complicating factor as well, that of menstruation. Vegetarians who do not eat any animal products other than milk are also at risk. Those who have low stomach HCL include patients on antacids, PPIs, and H2 blockers, as well as the elderly. Like with vitamin B12 and calcium, iron needs adequate HCL secretion for absorption.

With all of the aforementioned information listed, we need to put some things into perspective and arm ourselves with some data. Let's consider infants first. Healthy full term infants are born with a supply of iron that lasts 4-6 months. Given that information, there isn't even an RDA for infants 0-6 months of age. Beyond that, the iron in human breast milk is well absorbed. The American Academy of Pediatrics serves us well in recommending that breast milk be the exclusive food in the first six months of life. This is in part based on extensive data showing that cow's milk can cause intestinal bleeding in infants resulting in an iron deficiency at a time when growth is most important.

For infants beyond 6 months and prior to the introduction of heme iron foods, the data is mixed. One study found that infants who received breast milk exclusively for 9 months required an additional source of iron to not be deficient (3). Another trial tells us that infants breastfed exclusively for greater than 7 months were protected against iron deficiency, and exclusive breast-feeding for long periods was predictive of good iron status at 12 and 24 months (4). In yet another small study, infants who were exclusively fed breast milk for 8 or more months had normal hemoglobin and other iron measures when tested at ages 9-12 months. (5) Given wide variables in the composition of the mother's breast milk as a function of her diet, breast-feeding mothers may want to consider their iron intake. Possible internal bleeding may be caused by cow's milk, especially at early ages. The introduction of cereals may contribute to other GI issues, and their fortification with iron may be pro-oxidative, as you will soon see. Beyond this, cereal is not a food with which we evolved, and thus may cause digestive disturbances in the very young. For older children who are exposed to a varied diet, there are plenty of excellent sources of absorbable iron available in the American diet.

When you hear statistics from the World Health Organization (WHO) stating that iron deficiency is the number one nutritional disorder in the world and that 30% may have iron deficiency anemia, it makes you want to run out and buy iron supplements (6). But wait. We are not the rest of the world. Many other parts of the world do not have the access to animal proteins we do; many barely survive on a few staple items with minimal iron and absorption, and many suffer from parasites that cause internal bleeding.

If we return to our list of those at risk, we find it contains vegetarians, children, women of child-bearing age, and those with a compromised HCL output. In each of these cases, natural medicine, good food choices, and/or common sense offer up solutions. The vegetarian/omnivore debate is a high pitched and emotional debate, which we'll visit in the chapter on our ideal diet. Suffice it to say, although I like much of what vegetarianism brings to the table, I do not endorse the exclusion of all animal food sources. Children especially should have ready access to animal foods for their growing bodies. It's not until we get older that we need to modify our protein intake.

The Institute of Medicine informs us that vegetarians who exclude all animal products from their diet may need almost twice as much dietary iron each day as compared to non-vegetarians because of the lowest absorption rate for non-heme iron. It is true that vegetarians typically consume more fresh fruits that contain vitamin C to help with absorption, but they also consume more food constituents that bind up the iron which inhibits absorption.

People who have compromised HCL output are typically the elderly and those on drugs to treat heartburn or GERD. A provider in integrative medicine can help those on drugs to find the underlying cause of the disease and improve digestion. I know it sounds contradictory, but those with GERD usually have too little HCL, not too much. This is borne out by numerous success stories in natural medicine in treating these patients. Renowned integrative medicine practitioner Jonathan Wright explains in his article, "How to Accelerate Aging," that, "Since 1976, I've checked literally thousands of individuals complaining of heartburn and indigestion for stomach acid production using a commercially available, extremely precise, research-verified procedure. Over-acidity is almost never found, especially in those over age 35. The usual findings are under-acidity or normal acidity." The elderly are subject to the same diminishing of organ function we will all come to experience, although the function is in part a manner of how you live. Supplemental HCL is certainly one option that natural medicine brings to the table for these folks. In the end, much of your iron status is dependent on the foods you eat, and especially absorb. However, the goal is not to always have a high iron status either.

Just as children should eat protein, and women of child-bearing age should eat iron containing foods, adult men and post-menopausal women should rethink their iron and protein intakes. Supplemental iron should play little to no role for these two groups, if they are otherwise healthy. There is too much evidence to back this up. If you don't want to take my word for it, then take someone's you may trust. In a CNN piece by Elizabeth Cohen, four prominent figures in health were asked about what supplements they should take. Andrew Weil said that "men should not take iron unless they'd been diagnosed by a physician as having an iron deficiency anemia."

Why? Because iron is a double-edged sword and the body realizes this. In healthy people, iron is of little concern, but in cases of inflammation, excess iron causes oxidative damage. This is well underscored by the fact that oral iron supplementation causes flare-ups in those with rheumatoid arthritis. The body realizes the importance of controlling iron and has several mechanisms in place to do so. Albumin, ferritin, transferrin, digestive mechanisms, and lactoferrin all play a role in the management of iron.

It has been well proven that iron can be dangerous, and that it catalyzes oxidation. In other words, it provides the spark to light the fire. We know that iron helps to create the very potent and unstable superoxide and hydroxyl radicals. This isn't always a bad thing. Our immune system will produce the superoxide radical as a part of its anti-pathogenic defenses. It's kind of like the mobilized white blood cells are the soldier and the free radicals are the bullets shot at the enemy. As such, states of infection and inflammation produce the superoxide radical. As iron is not a problem in a healthy state, in conditions of inflammation, free radicals can fuel the fire by freeing up iron from its sequestered storage sites, ferritin. Whether your condition is cancer, rheumatoid arthritis, heart disease, or the common cold, we don't want too much iron released from an overabundance of free radicals.

In the case of the even more unstable hydroxyl radical, extensive oxidative damage may ensue. It can inactivate enzymes, causes DNA strands to break, and oxidize lipids. (7) It is estimated that a single initiated event, such as that of lipid oxidation, may create a chain of 10 to 15 other events before it is stopped, likely by vitamin E. So if you have a cell membrane, and that cell membrane is composed of numerous fatty acids, and this hydroxyl radical comes along, it and other free radicals can cause enough damage to oxidize the fatty acids in the membrane to such a degree that the cellular membrane fails. Since all the cells in our body possess a lipid membrane, this tissue destruction can occur anywhere.

Great indicators of the potential toxicity of iron are the proteins lactoferrin and ferritin. When the body is challenged during inflammation and/or infection, lactoferrin and ferritin will bind up more free iron from circulation in an attempt to control the situation. It can be confusing to practitioners because high ferritin numbers are usually associated with high iron stores, but can also signal disease. One example of this is from a trial that involved 1,675 adolescents when measured for serum ferritin in conjunction with or without an upper respiratory infection. The researchers found that there were significant differences in serum ferritin (bound iron) between the children who had a current or recent infection when compared to those who did not. (8) In other words, the kids who were sick, or recently sick, had an immune response which bound up more iron than normal to prevent the pathogen from getting a hold of it for its own use.

In a similar manner, a patient may have what's referred to as anemia of chronic disease. In this instance the disease has lasted for so long and is of such significant inflammation that the ferritin and lactoferrin are holding onto iron so well that transferrin capacity is significantly reduced. What happens is an ultimate decline in red blood cell production and its consequent "anemia" because of the combination of increased storage and sequestration of iron from ferritin and lactoferrin. Both overpower the ability of the reduced transferrin to transport iron to produce new red blood cells. This is amazing if you really think about it. The body recognizes how damaging free iron can be in disease, as it hides and holds onto iron so well, that it actually causes a deficiency in the body leading to anemia. Labs will often show a reduced serum iron level. A provider may make the mistake of recommending iron supplements but that will not help you fight your cancer or what have you. The supplements will be undoing what your body has worked so hard to achieve.

In a healthy state, the stored iron in the ferritin is not as much of a concern as it is in the inflamed person. It is the inevitable pathogen or other trigger, which can cause the release of iron. Pathogens battle with our body over access to iron in a war for resources. Iron is essential in their development, and evolution has helped us to cope with that need. We will sequester iron through various means, such as lactoferrin, transferrin, and ferritin. We will produce more lactoferrin and ferritin in inflammation, and transferrin will fill up more of its empty sites and bind up more free iron. But pathogens have ways of freeing up bound iron for their use. Although our defenses make the amount of iron available extremely low, the amount needed by pathogens is also exceedingly small. In instances such as a transfusion, where excess iron is dumped into the body, the conditions are ripe for pathogens and oxidative damage.

Another indicator of how toxic iron is to the body is overdose and death in children. Death has occurred from ingesting a dose as low as 200mg of iron, which is only about 20 times the RDA for children. I know of no other vitamin or mineral that has that effect at that dose. Symptoms of iron overload in adults are joint pain (particularly of the hip), abdominal pain, bronze skin, elevated liver enzymes, hair loss, frequent infections, and heart flutters. About a quarter of the time there are no overt symptoms at all.

One study took a look at the connection of the known GI side effects from oral non-heme iron therapy as it related to IBD. Based on other clinical observations that suggested iron exacerbates IBD in humans, these researchers induced colitis in rats and then administered iron therapy. They found that the iron induced intestinal inflammation, lipid peroxidation, and activation of pro-inflammatory cytokine pathways. (9) Not things you want in IBD. They postulated that since non-heme iron is not well absorbed, a significant amount makes its way to the lower GI, where the over-expressed immune system feeds off the iron producing potent free radicals. In the event you have IBD, and through that IBD you develop anemia, then taking supplements is not likely to be your best recourse. Simply upping your heme iron ingestion by eating any animal liver or other animal product will do the trick. The heme iron is absorbed much more quickly and further up the GI tract so as not to negatively impact the IBD as much. Another consideration for IBD, intestinal upset, or colon cancer is the iron content of your drinking water.

Have you ever wondered why women live longer than men on average? Men engage in riskier professions, drink more, seek less medical advice, and even drive faster, but that doesn't explain everything. One key factor, if not the leading factor, is the presence of iron. Iron is a pro-oxidant, and many researchers feel that aging is primarily due to the oxidation of the body. Women have a protective mechanism in place for much of their life known as menstruation. It is this concept that is at the core of this research.

Have you ever wondered why kids are giants these days compared to their size 50 years ago or more? One reason is that we started fortifying our foods with iron back in 1940. If you recall, iron is a growth promoter. That's why Scandinavians are larger people than the Vietnamese. It's not all iron, it's protein too, but what's in protein? Iron. Today we have other wonderful attributes to our food as well, which include hormones such as IGF-1. The Swedes caught onto this iron connection risk and stopped in 1995, after 47 years of fortification.

You may be familiar with the condition known as hemochromatosis. Hemochromatosis is a genetic iron overload condition that affects about 1 in 250 individuals of northern European descent. This disease is typically not diagnosed until excess iron stores have damaged an organ. It is very interesting to note the damage that can occur in untreated hemochromatosis. Cancer of the liver, damage to the heart, and arthritis are just three of several. These conditions line up closely with diseases that are present in our aging population. Given this link to high iron stores regardless of a hemochromatosis diagnosis, we'll investigate the connections. When detected, these patients are treated by drawing blood at regular intervals to keep down the iron levels. The goal of this chapter is to intelligently manage your iron level, dependent on your age and gender. This certainly applies to those with hemochromatosis, but does not imply that there is no concern for anyone else. Again, men and postmenopausal women should take particular note of this chapter.

CVD

It is estimated that excess iron accumulates in the blood at the rate of about 1 mg per day after full growth is achieved. (10) This accumulation varies, depending on diet, gender, and age, and is up for debate. For women who menstruate, iron losses help to compensate for iron gains, which keeps their circulating iron about half that of men. For men, there is no outlet for excess iron. Furthermore, some research shows that men's iron levels at age 45 are about equal to those of 70-year-old women, who on average have not had menses for 30 years. At age 45 men have a heart attack rate four times that of females while they also have four times the stored iron (11).

If we are to assume that one aspect of inflammation is the oxidation of LDL at the vascular endothelium, and this oxidized LDL plays a role in CVD, then we must consider the connection to pro-inflammatory iron. LDL by itself is only weakly atherogenic, but when it's oxidized it becomes strongly atherogenic. This oxidized LDL then attracts white blood cells and a series of events commences, which results in a plaque lesion on the endothelium. We know atherosclerotic lesions are rich in iron, and chelation therapy helps with atherosclerosis. LDL becomes oxidized in the presence of free radicals and in the absence of antioxidants. Your serum antioxidants can be dramatically reduced by continually eating oxidized fatty acids, such as deep-fried French fries. Free radicals, such as hydroxyl and superoxide, can be kicked off by inflammation. These combined with high iron levels and any other risks such as smoking and high cholesterol set you up for problems.

The impact of excess iron on CVD is not without debate, much like everything else in this book. However, there is sufficient evidence to suggest that iron promotes free radical production and tissue damage akin to rusting. These free radicals may oxidize cholesterol and inflame arteries, among other things. There are more studies than those I'll reference within this chapter, but these will give you a good flavor of the literature that is supportive of this iron theory.

In an Italian study known as the "Bruneck Study," serum ferritin concentrations were compared to the progression of carotid atherosclerosis over five years. They found that serum ferritin was one of the strongest predictors of atherosclerosis progression, and that this was particularly true for those with high LDL. (12) More specifically, they found that those who were iron deficient had a lower risk regardless of age, gender, or menopausal status. Those with a high iron burden constituted a higher risk for all, especially for high LDL, but also for low LDL status. This is in support of their theory that excess freed iron exerts its pro-oxidant effects on cholesterol, thus contributing to atherosclerosis. In addition, it supports the theory that women have a degree of protection conferred by menstruation, which can be lost in the years following menopause.

Whether we're researching iron and CVD, cancer, or another disease state, study protocols must take into consideration the fact that basic iron measurement parameters can be impacted in states of inflammation. In other words, if you're analyzing a bunch of patients in a study looking for differences in iron stores and disease incidence, it's important to know which of your patients may also have an infection, cancer, or liver disease. So when looking at transferrin, serum free iron, or even ferritin, all are proposed to potentially have errors since states of inflammation can alter these markers. This may in part explain why some of the trials support the iron hypothesis, and some do not.

Taking this into consideration, researchers looked at a subset of subjects from a previous trial who went on to have heart attacks. They compared the 99 men who had a heart attack during follow-up, which was on average 6.4 years, to 98 controls. This time they analyzed the transferrin receptor to ferritin ratio. Why and what's this? The transferrin receptor has been shown in other studies to be more indicative of iron needs in the body, while being independent of inflammation. So as the body needs more iron to make red blood cells, it produces more of this receptor to pick up iron for delivery to where it's needed. It makes sense given how the body works with negative feedback loops. So for this study, the higher your transferrin ratio, the more you need iron, and the lower the ratio the more likely your body has determined it has enough iron on hand. So what did these researchers find? They found that men in the lowest third (those who have plenty of iron) had three times the risk of a heart attack, while those in the middle third had twice the risk, both as compared to those in the upper third who had the highest ratio, or need for iron (13).

Another set of researchers took a look at women's risk for heart disease in relation to a hysterectomy, with preserved ovarian function. In this study, all of the hysterectomies were performed in these women before the age of 45. The average age of menopause is 51. Among the 112 women examined, there were five cases of confirmed coronary heart disease, which were defined as a heart attack or angina (14). When these statistics were compared to age-matched women from the Framingham Study without a hysterectomy, they found that those with a hysterectomy had five times the risk. Given that they still had ovarian function, which means they could still make estrogen, the results seem to point to factors directly attributable to the uterus itself. It is the loss of this regular shedding of iron from the body that is theorized to increase the risk of diseases attributable to iron's oxidative capacity, which is well established.

In a very similar study looking at the risk of developing heart disease, 369 hysterectomized women were evaluated according to the Framingham study criteria. At four years out, 25 were found to have coronary heart disease. The researchers calculated an increased risk of 3.3 times. (15)

Years later, the Framingham Study decided to look into this matter, since everyone seemed to be comparing results to their data. They looked at 2,873 women and found data to confirm the previous two studies. In fully intact women aged 45-54 who were pre-menopausal, not one heart related death was observed. In hysterectomized women of the same age group there were 10 such events observed. (16) They determined that the risk of new-onset coronary heart disease was 2.7 times that of non-hysterectomized women, and that this risk was the same regardless of whether ovaries were removed or not during the procedure. If you were to consider other possible risk factors for these women you might think that there was some habit or condition that predisposed them to ill-health and the need for their surgery. The Framingham researchers analyzed the data and found that this increase in risk was not attributable to estrogen use, smoking, cholesterol, blood pressure, and body weight. It is interesting to note the consistency in these studies that estrogen is seemingly not as protective as once thought, although it is to some degree, so long as it is not synthetic, as more recent studies have shown.

To even better understand the relationship between iron and health, we look to the extreme example of hereditary hemochromatosis (HH). The occurrence of HH in the population is only about 4 per thousand in those of European descent. They suffer from issues of iron absorption and storage, thus causing organ damage particularly to the liver, but also including the heart, joints, and pancreas. The increased risk in diseases sounds a lot like the diseases we discuss here for iron overload, which include diseases of the heart, arthritis, liver, and cancers, particularly that of the liver. There are two genes associated with HH, one is the HFE C282Y and the other is the HFE H63D. Should you inherit the mutation from either parent in one of those genes then you are what is referred to as a heterozygote. In this case you do not have HH, but you possess a single mutation that may increase your risk. Should you have both copies from your mom and dad, flawed in either of those two genes, then you have HH. To make matters even more complicated, if you have heterozygosity for both the 282 and 63, then that risk is high, which about equals the risk of having homozygosity for one. So why do I mention this genetic science babble, especially considering how rare HH is? It is true that HH is relatively rare, but people don't usually know it until damage has already occurred. Second, having just one mutation is not so rare, which puts you into the single heterozygosity group, a risk that runs at about 4% of the population (17). Third, this gives us an excellent model to consider iron overload in a unique population that may be a decade ahead of the rest of us in terms of iron deposition. So let's look at an interesting study.

Researchers in the Netherlands looked at 12,239 women aged 51-69, who they followed for an average of about 17 years. In this large group of subjects, they identified those who had a single HFE C282Y mutation. These women do not have HH, but do have a single mutation. They compared the mortality rates of the 282 heterozygotes to those without the mutation, and found some startling results. For the 282 group, the increased risk of death from heart attack was 1.5 times, and the increased risk in death from stroke was 2.4 times. (18) The most remarkable finding came when they looked at smoking and hypertension. They found that women who were smokers, who also had hypertension, and who were also heterozygous for 282 had almost 19 times the risk of death from CVD than those who had none of the three. Well, you could say that the smoking and hypertension must have accounted for most of that risk, right? Wrong. When they cut the data for women who were both smokers and hypertensive, but did not have the mutated gene, their risk was only 2 times that of women who had none of the three components. This is some really fascinating data. It not only provides more evidence of risk from iron overload, but also shows that an additional insult, in this case smoking, in some way accelerates the destructive processes.

These findings were supported by the Finns in a study looking at the same 282 gene, but this time in men. They found these heterozygous men to have a 2.3 fold increased risk for an acute heart attack as compared to controls. (19) It is of interest to note that most heterozygotes have stored iron well within what is considered to be the normal range. Another researcher found that heterozygotes had serum ferritin levels higher than normal in only 20% of the men, and 8% of the women. (20) This data actually serves to support the notion that the detrimental effects of iron are more closely linked to duration of exposure than to level of ferritin. One could reasonably assume that these heterozygotes attained a maximal iron plateau earlier in life than their counterparts.

Cancer

A recent trial found a strong link between cancer and iron stores in the body. Once again the thesis was that increased free radical induced oxidative damage initiated by the pro-oxidant iron would increase one's risk of cancer. Support for this arises from numerous trials looking at a wide variety of factors influencing body iron stores. In this trial, 1,277 patients were divided into two groups, one to donate blood every six months and one control group. After an average follow-up of 4.5 years, they found some interesting results. First, the phlebotomy group had a 37% reduction in their risk in overall cancer incidence. Beyond this note, for those who developed cancer within the blood donor group, it was found that they were less compliant with the study protocol, which means they donated less blood than those who did not get cancer. Another interesting finding was when all patients were examined, regardless of donation status, average ferritin levels were lower among all patients who did not develop cancer (76.4 ng/ml) as compared to all patients who did develop cancer (127.1 ng/ml). As one would expect, the average ferritin levels in the donor group plummeted as donations were given over the years. The researchers stated, "This study supports the hypothesis that levels of body iron stores represented by the serum ferritin level are associated with cancer risk and that lowering iron levels reduces cancer risk." (21) The question as to whether ferritin levels are a reliable guide to the estimation of disease risk seems to have been supported here.

Considering that colon cancer is touted as being highly linked to both iron consumption and stores, researchers took a look at these factors in 264 men and 98 postmenopausal women. They used ferritin levels as their marker for iron storage, and split the subjects up into quintiles (fifths) in order from lowest ferritin to highest. Colonoscopy and histology results were either normal, adenoma (think precancerous), or cancer of the colon. They found that adenoma risk for the third quintile was 3.8 times that of the first quintile, which is the group with the least amount of stored iron. In the fourth quintile the risk of adenoma was 5 times that of those in the first (22). It was interesting to note that when they controlled for all risk factors, the risk of adenoma in these groups was greater from iron than it was from smoking or even family history. Curiously, there was no significant difference between the fifth and first.

Animal data, in vitro data, and other human data suggest that there is a connection between iron and cancer. Among human studies, one study found that women with low iron defined as high iron binding capacity, had less than half the risk of lung cancer (23). Yet another looked at iron status and lung cancer and found that patients with lower ferritin levels had longer survival times (24). Yet another looked at cancer in men and found that those with markers that showed less body iron had a lower cancer rate than those with the highest levels (25). They went on to state, "These results are consistent with the hypothesis that high body iron stores increase the risk of cancer in men." Certainly we're not excluding women, as you've already seen they are not immune either, just at risk at a later age. For women I find it interesting to note that it has been shown that *breast cancer cells have 5-15 times more transferrin receptors than normal breast tissue.* (26) This makes perfect sense. The transferrin brings iron from point A to point B in the body. In cancer, which is an inflammatory condition, the body will cut down on the transfer of iron and free iron, and will store it away. A cancer cell will need more of these receptors to steal the reduced available iron from other normal cells, which also need it. This is why several iron chelating compounds have been shown to be beneficial in the treatment of cancer.

This next study is a bit of a stretch, but still yields some interesting data. Cancer incidence from blood transfusions has been studied several times now. There are several possible mechanisms behind cancer incidence and transfusion. There could be viral hepatitis, another carcinogenic transmissible agent, or excess iron. Many of these risks were much higher in years past, before the current stringent guidelines were enacted. The results vary according to the donor and time frame. For example, if your theory is that excess free iron from destroyed hemoglobin will cause a sudden influx to feed cancer cells then you should construct your trial to look for that. You will not see those results if the subjects received a transfusion as an infant, or even a pre-menopausal woman. You will also miss those results if you look at cancer incidence years after the transfusion. The cancer connection lies in a sudden burst of fuel for a cancer that is otherwise under control. Take prostate cancer, for example. Upon autopsy, most men have prostate cancer, but it has been controlled by the body so as not to become malignant. Should you compromise the system in place by providing fuel to the fire, you may get unwanted results. The time frame for analysis would have to be in the short run, as the body would cope with the excess iron over time by storing it.

With this in mind, a study from the Scandinavian blood banks was recently published in 2007. They took a look at 888,843 cancer-free recipients transfused after 1968. They were followed from the first registered transfusion until death, emigration, diagnosis of cancer, or the end of the study. In all of the years of follow-up, the risk of developing cancer was 1.45 times the average risk. But here's the kicker. When they looked at the first 6 months following the transfusion, the risk was over five times that of average (27). I realize there are several factors at play here, but some, like hepatitis, take longer than 6 months to cause cancer.

Thus, the iron hypothesis fits into this time index. This is not to say it's the only cause, but certainly may play a role.

This data seems to be supported by a study that looked at blood transfusions and surgery in tumors of the pancreas between 1998 and 2003. Of the 294 patients who underwent the surgery for tumors, 140 had received a blood transfusion. The median survival time for the transfusion group was 18 months compared to 24 months in the control group (28). Although this doesn't sound that impressive, it helps to illustrate the point. One must also consider the poor survival rate for pancreatic cancer. I am not saying that you shouldn't take a transfusion. The quality of the blood supply is much better today than in years past. What would be interesting is if a 12 month study was done today with our current standards to see how those results compare. Obviously, if you have an upcoming surgery or known need for blood, I highly recommend using your own.

If we know not to give supplemental iron in cancer, that our body restricts iron availability in cancer, to use drugs to chelate (bind up) iron for cancer treatment, and we know those with iron overload conditions such as HH develop more cancer, then doesn't it stand to reason that we should control our stores of iron in the hopes of starving a pre-malignant mass that is otherwise currently controlled by the body? Or for that matter, in the prevention of cancer, by reducing the number of free radicals, which can damage our DNA? If we apply simple reason to this theory it makes considerable sense. Whether its cancer, CVD, or something else, we wind up relying more on studies that may or may not be well constructed to validate or contradict this theory.

Blood Donors

There is no more effective way to reduce one's iron stores than by blood loss. There are supplements available that can chelate free iron in vivo, and help shuttle it out of the body. This is a slow process, and may be most useful in preventing an iron overload when starting from a pre-overload state. Blood donation is not only much quicker in reducing stores, it is also much cheaper, and you may very well help to save someone's life. With these dramatic iron losses in mind, the theory exists that those who donate blood should on average have lower iron stores, and with those lower stores they should present with better mortality and morbidity estimates attributable to conditions associated with iron overload. With this theory in mind, I have illustrated below several studies which looked at just that. These studies comprise many, but not all relating to this topic, but will provide you with a good basis.

In one study, frequent donors were compared to casual donors on average of ten years after the donation period from 1988-1990. Frequent donors were defined as those who donated more than one unit of blood each of those years, while casual donors were defined as those who only donated once during that three-year period. In the 2,260 subjects, it was found that those who were frequent donors were less likely to be taking antihypertensive and lipid drugs and were almost half as likely to have a severe cardiovascular event, to include death. (29) The authors concluded that, "Frequent and long-term whole blood donation is associated with a lower risk of cardiovascular events." Could these results possibly have been even more impressive had non-donors been compared to donors? In a similar study, subjects 40 and older with no apparent CVD were enrolled between 1985-1987 to measure the occurrence of cardiovascular events and the levels of blood donation. It was found that non-smoking men who donated blood had 2/3 the risk of a cardiovascular event over the course of the study. Relatively recent donations were found to be beneficial. In other words, don't rely on the blood you donated 10 years ago to reduce your risk for a lifetime. They also found that a high frequency of donations was not necessary for this benefit (30).

In another blood donor study, which was a cohort of the Finnish Kupio trial, donation data through the Red Cross was gathered on 2,682 subjects. This was matched up against all registered and verified possible heart attacks in this group over an average of 5.5 years. Of the 2,682 subjects, 153 had donated blood in the two years prior to their baseline data being collected. During this follow-up it was found that only one of the 153 donors had a heart attack, as compared to 226 of the 2529 non-donors. Statistically, this equates to an *86% reduction in risk of a heart attack* for the donors as compared to non donors (31).

In the spirit of full disclosure, and to confuse the hell out of you, I must present a donation trial that does not support the iron hypothesis. As a part of the Health Professional Follow-up Study, 51,529 subjects ages 40-75 were asked to report their total number of blood donations over the past 30 years. Average ferritin for non-donors was 187 ug/l, as compared to 64 ug/l for those who donated 30 or more times. As you can see, they found a very significant difference in ferritin values between these two groups. There were other subgroups, but I thought it appropriate to highlight the significant differences between these two groups. Given the marked difference in ferritin, and what we've seen in other trials, you would expect to see a difference in cardiac events. However, the researchers found no significant difference between any groups. Even more confusing was that men with high cholesterol did not appear to benefit from donation either. How can we explain these findings? Should we throw out the iron hypothesis? Even though ferritin values are tied to inflammation, these differences, I believe, are too great to be swayed by those numbers. These donors had significantly lower ferritin values as you would expect with their level of donation. This study involved a 30-year recall, which has its accuracy issues. In other words the men were asked how many donations they gave over all of those years. So we're dealing with estimates, but even if a guess was off by several donations, we are still talking about a hell of a lot more than non-donors.

It could be that there are differences between the trials. In the Finnish study, it has been shown that the subjects had higher cholesterol values and took significantly less aspirin and vitamin E than did the American counterparts. Since all of these factors weigh into cardiovascular risk, the Americans may have comparatively been doing more things right, and thus diminishing the negative impact of iron. If we compare our "failed study" to other American studies, it may be that these subjects hadn't donated in some time, re-emphasizing the results in the recent donation good results. It could be that there is something more to this than we are aware. This study of iron and its relation to disease is in its infancy, and we still have a lot to learn.

In regards to cancer and total mortality, a study out of Sweden and Denmark looked at 1,110,329 blood donors who were followed for up to 35 years from first donation to death, emigration, or end of study. They found that blood donors had a 30% lower risk of mortality (death) and 4% lower cancer incidence as compared to the control population. Consistent with other findings, they noted that more recent blood donors had a lower relative mortality than those who donated earlier. (32)

In another cancer and phlebotomy study, researchers recently analyzed the possible benefits of phlebotomy and low iron diets for the risk of progression to hepatocellular carcinoma in chronic hepatitis C patients. 35 patients with moderate or severe liver fibrosis, who either failed to respond to interferon or had conditions which prevented its use, underwent weekly phlebotomy until they reached a state of mild iron deficiency. They then went on a monthly maintenance course for 44-144 months, which also included a low iron diet. When they were compared to the 40 patients who declined this therapeutic approach, it was found that the phlebotomy group had half the risk of developing hepatocellular carcinoma. (33)

So let's put this all into perspective. This whole iron hypothesis began in 1981 when Jerome Sullivan, M.D., PhD, proposed that regular menstrual loss protected women from CVD, rather than their endogenous estrogen. As we have seen with the three studies that looked at hysterectomy and the risk of CVD, he seems to have a point. From his initial thesis, he kicked off years of debate and research, which continues to this day. The data is about evenly split. However, the data is either in support of, or just neutral, not contradictory.

What we do know is fairly substantial, and seems to support his theory when you look at the bulk of the good evidence. We know basic concepts, such as inflammation releases iron from stores and feeds the cycle, iron oxidizes LDL in vitro, serum ferritin levels in menstruating women are approximately half that of men and it takes about 10 years post menopause to make up the difference, chelators of iron protect tissue from oxidative damage, more men suffer from CVD disease at a younger age than women but this difference is roughly equal about 10 years after menopause, homozygous and heterozygous hemochromatosis patients suffer from the exact diseases one would attribute to iron overload, and ferritin is an acute phase reactant.

269

So here are my conclusions given what we know now.

- A diet high in heme iron over many years may bump up what would otherwise be considered a "maxed out" iron replete store.
- The negative consequences of a high iron load may take many years to have an effect. The number of years with a high iron load may have just as much importance as the degree of the iron load.
- Antioxidant status may help ameliorate the damage from released iron.
- Blood donation, iron chelation, and/or protein reduction is advisable for men over the age of 40 and women who do not menstruate.
- It may be beneficial to know one's risk for HH earlier rather than later.
- Be wary of "insults" to the body. Whether it is smoking, a blood transfusion, a disease, or another source of inflammation, the resultant free radical generation in an iron overload state may release so much iron from body stores in an unhealthy person that recovery could be compromised or forfeited.
- Growing children and menstruating women should on average not fear consuming more healthy heme-iron containing proteins relative to body weight.

With these considerations for men and women in the age groups I've identified as applicable, you should not be concerned about anemia. In fact, with our western diet it should be easy to see how a man or a postmenopausal woman can accumulate an excess of iron. The daily iron loss in adults is only about 1 mg per day. You could add another 1 mg or so if you sweat from exercise, work, or sauna. If we assume 50% absorption of one serving of beef, which is small by our standards, then you've met your daily losses right there. The risk for iron deficiency anemia is exceedingly small in these adults who are healthy. In fact, the NHANES III study shows us that 2% or less of men aged 20 or more and women aged 50 or more have iron deficiency anemia. Beyond that, the NHANES I data show us that about two-thirds of this mere 2% are attributable to chronic disease or inflammatory conditions. In yet another study, 62% of adults with iron deficiency anemia had gastrointestinal bleeding. (34) As you can see, your risk for anemia in gastrointestinal bleeding or chronic disease should be obvious to both yourself and your practitioner. However, for the vast majority, controlling your iron stores is good preventative and natural medicine.

If you feel you must take a supplement for your iron status, then consider the following information. I would encourage you to eat liver, but if you don't like the taste you could purchase supplements based on calves' liver. Liver is an excellent source of absorbable heme iron, and any supplement will likely come with vitamin C to boost absorption even more. Contrary to popular belief, much of the animal's toxins are not stored in the liver but in the fats, which is another reason to avoid animal fats. More importantly, heme iron is not associated with the side effects of non-heme supplementation. I would spread out the dosing during the day since the amount absorbed decreases with increasing dose. Your synthetic non-heme supplemental iron sources can cause nausea, flatulence, and diarrhea. These are indicators of the free radical effect that this source of iron has on the body.

Let's take a look at how you can absorb more of that dietary iron if you happen to be in an at-risk group. Analysis shows us that you can increase the absorption of iron from your foods with alcohol. In fact, alcohol is so good at improving iron absorption that it has been closely linked with iron overload. (35) Cheers. Vitamin C improves the absorption of non-heme iron, as does the inclusion of meat, fish, or poultry in the meal.

There are also components that impede iron absorption of which you should be aware. Tannins found in tea are one main agent, as are phytates found in legumes and whole grains such as soy and brown rice bran respectively. Dairy also inhibits iron absorption. The effects of calcium on iron absorption are debatable. Some of this can be used to your advantage if you want to control iron. Green tea, quercetin, milk thistle, and rice bran extract are some of the more potent scavengers of free iron.

If you think about it, we should have a reversal in this country of those who eat mostly meat. Men, by and large, eat red meat more often and in larger portions than women, yet it is the women who are losing the iron. Any child before the age of 18 or so, and any woman with an intact functional uterus should have few concerns about eating high quality meats, poultry, and fish. It is the men and postmenopausal women who should monitor their portions. As is the case at times, we have things backwards.

Likewise our focus on iron deficient anemia needs to be sharpened. There has been too much indiscriminant focus on supplemental iron and no attention paid towards iron toxicity and proper nutrition. Those in jeopardy of anemia could benefit from better nutritional support in the form of heme iron. Those who have a risk of developing hemochromatosis or general iron toxicity should have another set of nutritional standards. The point here is that the widespread enrichment of foods with iron should be reconsidered as was the case overseas. Instead, a more targeted approach is preferred.

According to the 2005 dietary guidelines for Americans, "Nutrient needs should be met primarily through consuming foods." I can't help but agree. Of course that's the crux of the problem. We consume a dead empty diet for the most part in this nation, and processed foods don't supply us with the nutrients we require for ideal health. In the end, many rely on supplementation for a wide variety of reasons. We have toxic exposure to chemical and heavy metals, we have disease states which may require select products, we want to optimize our health, combat pathogens, and much more. Supplements and whole herbs are here to stay, as they rightly should be. In the case of iron supplements, consider your less damaging options instead of the pro-oxidant effects of synthetic iron. In total, consider your iron load and its potential for oxidative stress. The pro-oxidant effects of iron have been well established by science and hopefully so in this chapter. It would seem there is something to this free radical theory of aging and damage after all. Iron is just the best way to illustrate that connection.

Chapter 10   Our Ideal Diet

So, what is our ideal diet? We could fill several rooms with literature debating this topic. It's certainly no wonder that you are confused as to what diet is best for your health, considering many bright researchers can't completely agree. In this chapter we'll consider our evolution, four "classic" books on the topic, vegetarianism vs omnivore, and other considerations. If it is at all possible to provide you with an abundance of facts and insight as to the proper nutrition for our bodies, then you'll finally be armed with the information necessary for yourself and your loved ones.

Before I blurt out what I perceive the answer to be, we must start with some theories and facts that will bring us back in time. Although researchers will often tell you things with certainty, I tend to take a more genuine approach. Many a doctor has been wrong telling a patient that they were certain from a seven minute appointment that your condition is because of X. Likewise, we are not completely certain of how we developed some two or more million years ago. I'm pretty sure our story from back then was not saved on a home video. With that said, let's review what we think we know.

It is thought that "humans" have been around for about 2.5 million years, give or take a day or two. It seems reasonable to assume that we descended from the primates. There was some combination of the ability to walk upright, which freed up the use of our hands, probably combined with nutritional changes that facilitated evolution. Our primate ancestors probably ate what today's primates eat, which is a mostly vegetable-based diet with minor amounts of animal protein. Considering that the brain needs enormous amounts of raw materials to grow and develop, a dietary change that involved more animal sources likely occurred. It is unlikely that the first generations were any good at hunting since this was yet to be learned. More likely, they were scavengers who ate bone marrow and perhaps brains protected with bone, which the more lethal predators could not access. There could have been an event much like our salmon runs in Alaska that lasted for hundreds of thousands of years and supplied excellent nutrition for the brain in quantities enough for both animals and man. These dietary changes led to the obvious physical changes of today.

273

As primates have protruding bellies capable of digesting complex carbohydrates for fuel, ours slimmed down to the point where they are about 40% smaller than those of a chimp, and our brains are about three times as large, in proportion.

The combination of hands and concentrated energy sources likely fueled the growth of their brains over many generations. At some point they went on to supplement their scavenging with hunting. Their first prey may have been fish and smaller animals. The lush tropical environment of Africa supplies vast sums of fresh fruits and vegetables as well, which was never abandoned. As the millennia passed, these people probably flourished by their standards, and feuded over food sources. This conflict combined with the curiosity of the developing brain may have led them to what was on the other side of that hill, and the next. More millennia passed and distant migrations began to separate these people. Varying geography may have brought varying vegetation and even seasons, but the realization that animal protein was a concentration source of nutrition never left the consciousness.

During all of this time scavenging, hunting, and foraging fruits, vegetables, roots, nuts, seeds, and animal proteins were probably upwards of 100% of the diet. Unlike us, they spent a lifetime in the open and could recognize root vegetables by their above ground components, knew which parts of any plant or animal were edible, and ate these things whole. Studies of their bones demonstrate that they were a strong and robust people, unlike some of the changes that had occurred following the Agricultural Revolution some 10,000 years ago. In fact, it has been shown that skeletal markers of reduced height, nutritional stress, and infection became more common at this time. (1,2) A must-read classic was written based on the fact that respected geneticists, paleoanthropologists, biologists, and evolutionary theorists agree that contemporary humans differ little genetically from our stone age ancestors. This book is called *The Paleo Diet*, and I recommend it for those who are interested.

The very premise of the book is that our modern diet should more closely resemble the diet from which our ancestors evolved. The logic makes *mostly* perfect sense to me. Our modern diet is far from a diet more in line with our genome, and goes a long way to explaining the ills of our society. Dr. Cordain establishes what you should eat by identifying what they did and didn't eat. This includes:

- No dairy.
- No cereal grains, which include wheat, corn, rice, barley, and more.
- No salt.
- No refined sugar (at best they had some honey).
- Wild, lean, animal protein.
- Non-starchy wild fruits and vegetables.
- A healthier ratio of fats.

With these concepts in mind, the diet allows for:

- All the lean meats, fish, and seafood you can eat.
- All the fruits and non-starchy vegetables you can eat.
- No cereals.
- No legumes (beans, lentils, peas, and peanuts).
- No dairy.
- No processed foods.

In my opinion, this philosophy is quite sound. He advocates a diet that is in the high 20th percentile in protein, low 30th percentile in carbohydrate, and high 30th percentile in fats. These ratios are not in agreement with other Paleolithic nutrition researchers. Others have shown over years of research that the estimated macronutrient intake of our distant ancestors was about mid-30th percentile in protein, low 40th percentile for carbohydrates, and low 20th percentile for fats. (3) Another discrepancy between the book and these other researchers is the inclusion of legumes (beans, peas) in the forager diet.

With that said, the premise is still the same. Eat a wide variety of unprocessed fruits, vegetables, lean meats, nuts, seeds, and legumes. This advice advocates more protein than you may be used to. The downside of this is that our domesticated livestock has about four times the fat content as does wild game, and the fatty acids present vary considerably as well. In a similar fashion, the wild vegetation of their day had more vitamins and minerals on average and much more fiber. Their fiber rich, protein rich, nutrient rich diet of the day probably can't be duplicated by the masses, but we can get close enough. I do have a couple points to mention for your consideration.

Point number one is that of practicality. Given our modern lifestyle, it is very hard to eat this way when out of the house. That's a challenge not just for this diet, but for anything else to be mentioned in this chapter. More importantly, the quality of our meats these days is very different from back then. If you've purchased free-range, grass-fed, drug-free beef online, as I have, you know how ridiculously expensive it is. The same is true for any online or local bison, deer, ostrich, or other meat. Today's meat supply is garbage. If we take beef, for example, we know that these animals are very sick at time of slaughter. We also know that the main cause of this is that they are being fed grains, which are NOT their natural food source. They should be eating grasses. The grains make them very ill, and thus require drugs just to stay alive so they can fatten up for slaughter. I recommend a great book on this called *The Omnivore's Dilemma*. These changes in their foods result in changes in their fat profile in the tissue. Instead of the lean healthy animals back in the day that had a much better fat profile, these sick, drugged-up animals have much more saturated and omega-6 fatty acids. I won't even get into all the toxins, such as pesticides, herbicides, fungicides, and more which concentrate in the fats of these animals. This makes for that tasty "corn-fed" New York strip steak on your plate, but it does your health no favors. So what I am saying here is: feel free to eat this way, but be prepared to fork over some serious cash in the process. As a compromise, seek out leaner cuts of proteins.

Wild caught fish, on the other hand, is unadulterated and in accordance with our needs. Fish should be a wonderful healthy alternative. The unfortunate fact is that our fish supply is highly questionable as well. Mercury is but one of many toxins concentrated in the fish we eat. Hell, pregnant women are discouraged from eating fish. Doesn't that tell you something? All toxins from our global manufacturing, farming, transportation, landscaping, and more wind up in one place, the water. These toxins are consumed gradually up the food chain, and ultimately concentrated in many of the fish we love to eat. Polar bears, killer whales, and humans concentrate these lipophillic toxins, as all are top predators. These toxins go on to affect birth defects, the nervous system, the reproductive systems, and every other system imaginable. For a great read on toxins in our environment I recommend *Detoxify of Die*, by Sherry Rogers, M.D.

My second point on the Paleo topic is that we don't really know about the long-term health of these people. We can infer that about 20% of them reached the age of 60 and beyond by studying more recent hunter-gatherers. (4) In my opinion, that might be a stretch, given the challenges of the day. Had they lived to our average age, we just don't know what chronic degenerative illnesses they may have developed, if any. Would their high protein diet have some ramifications on methylation, calcium balance, or iron overload? We think we know that they lived to around 30 on average, but that has nothing to do with diet. In the world of the "cave man" life was a bit more precarious than it is for us. Our big worries are traffic jams, paying bills, and many other more emotional stressors. These people had to worry about surviving another day. They could be eaten by a predator, or killed by another tribe. They could starve or freeze to death, or suffer from a traumatic accident. Either mom or baby may have died in childbirth, and in really unlucky cases, both did. They also had to fear pathogens. Whether by disease or infection, pathogens remained man's number one killer up until vaccinations. Since the abundance of fossil records will not find the longest lived Paleolithic inhabitants, we can only debate the issue.

The next best thing to going back in time to see how long and healthy our ancestors lived is to analyze how a similar culture lives today. If we could find a group of people who are immune from western influence and who live as closely to the way our ancestors lived as possible, then we might be able to form more educated opinions. Well, in 2009, it's unlikely we'll find anyone to fit this bill on our shrinking globe, but lucky for us, someone did back in the 1930s. His name was Dr. Weston Price, and his book, *Nutrition and Physical Degeneration,* is widely considered a classic. Dr. Price was a dentist, and his primary quest was to find the cause of tooth decay. In his journeys, he went to all corners of the globe. He visited the Swiss in an isolated valley, Gaelics on isolated islands, North American Eskimos and Indians, islands in the South Pacific, tribes in Africa, Aborigines and other tribes in Australia and New

Zealand, and isolated civilizations in Peru. For his day, the logistical achievements were as impressive as his contribution to nutrition.

The general premise was that if travelers, explorers, and scientists had noted that "savages" have on average excellent teeth, and while "civilized" people possess teeth in such terrible shape, then there must be a nutritional connection. It is well established that the American colonists had very poor teeth, best exemplified by George Washington's wooden teeth. Even today, fillings, bridges, dentures, and root canals are an everyday part of life in America. Contrary to the advanced society of the colonists, or even of today, for that matter, how can these primitive people avoid rampant tooth decay? In a society where there were no dentists, no toothpaste, no dental floss, how would their teeth fare? In each case, he compared the teeth of those in the group who had maintained their ancestral ways to those who had begun to adopt the foods and ways of the "western world". In every case he found that dental cavities were rare in those who maintained their ancestral whole-food nutrient-rich diet as compared to prolific cavities in those who adopted western foods. What were the western foods in question? White flour, sugars, and canned foods predominated the list in each instance around the globe. What were the ancestral foods?

- Isolated Swiss — Cow and goat dairy products, rye, meats, and vegetables
- Hebrides — Fish and other seafood, oats
- Eskimo — Salmon, seal oil, salmon eggs, kelp, nuts and berries
- American Indians — Moose, caribou, cranberries, and some vegetables
- Pacific islanders — Seafood, coconut, plants, fruits, and roots
- African tribes — Milk, meat, blood, vegetables, fish, roots, beans, cereals and fruits
- Aborigines — Kangaroo, fish, bird, wallabie, root, egg, berries, pea, rodents and seed
- Torres Islanders — Sea foods, fruits, roots, and greens
- Maori — Seafoods with a focus on shell fish, kelp, grubs, fern root, birds, vegetables, and fruit

- Peruvians   Fish, corn, bean, squash, llama, alpaca, potato, quinoa

What do all of these diets have in common? Not much other than the fact that they are unadulterated. The milk was raw, as were most of the other animal based foods. Organ meats were frequently consumed, as were other items that would make you nauseous. In fact, Dr Price found that the North American Indians had put a great emphasis on eating animal organs to the extent that much of the muscle meat (the part that we eat) was fed to the dogs. Fruits and vegetables were fresh and consumed as such. When they did have domesticated animals, they were not confined to a barn and were fed a diet in accordance with their make-up. The animals were free-ranging and ate fresh grass. As you can see, most cultures used no dairy, and most cultures had little to no reliance on cereal grains. Moving beyond nutrition, extreme physical activity was present in all cases.

I'm sure you wouldn't like to dine with the Aborigines on fresh rodent to include the internal organs. I don't think you would like to order any ground locusts in your favorite African restaurant, nor would you care for seal oil or fish eyes. The greatness of this book is that we as humans can survive healthfully off of a variety of foods, so long as they are fresh, unadulterated, quality, nutritious choices with some variety. If you pack your child's lunch for school, what do you put in there? A peanut butter and jelly sandwich on highly processed bread, a yogurt, some juice, and maybe a fruit or vegetable grown on the other side of the world with pesticides and herbicides banned for use in the U.S. for decades. In Dr. Price's book he found that the Maori were the most immune to dental caries (cavities) of all the people he researched. What did their kids have for lunch? Their parents didn't pack them a lunch at all. At lunchtime, the kids rushed to the beach. Half prepared bonfires, while the other half dove for a large species of lobster. Obviously this is totally irrelevant to today, but isn't that the point?

In addition to finding marked differences in cavities, he also found other significant health consequences, most notably tuberculosis. Over and again there was clear evidence that diet was not only related to dental health, but overall health. In fact, it was so bad in some instances that native populations had dramatically fallen since their exposure to western foods. You couldn't help but feel bad for these people.

If this is the ideal diet then why does it contrast with the Paleolithic diet a bit? Some of these peoples ate dairy, grains, and/or legumes. It is true that they all consumed animal proteins, and those proteins were more ideal than those of today. They also ate fresh fruits, roots, and vegetables in good quantities for the most part. Only the Pacific Islanders ate what would be considered the closest, if not identical to the Paleo diet. This makes sense since we come from the tropics anyhow, and there's a year round abundance of fruits, vegetables, fish, and roots for your delight. Dr. Price stated, "During these investigations of primitive races, I have been impressed with the superior quality of the human stock developed by nature wherever a liberal source of sea foods existed."

So what are the limitations in Dr. Price's book? In his focused research on the connection of diet to dental and general health, Dr Price took no data on longevity. Of course you can't do everything, and this would have likely been an impossible task since the written word was rarely used in most cultures and recordkeeping was generally absent in those that wrote. With that said, we have absolutely no evidence as to their life expectancy. As impressive as his research was, and as much insight as it gives us, we just don't know for a fact that these diets, or types of diets, are ideal for our long-term health and survival. Take the following two examples as cases in point.

Let's look at the Maori who hail from New Zealand. We will use them as an example since Dr Price had commented so favorably on their dental health. So what was their life span? Dr. Price doesn't make mention of it anywhere in his book. Our best indication of the Maori life-span comes from the time of initial contact with them. Captain Cook discovered New Zealand in 1769 and two sources estimate their expected longevity to be around 30-35. That doesn't sound so good. If you consider that at the same point in time the average life expectancy in "civilized" nations was around 25, then it sounds better. It sounds great if you consider that for Londoners in 1667, the estimate was 18 years old. (5) While hazards of conflict and accidents were likely similar, risk of disease and child bearing was probably greater in the western world, explaining the difference. Of course, I'm willing to guarantee the Maori had better teeth.

The fact is that we don't know how long these people could have lived in our safe environment of today while maintaining their old diets. My guess is that they'd die younger on average, particularly the men. Is this shocking? I'm just trying to present the unbiased facts. Their exceedingly high iron-methionine-sulfur diet would have limited their life expectancy. The native Maori diet had an iron intake of over 58 times that of the western diet that went on to replace it. Shellfish are quite high in iron, and this source was consumed frequently and would considerably add to their iron load. This also explains why they were large people.

Let's take a look at another one of these famous groups. This time we'll examine the Eskimos of Alaska. They went on to garner much attention given the fact that they eat a high fat diet but do not suffer from cardiovascular disease, hence your fish oil capsules. As Weston Price noted, they also do not suffer from malignancies. What do they suffer from? Osteoporosis. In a study on bone density from 1974, bone mineralization of Eskimos was compared to that of caucasions. Although bone mineral density (BMD) remained essentially equal through the thirties, significant differences became apparent in the decades to follow. (6) Eskimo women were shown to reach states of demineralization ten years sooner than their white counterparts, and it got worse from there. At about age 74, white women are shown to lose bone slower, by approximately half, while the higher Eskimo rate of loss continued. Vitamin D was ruled out because the diet of sealife with internal organs seems to provide plenty, especially evident in the fact that rickets was not seen in the children. The exceedingly high levels of protein intake were reasonably blamed for the loss in bone calcium.

Whether through Weston Price or other research, I cannot find any estimates on Eskimo longevity prior to the intrusion of the western world. It probably does not exist considering recordkeeping would be a challenge in a land dominated by ice. We can only guess at their average life expectancy, which I hazard to guess was not all that close to ours. Even if they were transported to the safety of our world, and yet maintained their native diet, I surmise that the lack of phytonutrients and other constituents would hinder their chances. Their exceedingly high protein diet with the accompanying high iron-methionine-sulfur content wouldn't help matters either.

The high protein diet of the Eskimos brings us to our next classic, which is the classical pro-vegan argument. I first read *Fit for Life* by Harvey Diamond as a teenager, and have since read his books several times. Just to be clear: the vegan eats no animal products, while other vegetarians may eat eggs, fish, dairy, or be a part-time vegetarian. Harvey references extensive research in support of his conclusions, and I agree with everything he says with one exception. Lets take a look at what we can agree upon.

In the non-food category he advocates fresh air, exercise, healthy relationships, good sleep and low stress. These elements are without a doubt crucial to the quality of health throughout your life, not only a part of the life extension component. All of these healthful goals played a significant role in Weston Price's work as well. For example, his stated requirements on sun exposure are quite accurate, which are supported by this chapter on vitamin D. Harvey goes on to write that "sunscreens are only necessary when you are in the sun for a prolonged period of time during the most intense hours." In regards to exercise he states, "If exercise is neglected, the body will become weak and all its physical powers will be diminished, but with regular exercise the entire system will be strengthened and invigorated."

In the "foods" category, Harvey sheds some light on things, and his points on water are dead-on. He informs us that our water supply is poor at best. He goes on to state:

"Tap water these days is more like soup, a chemical soup. Among the pollutants are soap, wood pulp, sulfuric acid, copper, arsenic, paint, pesticides, radioactive wastes, agricultural fertilizers, and chemicals from industries too numerous to mention. In addition there are inorganic minerals, mildly to highly toxic-sulpher, iron, gypsum, calcium, magnesium, lime, soda ash, fluorine, chlorine, etc. Moreover, further chemical pollutants are deliberately added to water supplies supposedly in an effort to purify the water and kill its bacteria. The only thing is, the chemicals are far more harmful than the bacteria they're supposed to kill."

He bashes chlorine and fluoride in water, and rightfully so. Ultimately the recommendation is for distilled water, which is clean but potentially acidic. If you're worried about robbing your body of minerals, he will argue that this is not a concern. If it makes you feel better, take a multi-mineral formula or get a water purifier that cleans and alkalinizes your water.

The bulk of his first book was dedicated to his principles of food combining, such as don't eat fruit with any solid foods. I won't get into all of that, and its efficacy can be debated, but we will focus on his urge to avoid animal products. It is in this arena where I agree in part, and disagree as well. Avoidance of proteins here in America today is not necessarily a terrible idea. We treat our animals quite poorly on average, and buying the product supports the system. Ok, I get it, but there's a way around that, which is also better for your health. The second argument is the poor quality of the meats, dairy, eggs, poultry, pork, and even some fish in our food supply. As covered in this book, these unhealthy animals fed an inappropriate diet are drugged up and fed to you and your children. It is likely true that the primary dietary cause of illness in this country is from the animal products we consume, especially when you consider the vast array of drugs, metals, and other toxins that accompany them.

To further impress upon you concerns about animal foods, simply reread my chapter on dairy. If for whatever amazing reason you can't believe me, then read Harvey's chapter on dairy. If you're still in disbelief, or your head's buried in the sand, then I suggest you do some research online through independent researchers. The sad fact is that the bacon, sausage, hamburger, cheese, milk, and more have been processed, over-cooked, contaminated, and otherwise fundamentally changed from what we evolved to eat. Even though what I say is true for almost all of our food supply, it doesn't mean that animal protein should be excluded from our diet, which brings us to the vegetarian versus omnivore debate.

Vegetarian vs Omnivore Debate

The purpose of this debate is to focus on our genomic nutritional needs. We must then discount any environmental and humanitarian issues, however valid they may be, in order to prove this point. We must also define vegan and vegetarian briefly. A vegan eats no animal products at all, in essence your purist form of vegetarian. A lacto-vegetarian will consume dairy products as their only animal source. The ovo-vegetarian will eat eggs, which is really moving away from vegetarianism and into omnivore. Others may eat some fish, or be "part time" vegetarians and consume various animal products on rare occasion. This all lend itself to too many variables with which to make a proper analysis, and thus I have chosen the pure vegan as the standard of comparison. Besides, all others are omnivores anyhow (discounting the ill-advised lacto-vegetarians). So then the simple question is: "Are we as humans meant to be vegans or omnivores?"

Despite the many fine arguments in support of vegans, the answer is very simple. We are meant to be omnivores. You can quote selected statistics, you can bury your heads in the sand, and you can rant and rave all you want, but you can't hide from the facts. My case can be made in many ways. You can look at our teeth, the anatomy and physiology of our GI tract, the number of nutrient deficiencies vegans can and do get, evolutionary data, longevity data, and common sense. I really only need one thing to truly make my point. That is vitamin B 12.

Vegetable products do not contain vitamin B12. The argument for brewer's yeast, fortified foods, and supplements doesn't hold water since we obviously did not evolve with these sources. Although our needs for B12 are relatively low, increased in pregnancy and infancy, a deficiency is nonetheless a serious matter. The anemia is not as detrimental as the irreversible neurologic damage. One interesting study illustrates the obvious shortcoming of the vegan diet by looking at B vitamins and homocysteine. If you recall homocysteine is essentially a free radical amino acid, indicative of CVD risk and more. This study looked at 32 vegans and 59 omnivores. As the vegan diet provides essentially no vitamin B12, and since B12 is the main determinant (arguable) of homocysteine levels in the blood, the researchers wanted to verify a connection. It was found that the serum B12 levels were significantly lower in the vegans, at 140 pmol/l as compared to 345 pmol/l for the omnivores. A B12 deficit was determined in 78% of the vegans and none of the omnivores. The vegans had an average homocysteine value of 15.79 umol/l while the omnivores averaged 10.19 umol/l. (7) This shows us that not only do vegans have lower vitamin B12 levels, but they also have an increased risk for CVD based on its effects on homocysteine. By the way, 15.79 is a high homocysteine number.

Weston Price came to the same conclusion. He states in his book, "As yet, I have not found a single group of primitive racial stock which was building and maintaining excellent bodies by living entirely on plant foods." Why is it that these people from around the globe, isolated from the rest of humanity, all came to rely extensively on animal foods, and parts of those animals we'd consider unappetizing for their nutrition? Why did none of them elect to become vegetarians? For even the few who consumed dairy, they too also ate animal meats. Clearly we were meant to consume animal sources. Thus our optimal health is tied to those sources. The real question is simply identifying those sources and *quantifying* them.

I endorse all poultry, meats, eggs, and seafoods wholeheartedly in their natural form. Animals who have lived in their natural environment, eating foods in line with their genetic needs, and free of drugs, disease, and virtual torture, are ideal for our consumption. The main obstacle in this equation is that these ideal foods are becoming increasingly rare, no pun intended. There is one animal source that does stand out above the others from a purely scientific viewpoint, and that is seafood, and fish more specifically. Fish is a great source of DHA, which is the superunsaturated fatty acid for which you take fish oil. Our brain matter is composed of a significant amount of DHA, which we cannot get from plant sources. It is true that we can convert its basic precursor alpha linolenic acid (LNA), into DHA ultimately, but it is widely thought that a percent of us have issues synthesizing DHA adequately in the quantities needed. This is why you'll see on numerous vegan websites advertisements for vegan DHA supplements from algae. But algae supplements weren't a part of our evolution either. Without animal sources to fuel brain development, we wouldn't be much different from our primate ancestors at all.

Another component of seafood is its iodine content. Not only is an iodine deficiency more likely with a vegan, it is quite prominent globally. It is estimated that approximately 30% or more of the global population has insufficient iodine intake. The remaining 70% or so consume iodized salt. If your soil has reasonable iodine content, then you could possibly get by living on prodigious amounts of certain vegetables. In one 1999 dietary and urinalysis study published in the *British Journal of Nutrition*, the researchers highlighted the potential danger of iodine deficiency disorders from strict vegetarian dietary practices, particularly in foods from iodine poor soils. (8) The simple fact is that our thyroid requirements for iodine highlight our connection to the sea. Why is it that we are most attracted to the ocean? Why is the most expensive real estate on the ocean despite high insurance and risk of death and destruction? We have a connection to the sea, which is borne out from our nutritional needs. Iodized salt was not a staple among our Paleolithic ancestors. Roaming wild game would consume varied and large sums of vegetation over large tracts of land to compensate. Domesticated animals and their human counterparts have to be supplemented. Granted that seaweed is the best source of iodine, which would fit the vegan model, but it contains no DHA or B12.

In addition to the B12, DHA, and iodine that fish supply in our diet, they also supply iron, but in more desirable quantities on average than land animals. It is likely a combination of fresh seafood consumption and several other factors that explains the longevity of various populations around the globe who consume fish based diets. Upon analysis of Weston price's book one can't help but notice that when access to seafood was available, none of these people consumed dairy. The isolated Swiss are probably the best example of dairy as a food of last resort. Without dairy, could they have subsisted on rye and animal protein once a week? Their diet was a function of their geography, and dairy played a large role given the harsh growing conditions and the unavailability of nutritious seafoods.

As further evidence that we are intended to eat animal protein, I bring you the long-lived people of Japan, Andorra, Italy and others. They eat the typical Medditeranean diet, which includes fish and lean meats along with vegetables, fruits, olive oil, and red wine. These people with their sunlight, low stress, seafood, healthy oils, exercise, and food in moderation repeatedly rank as long lived healthy people. These people are not vegetarians.

Vegetarians typically refer to various epidemiological studies noting that a vegan diet, or some form of vegetarian diet, shows improved mortality as compared to the standard American diet. This is not surprising since the standard American diet leaves a lot to be desired. That's not what I call setting your bar very high. In one such study, the California Adventists were shown to have a 7.3 year longer life expectancy for white men and 4.4 years for women. (9) Although several factors must be noted, the Adventists consumed diets ranging from simple avoidance of red meat to strict vegan. They get regular exercise, don't smoke, drink modestly, maintain more ideal body weights, and in general eat and live a healthier lifestyle. Even with all of that said, they had only ½ the U.S. rate of colon cancer, and very similar rates of breast and prostate cancer. Researchers estimate that they could gain another four years in life expectancy from modifying other factors. Considering that many are lacto-ovo-vegetarians, the elimination of the significant contribution of dairy to their diet would likely be a wise choice. This is evident in their rate of breast and prostate cancer. It is a whole lifestyle approach, not just the strict elimination of all animal proteins that extends longevity.

Sure we have inched up life expectancy, but at an enormous cost. We are now drugged up for many of those last years with a low quality of life and a cost to the healthcare system that is absolutely crushing. It is the avoidance of reasonable nutritional and quality of life measures that keeps us in the hole. We live at a faster pace, with more synthetic foods, and more stress. Mark my words, assuming that our current trends continue, and I believe that they will, you will soon begin to see a reversal of life expectancy in this country based on the principles in this book. Beyond that, you may also see a death blow to the U.S. economy if we maintain our current standards of practice and social commitments to the nation. Medical care for the elderly, healthcare for all, and drugs for all will benefit those in the healthcare field, but create an unsustainable trend to bankruptcy for the nation. With this doom and gloom forecast for the future, I bring you our last "classic" for your edification. Here's a population filled with healthy elderly who do not require medical care and still survive in this day and age. It is this island chain with its blend of most everything ideal for our genome that shows us that we can maintain a strong, vibrant life until very advanced age. It is their diet and lifestyle that we will try to emulate as best we can for our own health. It is here where we have a living laboratory with meticulous data, which enables scientists to witness and monitor as opposed to postulate and argue. It is the island chain of Okinawa and a trio of researchers who bring us *The Okinawa Program*.

I highly recommend you read this book. It is a synopsis of the ongoing "Okinawa Centenarian Study," which began in 1975. Centenarians are those who live to 100 years of age, and Okinawa has more per 100,000 inhabitants than anywhere else. This is no recent phenomenon since ancient Chinese documents describe the area as "the land of happy immortals." Unlike those unsubstantiated claims of longevity in the Caucasus Moutains of the Hunza, the Okinawans, in keeping with being meticulous Japanese, have kept reliable birth, marriage, and death statistics since 1879. Their low calorie, high plant based diet with many complex carbohydrates will be the focus in this section. This is not at all to discount their physical activity, purposeful life, free air, low stress, sunshine, and feeling of community.

Unlike the standard American Diet and the Paleo diets, this is a bit different, and more akin to the Mediterranean diet. While the Paleo diet recommends that protein consists of 19-35% of the diet, the Okinawans come in at about 10-20%, roughly half as much. Given less animal protein, the total fat content in the Okinawan program is 30% at a maximum, while the Paleo is 28-47%. Therefore, the carbohydrate load in the Okinawa diet is almost double, while the total calories are less. Although Dr. Cordain does not give a caloric guideline, she does state "eat until you're full," which is in contrast to the Okinawan "hara hachi bu" tradition of eating until you're 80% full. Unlike any of the previously mentioned valuable books, this is the only one that has a live multi-year observational clinical trial, encapsulating for us centuries of health-giving tradition, which may soon be lost forever. Who better to study than the longest lived and healthiest people on earth?

Do not discount the many similarities between these well presented books. These books are not trying to sell you a product. These authors are purists, and they present the facts as they believe them to be true, and it's up to you to make an educated decision. These aren't meant to be short-term fad diets but lifetime changes. These authors have no product line to sell you, just the truth as they see it. Let's now consolidate the common truths before we dive deeper into this book. Each book emphasizes:

- Plenty of fresh fruits and vegetables
- Plenty of exercise, low stress, and sunlight
- Three tout avoidance of too many saturated fats
- A reduction in Omega-6 fatty acid consumption (vegetable oils)
- An increase in Omega-3 fatty acid consumption (fish and flax)
- Increased mono-unsaturated fatty acids (olive oil)
- Avoidance of simple sugars, processed, trans-fat, fried, empty, dead foods

One could make the argument that their longevity is due to their genes, but this would not be factual. Three Japanese migration studies referenced in the book show that when Okinawans and Japanese abandon their traditional ways, they take on the same disease risks as their adopted country. Some will claim that genetics can influence your longevity by about a third. This may very well be true for individuals, as we know that some families tend to have good longevity while others do not. However, I question that statistic when applied to large groups of people as evidenced by the longevity of several other nations. Globally, we have several nations with longevity within one to two years of Okinawa. Some can even equal Okinawa, depending on who you reference. Since several other nations are right there in the ball park, and since Okinawans acquire the same diseases of their host nations in time, I don't see it as an Okinawan issue, but a human issue.

From a cardiovascular standpoint, the researchers found that the Okinawans had:

- Among the lowest homocysteine levels in the world
- Low total cholesterol with more HDL (good cholesterol)
- A healthy blood pressure
- Low obesity, diabetes, smoking, and stress

289

From a cancer viewpoint, the researchers found that the Okinawans get 80% fewer hormone-dependent cancers such as breast, ovarian, prostate, and colon. They also found that they had better bone mineralization with about half the rate of hip fracture as we have as Americans. How can that be if they consume essentially zero dairy products whatsoever? Among other connections to their bone health, such as a high calcium diet from plants, exercise, and sunlight, the researchers made note of the protein connection to bone loss. Their low protein diet in conjunction with these other considerations yields half the hip fracture rate, with no dairy.

So what do these people eat and do to have more 100+ year-olds than anyone else? Their diet and the way in which they prepare it is almost identical to the Mediteranean Diet, as well as the diet recommended in this book. They eat on average:

- Two to four servings of fruit a day
- Seven or more servings of vegetables a day
- Seven servings of grains a day
- Two servings of soy a day
- Omega-3 rich cold water fish at least 3 times a week
- Minimal dairy and meat

These foods are freshly harvested and caught. They live in a climate that provides them with an abundance of fresh fruits and vegetables. In fact, many garden well into their later years. When they cook, they do so as recommended in this book, with one exception. They stir-fry at a low temperature primarily with canola oil. They use cold-pressed canola oil as opposed to the canola oil mostly available to us here in the states. Canola oil is a new addition to their diet, for better or worse, since it wasn't developed until the 1980s. On flawed assumptions from animal data, the Canadians genetically modified rapeseed oil to make canola. If you elect to use canola instead of olive oil, I highly recommend you get a cold-pressed unrefined product.

What are their foods specifically? For grains they eat mostly white rice, which could be improved upon by substituting brown rice. They also use whole grain noodles made from buckwheat or wheat. Vegetables, legumes, and potatoes are among the most common foods in their diet. Their sweet potato traditionally rules the number one spot. The fruits consist of tangerines, papayas, watermelon, bananas, and pineapples. They consume small amounts of protein, usually fish, poultry, or pork. They also eat a variety of seaweed. Natural medicine plays a role in Okinawa, as it does officially in Japan, Germany, and other nations. Turmeric (curcumin) is one herb used to flavor for food and tea, and to treat ills.

Inevitably, when Japan's diet is discussed, the topic of soy comes up. This wonder-food may not be quite as wonderful as you think. It's certainly not hurting the Okinawans, but you have to dig deeper into the soy story.

We begin our story out of Manchuria some roughly 3,000 years ago. From this region comes a newly cultivated bean with interesting properties. The Chinese had been consuming rice, wheat, millet, and other crops for generations. This new bean of now modern fame was originally used as a fertilizer, to reintroduce nitrogen into the soil, like you would use today with some NPK fertilizer. Of course, commercial synthetic fertilizer wasn't available then, and since very few plants are nitrogen fixers, you can see how it earned its prominence.

What does one do with all the extra crop after you've enriched your soil? They learned early on, most likely through severe GI distress among other symptoms, that the soy bean wasn't meant to be eaten like any other. It took somewhere around 1,000 years to perfect techniques to make the undigestible, digestible. This was a boon, given its high amounts of protein and oil. As beef takes an extraordinary amount of land per pound of protein comparatively, soy is extremely efficient. This leads us to today. Our introduction to soy began by being all about the money, as usual. If one can grow more protein, more oil, and more overall calories more economically than the competition, then guess who has the upper hand? That's all well and good, given fairness and a quality product, but when distortion through marketing and lobbying is at play, the consumer suffers. The bottom-line money proponents have since found some new allies in the world of health and nutrition. However, not everyone in the field of wellness is so happy about the soybean.

A few years ago, Dr. Kaayla Daniel wrote a book on soy entitled, *The Whole Soy Story – the dark side of America's favorite health food.*" I can't do her book justice here, so if you're interested in getting her complete side of the story, you may want to inform yourself. In essence she links the soybean to a myriad of health issues due to a number of its characteristics, which include allergens, goitrogens, lectins, oligosaccharides, oxalates, phytates, isoflavones, protease inhibitors, and saponins. I believe Dr. Daniel brings up a great many relevant and interesting points in her extensively referenced book. Although one could label her book semi-alarmist, she does the public much service. She has also received a lot of flack, mostly from proponents of soy, not surprisingly. It's a shame that you, the consumer, will most often only hear one side of a story, and that side usually has a vested interest in your doing something with your money. So let's look at some of the basic truths on soy for you to make an educated decision.

Our first premise is that the soybean is loaded with anti-nutrients like no other. These anti-nutrients are the result of natural selection over millennia. Animals that would eat one kind of food would flourish, while others that relied on a different food source would not. For reasons of genetic circumstance and predatory food selection, the soybean's end result is something few animals can eat. We should learn from nature.

Asian cultures devised time-proven techniques for freeing up the nutrients in the soybean while diminishing its anti-nutrients. Products such as miso, natto, and tempeh undergo a process of soaking, cooking, and fermenting to turn this bean into something of use. Miso, for example, is paste used as a flavoring, but was originally used in food preservation. (10) It's fermentation process can take over one year. Natto and tempeh are both fermented products as well, as is soy sauce. It is the properly made soy-derived product that is what the Okinawan's enjoy.

Our second premise focuses on the American way. In our "I want it now, and I want it cheap" mentality, we have created many monsters unknowingly. One such monster is that of the soy industry. In the aim of bringing the America people what they want, Mosanto brings you the genetically modified soybean for 2/3 of the U.S. crop. If that doesn't much bother you then we'll consider the afforementioned soy products:

miso, tempeh, soy sauce, and natto. Each one of those products can be manufactured more efficiently just for you. It comes at a cost, however, but not measured in dollars. The highly heated, denatured, dead, soy may come with extra ingredients in the form of MSG and other flavorings, colorings, chemicals, and other industrial byproducts. If you haven't picked up one of several "rules of thumb" running through this book, it's simple. Seek out minimally processed foods! If you can't pronounce the ingredients and the food looks "synthetic" (fruit roll-up anyone?), then I'd encourage you to buy something else.

Another premise to consider is that we're offering up soy products that never existed before, and are NOT a part of anyone's longevity factors. Soybean oil had historically been used as kerosene and for other industrial purposes. (11) Today soybean oil has found its way into almost everything. Soybean oil plays no role in the Okinawan diet. The textured soy protein we use today to extend ground beef plays no role in any longevity program. The soy protein isolate that is found in numerous items and particularly in infant formulas also has no role. Like corn, some form of soy has found its way into almost every prepackaged food in America. If we want any perspective on soy, perhaps we should look at Asia.

Although the authors give slightly confusing figures at times, I'll try to consolidate as accurately as I can. They found that the Okinawans consume about three ounces of soy products per day, consisting mostly of miso and tofu. Three ounces is about half a medium apple. This is done in one to two servings per day. The Chinese consume less soy, on average. In either case, the numbers are probably far lower than you'd think, or than some of you may be consuming. If you are a vegetarian relying on soy for your primary source of protein, you may very well be blowing away these numbers. Keep in mind that all things should be in moderation. Whether its vitamin D, fish oil, soy, or exercise, there can be too much of a good thing. Don't fall into this soy burger, soy ice cream, soy everything American marketing hype. In the end, you may only be serving the financial interests of someone else.

Let's take another soy product, soy milk. I'd first like to start by saying that we need to drop this "need" for milk. Many people have switched away from cow's milk, and for good reason. Some have gone to soy milk. I've had many questions about rice milk. Why do we even need milk? Sure, you can put some in your coffee, mashed potatoes, or pumpkin pie, but these are minute amounts. We consume milk in this country at an astonishing rate. Please hear this: divorce yourself from the need for milk. Eat oatmeal or roots instead of cereal. Drink water instead of milk. There have been numerous reports on soy milk and side effects mainly attributed to the high phytoestrogen load. A high phytoestrogen load is just one of the many reasons to reconsider soy. Soy milk had historically only been a step in the process of making tofu. Okinawans unlikely consumed it with regularity until the late 1970s when the texture, taste, and marketing of soy milk increased its consumption. (12) Even more, the soy milk here in the states is a highly processed over-heated marketing phenomenon.

How about soy formula? According to the often quoted bulletin from the Swiss Federal Health Service, infants drinking soy formula receive the equivalent of one-fourth of a birth control pill, or more, every day. When an infant's weight is taken into consideration as compared to women for whom the drug is intended, it equates to a dose of three to five birth control pills a day. If you're a woman, I wonder if that sounds appealing. A study was conducted looking at the isoflavone composition of 25 randomly selected samples of infant soy formula representing five major brands. Isoflavone is for all intents and purposes equivalent to phytoestrogen. Twenty-one 4-month-old infants were split evenly into groups receiving soy formula, cow's milk, or breast milk. They found that the isoflavone content was similar among the five brands, and was dependent on the amount of soy protein isolate used. The researchers concluded that the circulating concentrations of isoflavones in the seven infants fed the soy-based formula were 13,000 to 22,000 times higher than plasma estradiol concentrations in early life, and may be sufficient to exert biological effects. (13) When you compare the range of isoflavones in the serum of Japanese adults, which is 40-240 ng/ml, to the infants in this last study, who had an average of 980 ng/ml, the issue becomes a no-brainer. In further admonishment of our unnatural use of soy, the British Department of Health issued a warning that the phytoestrogens found in soy-based infant formulas could adversely affect infant health.

If you're a soy proponent and you tout the fact that soy is good for reducing menopausal symptoms, as experienced by the Japanese, then you're attesting to the phytoestrogen content. If big pharma has seen it in their wisdom to source their natural estrogen for transdermal hormone replacement therapy from soybeans, then maybe there's some estrogenic potential in them there beans. So, if we can admit soybeans have estrogenic qualities, then should we be giving it to anyone who's not fully mature, especially infants? According to the Committee for Toxicity's 444 page publication on phytoestrogens, soy flour is sky high. Soy protein isolate, the stuff in infant formula was half of flour, but twice that of miso, tempeh, and tofu. Given these facts, I only think it's prudent to temper any soy given to your children. As far as breast-feeding is concerned, it doesn't appear to be a significant issue as very little seems to make its way through the breast milk, and that little bit is probably protective for the infant. (14) If breast milk is not an option for your baby, your options aren't fantastic. Cow's milk, soy milk, goat milk, hydrolyzed formulas, and amino acids based formulas are your options. I'd measure them out and decide as to what's best for your child.

Soy is not a total loss. I am not here to bash soy altogether, just its excess and perturbation. Soy serves as the primary source for the supplement phosphatidylcholine, as discussed in the chapter on IBD, as well as vitamin E and other supplements. Phytates, which are present in soy and in brown rice, are used to treat cancer and heavy metal toxicity via their sequestering ability. Soy phytoestrogens when used properly can treat the symptoms of menopause. We can theorize that Okinawan women have stronger bones than Americans for many reasons, one of them being a higher estrogen load postmenopausally. We can theorize that Okinawan men and women have lower rates of hormone dependent cancers for many reasons, one of them being attributed to the phytoestrogens. In a nut-shell, the weaker phytoestrogen occupies the estrogen receptor thus blocking the effects induced by the stronger endogenous estrogen. It's a nice compromise for women. These estrogens in reasonable quantities are weak enough to help prior to menopause, but strong enough to help after menopause.

You must realize that the success of the Okinawans is not solely attributable to soy. Do not fall into the one-answer miracle in a bottle super solution that everyone with a vested financial interest wants you to follow. Soy consumption is a part of a much larger picture. They consume a varied diet and excellent foods in good ratios and small portions while avoiding much of the disease causing foods we ingest. They also get plenty of exercise, fresh air, and sunshine. Other long-lived peoples don't eat soy at all. Several other nations are within a year of the Okinawan's average longevity, and although the dietary principles are the same, there's no soy on their menu. Soy does have its place in your diet if you want it to; it just needs its proper place. You may want to consider buying only certain organic whole soy products that are manufactured in accordance with proper traditional-based techniques.

After all of this, what standards are we to use in establishing a healthy diet, or the healthiest diet possible? We've covered what these four books have in common. We can easily pick out the fact that fruits and vegetables are emphasized in every book. In today's world we are fortunate to be able to drive a few minutes to a store and buy these less than perfect fruits and vegetables at any time of the year. In this way, we continue to get minerals, vitamins, and phytonutrients year round. Try to shoot for an even blend of cooked versus raw vegetables as well. Some vegetables are obviously best cooked like the sweet potato, and other are obviously best raw like lettuce. In the end, eat as much of these phytonutrient-rich foods as you please without regard to calories, sugars, or any of that other crap.

What about the differences? One book advocates more lean protein. Another advocates almost anything so long as its unadulterated, to include dairy. One rejects animal protein. The last advocates soy to a degree. What is the final answer? I'm sure you can already guess, but we'll review anyhow. Whether your diet is Mediterranean based, Okinawa based, or however you want to label it, it should contain these same principles.

- Plenty of fresh fruits and vegetables
- Avoidance of too many saturated fats, and no hydrogenated oils
- A reduction in Omega-6 fatty acid consumption (vegetable oils)
- A moderate increase in Omega-3 fatty acid consumption (fish and flax)
- Increased mono-unsaturated fatty acids (olive oil)

- Avoidance of simple sugars, processed, fried, trans-fat, empty, dead foods
- Enjoy nuts, seeds and legumes
- Eat plenty of cold-water fish, hopefully it's toxin free
- Other animal proteins should ideally be free range, drug free, and fed correctly
- Consume protein in a limited quantity, think half of what you're eating now
- If you want soy, eat it in moderation, and ensure its quality
- Cook at low temperature with extra virgin olive or coconut oil
- Some whole grains are better than others, food preparation may matter

Assuming you're not allergic to beans, nuts, seeds, peas, lentils, or peanuts, I see no reason why they can't occupy a reasonable portion of your diet. Take flax seed, for example. Flax (Linum usitatissimum) is grown in every part of the world except for the tropics and arctic. It's an annual, with gold or brown seeds, both equally nutritious. Flax has been cultivated since at least 5,000 BC for its fiber, oil, nutritive, and health benefits. The emperor Charlemagne considered it so important to health that he passed laws requiring its consumption. For the purposes of this argument, we can break up flax's health benefits into two categories. Those attributed to the oil, and those to the rest of the seed. A sample of 100 grams of seed will yield about 35 grams of oil, 26 grams of protein, 14 grams of fiber, 12 grams of mucilage, 4 grams of minerals, and 9 grams of water. It is also the richest known source of lignans.

Lignins are a kind of insoluble fiber. Lignans have anti-viral, anti-fungal, anti-bacterial, and anti-cancer properties. The gut metabolizes them into their active molecular form, that of a phytoestrogen. For example, the lignan enterolactone is a moderate inhibitor of estrogen synthetase, which is an enzyme that plays a role in estrogen synthesis. In other words, the body senses the presence of more estrogen, and reduces the enzymes necessary in the production of the more powerful endogenous estrogens, theoretically resulting in lowered rates of estrogen dependent cancers. There are other kinds of lignans; for example, the flavolignans from milk thistle have hepatotoprotective effects by gearing up the cytochrome P450 activity. Flax contains 100 times the quantity of lignans as compared to the next best source, which is wheat bran.

Mucilages are water-soluble polysaccharides able to absorb about 20 times their dry volume, adding to fecal bulk, ultimately helping with constipation, which affects about 1/3 of Americans. Millions of physician visits were the result of constipation, and the annual sales of OTC laxatives is almost $1 billion. Think of the healthcare cost savings alone from alleviation of chronic constipation. They also decrease cholesterol by decreasing absorption from food, and by preventing the resorption of bile acids. Lastly, it acts as a local demulcent while in contact with mucous membranes, coating, soothing, and protecting irritated surfaces of the GI tract, which is quite useful in a number of disease states. Other mucilage sources include marshmallow root and leaf, slippery elm bark, fenugreek, and comfrey root and leaf.

Fiber acts in a similar fashion to mucilages, and fiber has a number of the same benefits. It adds to the bulk of the stool, helping to clear metabolic wastes, and decrease transit time. It feeds the healthful bacteria within the gut, and in turn they produce some of our vitamins, keep down pathogens, help in detoxification (i.e. decreasing beta-glucoronidase activity), and a multitude of other functions. Additionally, the fiber (indigestible cellulose) lowers serum cholesterol in the same fashions as the mucilages.

The oil is the central constituent that receives the most attention. Flax oil is the richest known source of alpha-linolenic acid (LNA), with over 50% of its fatty acids consisting of LNA, the remainder a mix of monounsaturated and saturated fatty acids. LNA is an essential fatty acid. The body can in most cases efficiently convert LNA to EPA and DHA over a few steps. So, LNA is the basis from which all of these important fatty acids can potentially be derived. LNA strongly attracts oxygen and light, which are the keys to their importance, and the downfall to their instability. The omega-3 fatty acid in flax, alpha-linolenic, is a very unstable oil. For this reason, I do not recommend buying it bottled in a store. Very simply buy the whole seed in a bag, refrigerate, and use as needed. When ready, throw the requisite amount into a coffee grinder, and grind away. Those little shells are the best way of preserving those oils. This way, you'll be able to digest all of the benefits of flax seed, and not just a partly rancid oil with fewer benefits.

Deficiencies in LNA number so many, that they will not be listed. So, how do they help with the diseases of the day? They increase our metabolic rate, aiding in fat loss. They aid in oxygen transfer in the lungs, within the cells, and essentially everywhere else. LNA is a part of the cellular membrane, as well as the membranes of the organelles. LNA facilitates the conversion of lactic acid to water and carbon dioxide. LNA improves skin quality, reduces inflammation, enhances the stability of cell division, speeds healing, reduces platelet stickiness and blood pressure, and is required for brain development and virtually every other process in our body. As you can see the oil of flax is valuable to our health, but the whole food offers up even more benefits.

Please don't start eating vast amounts of ground flax seed. According to Dr Artemis Simopoulos, you should eat no more than three to four tablespoons per day since flax has chemicals that can interfere with your thyroid gland. Again, moderation is key, just as it is for soy, which can also interfere with your thyroid. There is fairly extensive data linking soy consumption to thyroid issues in adults and infants. As we already know, estrogens impede the thyroid, which is why most thyroid patients are women. If you are hypothyroid, it may be sound advice to avoid soy, and limit your flax.

As for protein, seafood is far and away the number one recommended animal protein in this book. This assumes it is fresh and contaminant-free. Cold-water fish are probably better options. Some fish are farm-raised, which I do not recommend. Basically, this is the equivalent to our poor domesticated animals. The fish are fed unnatural feed, drugs are poured into the pens to prevent disease, and color is even added to the salmon. If your salmon says wild caught, then you're safe. If it's farm raised or says "Atlantic" then I suggest you avoid it. Other farm-raised fish are usually trout, catfish and talapia, to name a few. If the meat and poultry says organic, that doesn't mean it's the best. They are certainly better than the other stuff in the store, but not ideal. Organic just means no genetic modification, no drugs, and no herbicides/pesticides. The animal can still be getting the wrong feed. You can still feed a steer organic corn grain, and make it sick.

As far as oils go, the answer is pretty clear-cut. This no-name dietary program of mine allows for the use of only two oils for cooking or flavor, and they are extra virgin olive oil and extra virgin coconut oil. Should you have any doubts about this conclusion, I recommend an excellent, and reasonably technical book. Read *Fats that Heal Fats that Kill*, by Udo Erasmus. When cooking with these oils you should saute or stir-fry in a pan at the lowest temperature possible to cook the food. We don't want to overheat these oils and denature them. The settings on your stove-top will probably equate to either #3 or #4.

If you haven't picked up on this yet, "Get rid of the dairy products!" Minor amounts of dairy from organic free range animals in those without allergy are OK in small amounts. Don't get too neurotic, but try to eliminate dairy products as much as possible. I know ice cream tastes great. Just don't buy it at the store until you get on track with your diet and any illnesses you may have.

What else should be eliminated? For optimal health, you should consider the following:

- No sugars
- No liquids other than clean water, home-made juice
- No processed salt (some sea salt is fine)
- No processed, preserved, chemical laden foods
- No deep fried foods
- Reduce corn consumption
- Reduce the quantity of food consumed at each meal
- Reduce canned foods
- Reduce white flour as much as possible

With that said, let's discuss white flour for a bit. White flour permeates our entire food supply. It plays a role in pasta, pizza, sandwiches, cookies, cakes, breads, and more. As we saw in Weston Price's book, white flour along with canned foods and sugars cause rampant tooth decay in quick order. Obviously, it's almost impossible to avoid it entirely, so just try to reduce it. Perhaps relegating its use to occasional pasta or a sandwich may be best.

I don't want you to get hung up in counting calories or trying to calculate what percent of your meal is coming from protein, fats, and carbohydrates. If you're exercising properly then it all becomes fairly irrelevant anyhow. If you're not exercising then use good judgment. Keep the ratios and portions reasonable. Proverbs from Okinawa and India advise you to stop eating shortly before you're full. This is likely sound advice since we know that in humans and animals one of the strongest factors in life extension is controlling for caloric intake. Be creative with your cooking, but cook nonetheless. Try not to buy your foods pre-made. Go through with the effort of the buying, cooking, and cleaning, as unappealing as that may sound. In the end it will pay dividends for your weight, health, and in your wallet.

The western world has done an amazing job over the past 200 years or so in improving life expectancy. As recently as 1900 the average life expectancy here in the U.S. was only 49 years old. You must realize that this is an average. Some people, like President John Adams, lived into their 90s, while others died at birth. With the advent of vaccinations, sanitization, and other medical and civil improvements we've extended life expectancy into the high 70s. We all assume we'll make it; that's why we have 401Ks and speak of retirement. Although each day could be our last, here in America we all plan to live a full life. It comes as a shock to us when someone doesn't, but this is very different from the rest of human history, and many places around the globe today.

Although the purpose of this book is to save you money in your healthcare, a nice benefit would be increased longevity. Once you sift through the clutter in the data, two basic things smack you in the face. You can expect to live a reasonable time in reasonable health within a secure nation with decent healthcare without going overboard on dietary measures. Hopefully your later years will be healthy and active, unlike so many older folks I hear from who say, "I'm finally retired, and look at me now. All I do is go from doctor to doctor. Don't get old." I don't think this sounds appealing to anyone.

The other option is to try to control for as many health factors as you can, and hopefully enjoy the second half of your life. The Okinawans are special, but so are other pockets of peoples around the globe who follow these basic principles. Following the dietary recommendations, physician/patient guidelines, and the use of proper integrative and preventative medicine as outlined in this book should give you the best chance to live a long, healthy life.

Chapter 11   Supplement Quality

Supplements have great potential to help with existing conditions, or in preventative care. There is also great potential for you to spend sums of money with no results. There are many really good "stories" out in the market place pushing a certain product or line. Some of these stories are more accurate than others. Whom can you trust, and what are you to believe? How does the average consumer discern one product on the shelf from another in the treatment of their own ailments?

The supplement industry has many players. These players will work through various avenues to put product on the shelf for your purchase. There are generally three separate categories from which you can purchase a supplement. You can buy in a retail setting in a store or over the internet; you can buy through a practitioner of natural medicine; or you can buy through a multi-level marketing program. There are raw materials vendors, distributors, retailers, manufacturers, and more.

What you're most familiar with is the manufacturer. These are the companies that have their product on a shelf for sale with their name on the label. There are many of these players in natural medicine. Manufacturers generally buy bulk ingredients from a wide array of raw materials vendors. They will then go on to blend, encapsulate, or package products in some way for resale. The federal government has implemented dietary supplement Good Manufacturing Practices (GMP's) on the industry, but there are still loopholes within the policy. With that said, most manufacturers make a good product, but there can be variances. It is within these variances where you can be spending money needlessly.

I generally classify supplements into three categories, but this is not all-inclusive. On the first tier you have what's called true or relative commodities. A true commodity is a product made by one single source globally, but sold under different labels or different names. Whether it's from one label at one price to a different label at a different price, they are all the same, and you can in this case shop exclusively on price. Why is this the case? Let's say you've developed a product that has good clinical data to support its use. Maybe your herb is more potent, your delivery technology is better, or the way you manufacture this whole new product is patentable. Your company goes out for a few years and sells all that it can on its own, but at some point your sales plateau, at which time you offer up rights to sell your product under various other labels at whatever price they want to charge. So, in the end, two or more products with different prices and labels may be exactly the same.

In a relative commodity, it's slightly different, but the gist is still the same. Products such as DHEA, 5-HTP, acetyl-l-carnitine, calcium-d-glucarate, vitamin D and many more are essentially all the same. These products are typically made within a controlled, usually enzymatic reaction yielding huge quantities of uniform raw material. The manufacturer may offer up a different delivery system, which may or may not have added benefits, and they may formulate with more benign flow agents, fillers, and binders in the product, but in the end, if the label says 25mg of DHEA then there are usually 25mg of active DHEA in the capsule. For example, to my knowledge there are only three manufacturers globally for acetyl-l-carnitine, one of which is a pharmaceutical company. They will sell the raw materials to any given supplement manufacturer to package and sell to you. You can find analyses of supplements on a website called **ConsumerLab.com**. They typically test to verify label claims and heavy metals in retail products, but at times will perform other tests when applicable. In their testing, most manufacturers will "pass" label claim on their tests with these relative commodities.

On a higher level you have what I term herbal blends. These can be a blend of many ingredients, some of which are herbs, usually designed for a given condition, such as prostate health, liver detoxification, and so on. This tier requires a higher level of oversight, as herbs are not made like our first tier in a well-controlled laboratory environment. Not only are there many variables in the herb itself, but there may be toxins, such as pesticides, herbicides, solvents, and other "fun" ingredients you should not be ingesting. Here is where a relative lack of industry oversight can have a significant impact on your success and your wallet. There are many excellent manufacturers who bring you quality products, but there are many others concerned about meeting the letter of the law, but not the spirit of the law. In a moment, I will provide you with numerous examples of flawed products. I want you to appreciate that all items on the shelf are not created equal.

The last tier I will mention is what I refer to as the "hard to make stuff." The best example of this is probiotics. In my opinion, this is probably the most difficult product to make in the industry. To begin, even though the probiotic strain may be the same, there are differences within the strain. Let's take lactobacillus acidophilus, the most well known strain. These bacteria can be selectively bred to be hardier in acid resistance and temperature just to name two qualities. Likewise, a raw materials vendor will charge more money to a manufacturer for the hardier strains. You have to consider stability during manufacturing, the shelf-life, and the survivability in passing through the acidic stomach as well. There will be more on this in the chapter on probiotics, but suffice it to say, these guys are tough to make, keep alive, and get to where they need to be.

There are many great stories in the industry, much like any other industry. Some things are gimmicks, some are founded in truth. Some products are made better than others for a variety of reasons. Some products you should strongly consider as a part of your daily regimen, and some are a total waste of money. Even with many good products and manufacturers out there, this industry deservedly has a bad name for several reasons, and it's something that irks me. I believe natural medicine has a high likelihood of success with the right diagnosis, with certain conditions, using the right products at the correct dose, and with other incorporated measures, such as dietary changes.

Unfortunately, many of you have purchased products off the shelf, with no results. "That was a waste of money" is the usual retort. Let's look at the many obstacles you have in treating yourself with natural medicine, reinforcing the need for someone with knowledge and integrity to assist you in your endeavor. We will dedicate this chapter to four major topics: manufacturing, labels, unsupported efficacy, and independent lab results. I will hopefully give you enough knowledge to make more intelligent decisions. If you continue to spend $10, $20, or more a month on supplements that aren't well made, or aren't appropriate for your condition or goals, then this section is well worth it.

What are the potential reasons that natural medicine will fail you?

- You may only be taking one product for a complex condition that may require several. Conditions frequently require more than one supplement for various reasons.
- The product you purchased may not contain the ingredient or potency listed on the label.
- The product that you are taking has not been shown to have any efficacy in independent well-built clinical trials either for the condition in which you are using it or for any condition at all.
- The product contains a nutrient that should work for the given condition, but the form or delivery of the nutrient is wrong for whatever reason.
- Your diagnosis is wrong.
- You have chosen the wrong product or dose for your condition.
- The patient doesn't comply with the treatment protocol.
- There is no natural remedy effective for the condition.
- Patient variability. Some things work in some people and not in others.
- You may have nutritional factors, such as deficiencies or allergies, which may complicate the situation.
- You may not be absorbing the nutrients, as agents such as magnesium stearate inhibit this process.
- You may have an undiagnosed issue.

Of the reasons I defined above, this chapter will only address those related to product quality. I get questions all the time on what products to take. As consumers, we look for direction in our purchases. Most people who take supplements believe that they are of some value to their health. In 1990, a Harvard based survey found that about 33% of Americans were utilizing some form of alternative medicine. In 2002, a government survey found that number had grown to 36%, and again in 2007 to 38%. Patients with insomnia, pain, anxiety, and chronic diseases are usually placed by their doctor into a misdiagnosis basket, such as IBS and Chronic Fatigue/Fibromyalgia. Many others use natural medicine for a variety of other issues. Why don't more people? Well, to this day the vast majority look at natural medicine as a "last resort" when modern medicine has failed. They also justifiably view it with skepticism. The whole paradigm has to shift. Natural medicine should be viewed as either a form of preventative medicine, part of an integrative approach, a sole approach, or of no use, depending on the situation. Until we see solid clinical results, an industry with excellent quality control, relative consensus on treatment protocols, and an overall higher quality of care, this usage number will probably not go much beyond 50%.

There are thousands of brand names, and tens of thousands of individual products, so addressing each one is impossible. Realize that at all times someone is trying to separate you from your money. Some offer up a valid product in return, and some don't. Manufacturing, raw materials, and quality control can vary quite substantially, producing products from efficacious to useless to downright harmful. In 1994, Congress passed the Dietary Supplement Health and Education Act (DSHEA) to regulate supplements, which was an attempt to implement quality control. In 2007, the FDA announced what is referred to as the "Final Rule," which is an updated list of measures on quality control in the industry. The rule is meant to ensure that dietary supplements are produced under quality control, they do not contain impurities or contaminants, the products are accurately labeled, and a measure is in place for the reporting of adverse events. It was phased in over three years, and the last phase of implementation was in June of 2010.

The "Final Rule" is a move in the right direction, that is for sure. This industry needs quality control for the benefit of all, at the expense of the few who are out for the quick buck. However, as mentioned, it does have loopholes. Let's first start by looking at a number of examples why standardized quality control is needed for the betterment of the industry, and for the health of America.

A Canadian study published in the *Journal of Natural Products* in 1991 found that no North American feverfew product that was analyzed contained the recommended minimal amount of 0.2% parthenolide believed to be required for effectiveness. Feverfew is frequently used for migraines, and parthenolide is the natural compound for which the product is standardized.

The *Washington Post* in 2006 posted the results from a *Consumer Reports* analysis of 18 multivitamins. They found that nearly half of the tested brands failed to contain the labeled amount of at least one nutrient, and several did not dissolve adequately.

A study lead by a UC Davis public health expert found 8 out of 9 herbal kelp supplements had higher than acceptable arsenic levels.

A study published in the *American Journal of Clinical Nutrition* in 2001 found that of the ginseng products tested, they contained from 12% to 328% of the active ingredient listed on the bottle. A previous ginseng study from 1979 found that 24% had no ginseng at all.

ConsumerLab.com reported on seven garlic products that failed a round of testing. The cause of failure was predominantly related to a lack of the active compound allicin. In each instance the products only yielded a fraction of the label claim, or a fraction of what should have been present for the given product. One claimed to provide 25,000 ug of allicin, but only yielded 63 ug, while another had no allicin at all.

In a study out of Seattle, lactobacillus supplements were analyzed from 20 manufacturers. The researchers found that only one brand had a match for what was in the pill as compared to their label claim. 30% had contaminants. 20% had no growth of the probiotics, implying the beneficial bacteria were dead, and consequently would be of no benefit when taken.

An analysis of ginkgo biloba from Environmental Nutrition in 2003 found that only 22% of the gingko products tested met quality standards. Gingko is a very popular herb used to help with cognitive function.

When 59 retail echinacea products were analyzed for label claim versus content, the results weren't pretty here either. Published in 2003 in the *Archives of Internal Medicine*, it was shown that 6 contained no measurable echinacea, and only 31 of the 59 had assay results that were "consistent" with the label claim.

In 2003 the FDA cited that 5 of 18 soy and/or red clover products contained only 50-80% of the quantity of isoflavones stated on the label. In a separate analysis, they stated that 8 out of 25 probiotic products analyzed contained less than 1% of the good bacteria claimed on the label, which was still alive and viable.

Here's another interesting analysis from **ConsumerLab.com**. They looked at glucosamine and/or chondroitin products and failed a number for mostly lacking ingredients as compared to label claim. One contained only 51% of its claimed chondroitin although it claimed to be "manufactured under strict quality control to ensure the optimum in purity, potency, and reliability." Another had no detectable chondroitin despite claiming to be "the highest quality chondroitin sulfate supplement ever developed." Yet another contained only 8% of its claimed chondroitin, while two others fell short on label claim. The last defect failed because the product did not disintegrate in the allotted amount of time.

A study published in the *Journal of AOAC International* in 2007 found that 35% of the bilberry products sold in the U.S. did not match their label claim, and 10% didn't even contain the active principal. Commentary on bilberry published in the *Alternative Medicine Review* in 2007 by Al Czap at Thorne Research notes that an independent lab states, "Many of the bilberry samples they have analyzed contained inactive ingredients colored with synthetic dyes."

Rick Liva of Vital Nutrients published lab results from his experience in the journal *IMCJ* back in 2008 lab results from his experience. These were all analyses on individual raw materials to be used in manufacturing supplements. This is an example of a proper screening process where quality control measures help ensure a better product. He showed that one particular bilberry extract failed to pass the identity test, three batches of black currant seed oil were rancid, an organic wild yam root and a milk thistle extract had a high aflatoxin content, a curcumin extract, 2 milk thistle extracts, and one DIM raw material each contained a toxic solvent, as well as other raw materials that did not meet the raw material label claims.

To continue with probiotics we'll reference a **ConsumerLab.com** analysis. They found that four failed a test due to low probiotic counts. Three contained significantly less viable probiotics than the label claimed, and one didn't even make a label claim for dose, but the amount was essentially useless therapeutically.

ConsumerLab.com looked at 10 St. John's Wort products, and only three passed. Of the seven that failed, three did not comply with label regulations stating herb part used, two had less herb than label claim, and two failed due to heavy metal contamination. One exceeded the World health Organization (WHO) levels for cadmium by over 100% even though it was organically grown.

Let's talk a bit about heavy metals, particularly lead. The FDA does not set the standards for toxic metal content in dietary supplements, but instead leaves that up to the manufacturer. I think this qualifies as a hole in the "Final Rule". Seemingly their general policy statement in regards to lead is to reduce lead levels to the lowest amount that is practicable in manufacturing. The FDA does set guidelines that are <u>not</u> legally binding for a few products, such as no more than 750 ug of lead per daily serving in calcium. As an additional reference, the FDA sets a standard of no more than 5 ug of lead per liter of bottled water. A different agency, the EPA, sets a standard of no more than 15 ug of lead per liter of drinking water, three times as much. In Canada, they have set a daily limit based on weight. So, for an average person weighing in at about 60 kg, the limit would be placed at 17.4 ug/day. There are many other rules and guidelines for products based on consumer attributes, such as age, weight, or gender.

So, as you can see, it can get quite confusing. The state of California has not surprisingly imposed the strictest standards. Their law, referred to as Prop 65, allows for lead levels only up to 0.5 ug per daily serving. One could consider the California law a bit extreme, but no one wants to ingest more lead than they have to. Since it's really the only hard reference point to use, we'll refer to it in the following reports. Keep in mind that the FDA policy seems to be for manufacturers to reduce the amount of lead to the lowest amount practicable. Considering that a 2008 FDA analysis on 324 multivitamins yielded an average lead content of .576 ug/day, it seems quite possible that the Prop 65 guidelines can be reasonably met. This Prop 65 allowance is achievable, considering for each failure I can find due to heavy metal toxicity, there are even more products that passed.

Consumerlab.com tested 13 gingko products, and seven failed. Three failed due to lead toxicity. Lead limits were set at 0.5 ug in a daily serving, in accordance with the State of California standards. One had 16.6 ug, one ranged upwards of 12.1 ug, and another had upwards of 1.68 ug per daily serving..

Published in 2004 in *JAMA*, researchers Robert Saper and others looked at 70 Ayurvedic medicines available through retail outlets in the greater Boston area. Ayurvedic medicine is India's version of natural medicine, although it's more first line therapy than over here. The researchers found that 20% of the tested products contained the heavy metals lead, mercury, and/or arsenic. The range of lead seen was from 5 ug to 37,000 ug per daily serving, with an average of 40 ug.

In a follow-up to this analysis, the same researchers looked at Ayurvedic products available on the internet. In 2008 they published this round of information, which was as unflattering as the first. Of the 193 products tested, almost 21% were found to have detectable levels of lead, mercury, or arsenic. They concluded that several of these products could result in **lead and/or mercury ingestions 100 to 100,000 times greater than acceptable limits**. By the way, these products were not just made in India, they were also made here in the U.S.A.

I could go on all day writing this stuff. There are countless examples of products that do not pass muster for various reasons. This upsets many of us who are passionate in this industry, because it is a discredit to our field and inhibits the potential benefit of this medicine in its proper use. So now that you are sufficiently annoyed at the fact that you may have been wasting good money on natural products, I'm going to add more fuel to this fire. I expose this not to bash natural medicine, because as you've hopefully figured out by now, I wholeheartedly support its proper use. I mention this to best inform you for your health and financial decisions, and perhaps some greater industry quality may even come of it.

I recommend that you join **ConsumerLab.com** to be informed. The paltry annual fee of $29.95 is well worth the money. Will this guarantee you success in your therapy? Absolutely not. As you read earlier, there are a wide variety of reasons for a given protocol to fail. Their analyses are very limited and their business model questioned within the industry, but they are the only game in town supplying you with any data with which to form an opinion. For now, we'll continue to focus on product quality.

Let's say you want to buy a supplement to treat a given condition. You do your research and you've determined that the manufacturer has put into the bottle what they say is on the label. Let's say the product you seek is CoQ10, and if you buy the dry powdered form, the manufacturer may have satisfied the heavy metal and form/dosing requirements. However, you are unaware that the absorption of the dry form of CoQ10 is minimal, and the product is all but useless. So let me repeat, although the product contains what it claims, and has no other quality issues, this inexpensive form of CoQ10 is money not well spent, as dry powdered CoQ10 has terrible absorption within the GI tract. This is why manufacturers these days are pairing the CoQ10 with some type of lipid to increase absorption within the GI tract. This all falls under the umbrella of delivery technologies, which you can't reasonably be expected to know.

On a side note, some raw materials vendors use propylene glycol in the manufacturing process of their CoQ10. You may better know propylene glycol as antifreeze. It's a neurotoxin, and this is ironic and unfortunate, as CoQ10 has uses in neurological conditions.

There are a whole host of tests to be run on raw materials, which work their way into a manufacturer's doorway. To complicate things further, most companies don't even manufacture their own products. Most products are contracted out, so the manufacturer has no direct oversight over quality control. For example, a company selling a line of supplements may contract out the encapsulation, bottling, labeling, or everything to the lowest bidder. You then rely on the contract manufacturer's word, if it's even given, as to the quality of the product going out under that company's name. So when you read that your bottle says something to the effect of "quality and GMPs", I'm sure it does. They all do. So if all the labels claim such great quality controls, then how was I able to generate so many flawed examples, which was a fraction of those known to me?

Published in the *Alternative Medicine Review* in 2007, Al Czap from Thorne Research oversaw an interesting quality control test of a competitor. The manufacturer in question touts that they can supply a certificate of analysis from an independent laboratory on every one of their products manufactured. So, he had a pharmacist purchase a multivitamin-mineral from said company. The pharmacist then divided the contents of one bottle into two different bottles and created his own labeling. He changed the dose of three of the vitamins on one label, while the product remained the same. He sent these two bottles back to the independent lab for label verification, although in one of the two bottles the label was inaccurate. The lab confirmed almost exactly the levels he claimed on the label, even though they were significantly altered from the actual contents. Did the lab even perform the analysis? Is something wrong in the lab? What does this say about the quality of the supplement line that touts the use of this lab to verify its products?

This list of more flawed products and methods could go on like the last, but I think you get the point. Deciphering fact from fiction between products and manufactures is time consuming. Many providers who are too busy managing all of the other aspects of their business usually take the word of the manufacturer, an ad, or a sales person. Practitioners have the added benefit of knowing what has worked in the past clinically versus the one time user. Practitioners justifiably stick with time tested products, but this doesn't preclude them from trying new products, for better or worse.

Let's get back to these labs providing verification of product quality. There currently exists no federally mandated standardization for these labs that assure quality. This is not to say they are all bad or useless. So how should we bring all labs into the fold? I am not a big fan of the federal government, but one of the few things they should be doing is protecting the consumer. So as you see, it's a tricky path out there. The industry is self-regulating from the supplier, to the manufacturer, to the independent labs. You hope to find a product or two that is able to surpass these potential missteps. And yes, there are even more considerations as well.

Your better manufacturers will perform what is called a dissolution test, which tests to see if the finished product breaks apart within an allotted amount of time within the GI tract so that it can be absorbed. Disintegration can depend on the pH of your GI tract, binders, and the time of exposure. So if a given product does not break apart as it should, then in the best case scenario you won't absorb the nutrients. In a bad scenario, you could have one of these little guys lodge into the orifice of the appendiceal remnant (the entry way of the appendix).

Beyond dissolution and the other aforementioned issues, we need to concern ourselves with other components of quality control. So far we've covered identification of the active component and whether it is at the dose listed on the label, heavy metal screening, dissolution, and labeling compliance. Briefly touched on much earlier were other components to consider. Microbiology screening tests for bacteria, fungi, and parasites. Aflatoxin tests look for toxins left behind by members of the fungi world, which can be carcinogenic. Solvents are used extensively to concentrate standardized doses, and being toxic, should also be screened. Likewise, fungicides, herbicides and pesticides should be screened. We should round this out with shelf life testing, which is most applicable in the example of probiotics. If I were you, I'd shy away from a probioitic that gives you a CFU count based on the time of manufacture, and instead look for a product that ensures a given count to the time of expiration.

Should you want to take things further, you may want a product that comes from a facility that cleans its equipment after every batch, and perhaps has separate ventilation. If you are sensitive to anything that could cross contaminate from another batch on the same line, I'd take that into consideration. Another area with which to invest some time is that of fillers, binders, capsule/gelcap constituents, flow agents, lubricants, colorants, preservatives, and more. These "extra" ingredients can affect absorption, tolerability, and/or toxicity of your product.

Binders, fillers, and lubricants are excipients. These are used to ensure consistency of product. Magnesium stearate, which is made of magnesium and stearic acid (a fat), is used as an inexpensive lubricant to ensure that the raw material does not stick to the machinery. This ensures a consistent product for you to consume. Tablets cannot be manufactured without these excipients, but capsules can. These substances may come from corn, wheat, or dairy. Should you be sensitive to any of these, then your experience may be more than what you had hoped for. A better philosophy may be to add excipients that serve their role, but also act synergistically with the active ingredients in the product. Even better would be to avoid them altogether, which is why I use capsules as much as possible.

I'm assuming you've now gathered that all products on the shelf are not created equal. Why is that? The answer is the same as it is for so many other things in life--money. These steps come at a cost. Have you heard the phrase, "You get what you pay for"? That is mostly true in this industry. Of course, there's some overpriced crap out there too. So do your due diligence, and spend your money wisely. You have to understand that many products are built as inexpensively as possible because that is how most of you spend your money. You have to realize that your shopping habits are a part of sales and marketing. The powers that be calculate what percent of you will buy the cheapest bottle, how many will settle in the middle, and who will reach for the pricey stuff. So in effect, much of the cheap stuff is on the shelf because that's how many people shop. Some is OK for use, but some is not.

Picture yourself in a store, and you're reading labels, and all you know is you want 100 mg of CoQ10. You may more often than not pick the least expensive product on the shelf, figuring they all say the same thing. They all are unlikely the same, and although there may be no real differences among the real cheap stuff, there may be significant ones as you go up the ladder in price. This is why there is a need to be an educated consumer, as you are shopping for your healthcare, but with minimal direction.

So how should you go about determining a quality product from the rest? It's hard to rely on asking many folks, since they either don't know or have a vested interest. So what should you do? Here are some basic questions to ask.

- I suggest you join **ConsumerLab.com**. At the very least they will clue you in as to whether the product you are considering buying has the appropriate amount of active ingredient as shown on the label, its potential for heavy metal contamination, and a few other tidbits dependent on product.

- Find out if the company in question makes their own stuff. Only about 3% do. If they do, then they probably have their own lab for quality control, but you should verify that. If they use an outside lab, inquire about them. Hop on any relevant websites, and don't be afraid to call a manufacturer.

- Do you meet all of the Final Rule requirements, or do you exceed them? If so, then how?

- Have you been independently certified for cGMP compliance? By whom? If so when was the last time? Can you refer me to any independent testing agencies?

- When testing raw materials, do you test every lot for identification, potency, microbiology, heavy metals, toxins, shelf-life, and dissolution?

- Find a healthfood store with a knowledgeable attendant. Let common sense help you. If you have a teenager telling you to take something, maybe you should find out more. Ask for credentials. Ask for any clinical data to support its use. They may even have a computer up and running, and the employee or owner can show you how to work Pubmed. They may have books for your reference, or can suggest articles to read.

- If you're working with a practitioner, ask them how they screen the products they carry. Do their manufacturers have QA/QC on their own products, or do they just take the word of a contractor?

Beyond these points, you will want to consider the ingredients. If you are a strict vegetarian, you may want to take special notice of the materials used to make gelcaps and capsules. They are usually made from gelatin, which comes from animal parts. You may want to look for additional ingredients that may be allergenic. I like to see as few "other ingredients" as possible. If you have hypochlorhydria (low stomach acid) you may want to keep away from the words stearic/stearate. Look for natural colorants, such as beet, as opposed to synthetics. You may want to choose a line that utilizes a number of capsule sizes, which will decrease the fillers needed. If there are numerous "other ingredients," and if you can't pronounce the names, then look elsewhere.

Beyond the ingredients, you'll want to consider clinical efficacy. What is this term clinical efficacy? It means that a given product or ingredient has been studied in a clinical trial and proven to be valid to a certain degree for a given disease state. So what does that mean? Well, we could take just about any ingredient. Let's take 5-HTP, which is a precursor to serotonin, which is in turn a precursor to melatonin. In 1991, Swiss researchers, Poldinger and others published in *Psychopathology* a trial in which they compared 5-HTP at 100mg to an SSRI called Luvox at 50mg, three times a day for six weeks for depression. The improvement in the 5-HTP arm was 61% as compared to 56% for the drug. So in this instance, 5-HTP was compared to a drug in a controlled clinical trial, which was published in what's called a peer-reviewed journal. The theory behind these peer-reviewed journals is that its rigorous requirements for admission imply only quality trials are published, but this is not always the case. 5-HTP has many other trials to attest for its reasonable efficacy.

5-HTP is a relative-commodity single ingredient widely available, and so the data on it would apply to all standard 5-HTP products across the marketplace. This is an instance where the ingredient had been studied, and not the actual product itself. Beyond this you could take into consideration the bulk of all the clinical data, trial quality, and so on to determine a trend, but that's a bit much for now.

Researchers could also conduct a study on an individual product, which may or may not be patented, such as a brand of fish oil, a brand of CoQ10, a brand of probiotic, or a branded blend of ingredients. That trial would tend to support that general ingredient as a whole, but with more specificity of support for the actual product itself, especially if it is unique.

Try not to fall into the trap of using a product with no data in its support. Although there are many ingredients, and many products that have clinical data to support their use, there are also a number of ingredients available to you that do not have support in the data. These ingredients survive off of heresay. My uncle's friend's cousin used product X and got great results. Well, could the results have come from something else? This is why we measure potential medicines in clinical trials. Clinical trials are certainly not perfect; in fact they can have several flaws. However, heresay has even more flaws.

So in your search for clinical data that may or may not validate a product you are considering for a given disease state, here are some steps that may help. To begin, in 1994 the Dietary and Supplement Health and Education Act (DSHEA) allowed what are called structure-function claims. These mild claims are what you see on bottles where a product claims to help a particular body function. In regards to the more hard-hitting clinical data, which allows drugs to make disease state claims, the following apply for supplements.

In short, retailers, manufacturers, and distributors are permitted to distribute educational information written by an unvested third party that makes claims for natural substances, as long as the information is balanced, accurate, and does not mention a particular brand name. That may sound restrictive to you, but there is plenty of clinical data out there on natural substances. Some of it supports its use. Some of it does not. So how do you come by this information? Ask for it. If you're buying products from your provider, ask for products that have been clinically validated as much as possible. Then ask for the data, which could be supplied by the manufacturer. If you are in a retail setting, do the same. Companies are more than happy to supply data that supports the use of their product, whether it's a commodity-like product like 5-HTP, and especially when it's proprietary.

A word of caution on the proprietary items. The research can often be sponsored in obvious, or less obvious ways by the company that sells it. This may or may not skew the data. Should your quest for valid data fail, then there is yet another wonderful website to come to your aid. Housed at the NIH, **PubMed.com** is a website that carries as much clinical data as you can handle, and is available to you free of charge, sort of. You can conduct searches off of key words relevant to your needs, or perform more advanced ones. Depending on your search, you could get hundreds of articles. This is the core research. This is the stuff you hear referenced in the news when some talking head states, "Such and such a drug has been found to reduce the number of deaths from disease X." The study may show a drug is harmful as well, which may lead to its recall. The same applies for natural medicine, and a host of others that require validation. You may be able to print off the complete trial "full text" for free, or you may have to order it and pay. It will take you a while to get the hang of it, but when you do it is quite valuable. Website: **www.ncbi.nlm.nih.gov/pubmed/** or just type **pubmed.com** into your searchbox and select the first option. Keep in mind that some of these studies are in animals, and some are in vitro. Some are very dense, and some easy to read. Some are poorly constructed, and some are well done. The site will even give you similar papers listed to the far right, to aid you in your search. I highly recommend you spend time reading from this website, to aid you in your endeavors.

On a different note, if you are seeing a practitioner of natural medicine, and you're buying your supplements through them, the costs can become quite high. You have a few options at your disposal. You could ask the practitioner to "work with you". Many will. I'd rather see you on more supplements for less money to get you the proper results. In the end, this is a mostly referral-based business. Your success = practitioner success. Also, consider that some products are relative commodities. Ribose, betaine HCL, most B vitamins, ascorbic acid (a form of vitamin C), bromelain, GABA, lipoic acid, NAC, TMG, and calcium citrate are others in addition to those I've already mentioned to you.

So now that you're armed with all this information, you're in a store looking at the shelves and you are completely overwhelmed with your choices. Where do you start? How do you decide what you're willing to spend money on? For all intents and purposes, let's assume that all of your choices have in the bottle exactly what they claim on the label. Let's also assume that all of your choices met all of the quality standards set forth earlier in the chapter in regards to heavy metals, toxins, etc. So now we've boiled this scenario down to just a few last considerations, centering mostly around price. We'll look next at dosing, delivery, and patented ingredients.

Dosing

We'll discard any differences in taste, pill burden (the number of pills per day), texture, and form (liquid vs solid, powder vs pill, pill size) as these differences are obvious. So, let's begin with our system of weights. You see little letters, such as g or mg, after your ingredient; what do they mean? "g" stands for gram; "mg" stands for milligram, or 1/1000 of a gram. So if you had an ingredient at 500mg, that would be ½ of a gram. So, 1,000mg = 1 gram. "ug" or "mcg" are both considered to be micrograms, or one-millionth of a gram.

Also pay attention to the serving size. Manufacturers can throw you on this one quite easily, making you think you're getting more for your money. The serving size is the quantity of product and depends on the form needed to provide you with the dose on the label. It may take one or more pills to get you the dose stated on the label. You must also factor in the total number of pills in the container. This will help you to do some conversions to compare products on an even scale. You have to perform these conversions if you want to save some money assuming all other things are created equal.

Same single ingredients are the easiest to compare, and so we'll do a couple real-world examples now. Which would you rather purchase, assuming all else is equal?

Brand X 30mg CoQ10, 90 in a bottle (count), serving size (ss) =1, price = $14.95
Or
Brand Y 30mg CoQ10, 60 in a bottle (count), serving size (ss) =1, price = $8.50
You first need to calculate how many total mg you're getting in a bottle.
Brand X – multiply 30(mg)x90(count)=2,700mg in total in the bottle
Brand Y – multiply 30(mg)x60(count)=1,800mg in total in the bottle
Now divide, to calculate how many mg you get for a dollar
Brand X – 2,700/14.95=180mg/$
Brand Y – 1,800/8.50=212mg/$

So, with all other considerations being equal, brand Y is a better buy, since you get 32mg more per dollar spent on the bottle. Now let's do something a little more complicated. The same assumptions apply. This time we'll work with chaste tree berry extract, which is used for issues pertaining to menstruation. Which would you rather buy?

Brand A offers 225mg standardized to 0.5% agnusides, count=60, ss=1, price=$11

Brand B offers 750mg standardized to 0.5% agnusides, count=120, ss=2, price=$22.50

The 0.5% agnusides is the degree to which the product is standardized based on a particular molecule to which its efficacy is associated. In this example, they are both of the same concentration, so that's a wash. We have two different variables this time, the dosing is different per serving size, and the serving size is different. We still have to find out how many mg we get for one dollar.

Brand A – 225(mg)x60(count)=13,500 total mg in the bottle

Brand B – convert the dose of 750mg with a ss=2 into a dose for one capsule, which is 750/2=375. So you get 375mg/capsule. Now multiply the total count 120x375=45,000 total mg in the bottle.

Now calculate the mg per dollar
Brand A – 13,500/11=1,227, you get 1,227mg/$
Brand B – 45,000/22.50=2,000, you get 2,000mg/$

Obviously, Brand B is a better buy since you get considerably more mg per dollar of active ingredient. You can use this for a wide array of products available. Some calculations get trickier based on different concentrations, multiple ingredients, and other factors.

Briefly, concentrations can vary dependent on the ingredient. Let's take the enormous and complex field of herbs, and boil it down to a simple analysis on dose. We'll skip the debates on whether or not to use the whole herb or a part thereof. We'll just give you the most relevant information for a decision when comparing bottles. You may see numbers on labels that look like this, 50:1. This ratio of dry herb in a capsule means that it took 50 parts of crude herb to make one part of the concentrate. So an herb concentrate at a strength of 50:1 is more potent than an herb at 5:1. In tinctures, the numbers are the other way. A 1:5 ratio means 1 part (gram) of herb to 5 parts (ml) medium, usually grain alcohol. A 1:10 tincture takes 10 ml to yield 1 gram of herb. So a 1:5 tincture would be stronger. Fresh herb preparations are a bit different since fresh herb still has water, and is therefore less potent per unit weight. As you can guess, if you solely look at the overall dose of 500mg of herb, for example, and you miss out on the concentration component, you may have lost out on a better deal.

Delivery

It doesn't do much good to buy a product that is not absorbed well, or at all. In most cases, to get a health benefit from whatever you may be taking, it must be absorbed within the GI tract. With demulcent herbs the goal is to coat the GI tract to help an inflamed state, and therefore absorption is not an issue. The vast majority of what you take needs to get into the body to do its work. Realize you're taking something that is usually not packaged the way mother nature does, and therefore is not the same as what the body is used to. Magnesium is at the center of the chlorophyll atom, which provides a wonderful opportunity to cross the intestinal wall. Magnesium supplements are still absorbed, but to varying degrees.

Those who bring you your supplements realize this. Some make the effort to supply you with products that can be absorbed, and some don't. Providing you with a quality product made in an exacting facility comes at a cost. Companies are aware that many of you will gravitate to the lowest cost products. Once again, the consumer may not be aware of product variability, through no real fault of their own, and yet buys something that may not help in their endeavors. If they don't get better, they may tell others that natural medicine has no merit, and return to their drugs.

Many manufacturers are complexing or binding the active ingredient with something that is more absorbable. We previously covered CoQ10, and how the powder is not absorbed well, and how you're now seeing more CoQ10 bound to fatty acids for better absorption. In fact the absorption of dry CoQ10 is so bad, that manufacturers use it as a comparitor in tests to show how well their new CoQ10 is absorbed. Absorption is an issue for other things as well. A company called Indena claims that flavonoids are so poorly absorbed that rarely does more than 10% of an administered dose reach the blood. They have developed and patented what's called phytosome technology, whereby the active ingredient is complexed with phosphatidylcholine to enhance absorption. In their ginkgo product, they produced 2-4 times the blood levels as the non-phytosome herb, and in the green tea comparison theirs showed twice the blood concentration.

Similarly this has been done with an ingredient known as DIM (diindolylmethane). DIM is primarily used in hormone management, in the hopes of preventing or treating hormone dependent cancers, particularly those dependent on estrogren. A company called BioResponse has done virtually the same thing with their product. They go on to show drastic differences in absorption between their and other DIM products without the added benefit of an emulsified technology. They also claim that all clinical trials have only used their formulation.

You can research these product differences by hopping onto the internet. If you see a registered ingredient on the label, then that raw material is owned and sourced by one vendor. They will have details on their website attesting to the benefits of their unique ingredient, and may even list references to clinical data. So let's look at a few of these guys.

Patented Ingredients

In some cases you will come across ingredients that are identical from the original source. You will usually see an indication next to the ingredient to denote a registration or trademark. Additionally, sometimes there is only one global supplier for that ingredient. When you see these licensed products, they are unique in their manufacturing, and usually have some clinical data to attest to their efficacy. The data may or may not be unbiased.

Our first example is Petadolex. Petadolex contains the herb butterbur in a gelcap. It is owned by a company named Weber and Weber. They state on their website that it has been proven to reduce migraine attacks by 62%. On the shelf, all Petadolex is their Petadolex, regardless of price and label. They make the softgel. Other companies just put their label on it. However, all butterbur is not Petadolex.

OptiMSM is owned by Bergstrom Nutrition. They have a unique product through their own manufacturing process, with the subsequent research, and thus have licensed worldwide patents. MSM consists of sulfur and methyl nutrients typically associated with joint repair. If you hit the "where to buy" button on their website, they will list a number of the biggest names in supplements. They sell their raw material in bulk to these companies, which in turn bottle it up and re-sell to you. Again, all OptiMSM is the same regardless of label, but all MSM is not OptiMSM.

Suntheanine is owned by Taiyo International. They have their own process to manufacture L-Theanine for your consumption. They claim that it stimulates alpha waves in the brain, which are associated with a relaxed, but alert state. They too have their own data for your reference. On their website, some of the biggest names in retail supplements scroll on their home page, names you'll recognize. Once again, Suntheanine is Suntheanine regardless of the label, but not all theanine is Suntheanine.

I'll give you one last example. Ostivone is the registered name for a man-made isoflavone called ipriflavone. They claim that it is the only non-hormonal nutrient shown to stimulate the formation of new bone cells and inhibit the loss of healthy bone when taken with calcium. It is owned by a company called TSI Health Sciences. If bone health is a concern for you, and you see different products on the shelf with the ingredient Ostivone, then all other things being equal, calculate your "best buy" scenario accordingly.

I could provide you with more examples, but I think you get the point. I had no agenda in using these in particular. I do not use them as an endorsement, nor as an example of something to avoid. I only illustrate them for you so that you can understand some of the intricacies of the field, so you can make the best decisions for yourself. Manufacturers have to buy their raw materials somewhere, as they don't make their own raw materials. They purchased them from a number of vendors. I hope I've highlighted a way for you to determine ingredients that can be universal across several lines, thus helping to clarify your purchasing decision process.

I won't torture you with extending this list any further. We could spend a day just on herbs alone. You're not going to know if the plant was in good health at the time of harvest, if it was harvested at the right time, or if the drying process was correct. They may or may not tell you what part of the plant was used in the formulation, which can make a world of difference. You won't know how long the herb was exposed to air, light, irradiation, and/or heat, which all contribute to degradation of the product. For herbs alone, you won't know these and many more pieces of the puzzle.

I am aware that this is a bit overwhelming. I'm sure you're frustrated not knowing whom to trust, and the amount of effort it may take on your part. Again, realize that there are many good companies out there. It would be a shame if your first forays into natural medicine were failures. If buying through retail, try to follow some of the aforementioned guidelines. If working with a good practitioner of natural medicine, they should be working with companies who espouse good practices, and who hopefully follow through on their claims. In the end, it's your health and your money, and hopefully you are on track to be your primary advocate in these matters.

In the spirit of supplement quality and efficacy, we'll look into supplements over the next four chapters. You will be pounded over the head with information, which should help you to make the most informed decisions for your health. Of the numerous supplements to review, I addressed these four for several different reasons. In the end, they are all high on the list for the vast majority of Americans to consider taking.

Chapter 12   Vitamin D

Vitamin D is currently the "big thing". But, who really needs vitamin D and how much of it? Do you know your vitamin D status? Are your levels optimal for health? As with numerous nutrients, there are values in place to stave off disease, and then there are optimal values for health. There is a gray area in between for many nutrients, if not all. Vitamin D is no exception. Chances are pretty good that you are deficient. A European study reported in 1992 that 40% of young healthy adults were vitamin D deficient during the winter. (1) In another European study, 56.7% of post-menopausal Hungarian women were found to be deficient during the winter. (2) A Finnish study analyzed vitamin D in 193 girls ages 10-12. They found 78% of the girls were suboptimal. 32% of these girls had levels equal to or less than 10, classifying them as deficient, while the remaining 46% had insufficient levels topping out at 16. (3). In yet another trial, 52% of adolescent children of color were vitamin D deficient here in the states. In Boston, 32% of adults age 18-29 tested at the Boston Medical Center, were also deficient. (4) Suffice it to say, there are many of us with insufficient vitamin D levels for optimal health, so let's first get some background on this popular supplement.

Vitamin D is not even a vitamin. In its active form it is a steroid hormone. This misnomer is a vestige of the past, when the vitamin was discovered before it was known we could synthesize it. We cannot synthesize vitamins, and thus need them from our diet. We can get vitamin D from the diet as well; however, the primary source is the sun. Upon UVB ray sun exposure, a cholesterol precursor (7-dehydrocholesterol) within the skin gets "activated" into the pre-vitamin cholecalciferol. We ingest this same cholecalciferol in the form of vitamin D supplementation. It then readily undergoes what is called a hydroxylation in the liver to produce 25(OH)D, aka calcidiol. This process is seemingly not well regulated, so in other words, the more D you ingest, the more 25(OH)D you'll have in the body. The next hydroxylation in the kidneys yields the systemically active 1,25(OH)2D (calcitriol). This process is tightly regulated. This is all good. Systemically we want the active D to be kept within a fine margin so that we don't get calcification of soft tissue, but we also want optimal 25(OH)D for our many tissues to use for themselves for various health reasons, which we'll cover in a moment.

Take from this preceding paragraph a few things. There are two forms of vitamin D with which we will concern ourselves: the active form, which we'll call 1,25(OH)2D, and the precursor to the active form, 25(OH)D. Impairment of the functioning of either the liver or kidneys may inhibit your active D synthesis. We need sunlight or supplementation, because dietary sources are, for all practical purposes, not enough. Sunlight through windows doesn't count. The big hitters from the diet come from sardines, mackerel, tuna, and salmon. Wild salmon provides significantly more vitamin D than farm-raised, about 981IU from one 3.5 oz serving. Researcher Michael Holick has found that farm raised salmon may only contain 10-25% of the vitamin D in wild caught salmon. This is only one of several areas in which farm raised salmon is inferior. As Weston Price mentions in his work, "With the *remote possibility* of egg yolk, butter, cream, liver, and fish it is manifestly impossible to obtain any amount of vitamin D worthy of mention from common foods."

Let's consider our ancestors, and use some common sense for a moment. Assuming we can reasonably agree that our ancestors originated in warmer climates, possibly Africa, then we can establish our foundation. Over hundreds of thousands of years our forebearers were exposed to plenty of sunlight, much more sun than we get here in the states. They spent their lives outside, while we mostly don't. When we do get sun, we have been trained to go nuts with sunscreen. An SPF of 15 will decrease your ability to make vitamin D by 99%. They didn't wear clothes, while we do. For those who migrated to colder climates, a gradual sensitization of the skin to sunlight occurred in the form of lighter color. These people too, spent much time outside in the sun, and as you move up in latitude, the color of skin evolved to be more sensitive. Given our lifestyles, most of us are not getting the sunlight we were programmed to get throughout our evolution. This explains why people of darker skin need an estimated 5-10 times more time in the sunlight to synthesize D, according to researcher Michael Holick. For example, Africans who had nearly constant exposure to the sun evolved a combination of dermatological genes that protected them from the rays of the sun, while still making enough vitamin D. The ancestors who migrated from the continent, particularly to colder climates, required less skin protective features, and more attributes to make the most of D production when they did get sun.

Until recently, vitamin D was only discussed when addressing rickets, and consequently bone mineralization. An amazing amount of relatively recent research on vitamin D has shed a great deal of light on its importance in many other facets of our health. It really only stands to reason, doesn't it? Who doesn't like a sunny day? Who doesn't like the warmth of the sun on their skin? Don't we look forward to the summer more than the winter, at least most of us? The sun is the source of virtually all energy. Without it, almost nothing would live. It gives us life, which is probably why it has been revered throughout human history. So now let's understand from a technical level what it does for us, and how the use of vitamin D can save us money in our healthcare, and by the way, improve our quality of life.

If you've had your D levels checked, what they are checking, or should be checking, is the 25(OH)D levels, which is a better indicator than the active 1,25(OH)2 D for several reasons. The result may be reported in either ng/ml (nanograms per milliliter) or nmol/l (nanomoles per liter). For this chapter, we will be referring to the ng/ml numbers. There is no established standard reference range for your D labs, but the minimum for ideal is considered to be greater or equal to 30-32 ng/ml by many researchers. A number of other researchers agree with the afforementioned minimum of 30, but with more recommended dependent on disease states. Others recommend levels into the 40s, 50s, and even higher. It's safe to say that two things are clear. The experts can't agree on a desirable value, but they all agree that the current governmental recommended intakes are way too low. I think a great indicator of an ideal value is yielded from at least three trials looking at D levels in people living and working in a sun rich environment. They found D levels from 54-65. This was D from the sun. So if you transplant us to the tropics from which we came, we could theoretically synthesize this much D outside of supplementation. Ultimately, optimal D levels will vary depending on whom you're talking to, and should vary on genetic contributions as well.

What does vitamin D do in regards to calcium? Its primary role is to aid in the absorption of calcium in the intestines. But, it also tells the kidneys not to excrete as much calcium, and it stimulates osteoblasts, which are cells that build bone. Through this calcium role, it controls parathyroid hormone (PTH), which we'll later learn is a good thing. This makes sense, since the role of PTH is to put calcium into the blood from the bone.

At very high doses, and possibly also in the absence of dietary calcium, vitamin D can pull calcium from the bone. A high PTH would stimulate the kidneys to produce active D, because the parathyroid was sensing a low calcium level. So the body reads exceptionally high D levels as a need to dump calcium into the blood. These levels are way above what's reasonable, but I just mention it to illustrate that there can be too much of a good thing.

Interestingly, it has been found that <u>most cells and tissues in the body have vitamin D receptors, not just bone</u>. In other words, there is a spot on the cellular membrane where the vitamin can bind to the cell with the end result being some type of modification in cell function. These organs include the heart, stomach, thyroid, adrenals, and more. There is another really fascinating piece of information from a number of researchers showing that inactive 25-D can be converted to active 1,25-D in various tissues and cells; thus they possess the enzymes necessary to do so. Remember we said earlier that this was done in the kidneys. <u>This ability to make active D locally</u> has also been found in the brain, pancreas, breast, macrophages (part of our immune system), epidermis, parathyroid, and intestine. Said another way, vitamin D has systemic effects in ways we never understood with the ability to positively impact our health. Your body does not have to wait for the kidneys to make more active D. Instead, numerous organs in your body can make their own, utilizing an increased level of inactive D, from the sun, diet, or supplements. So, let's look at some interesting studies.

It would appear from the research, that vitamin D has possible uses in both diabetes type 1 and 2, musculoskeletal pain, cardiovascular disease, osteoporosis, fertility, certain cancers, psoriasis, fibromyalgia, menstrual migraines, and more. I will touch on a few of these disease states below. Understand there is much more data, but I tried to identify some of the strongest correlations between disease and vitamin D administration/deficiency.

Diabetes

The incidence of type 2 diabetes in the United States is astronomical, and getting worse. Due to our very poor diet, and sedentary lifestyles, here in the states we have more than 1 million new cases diagnosed per year. As a total, about 7% or some 21 million Americans are affected by this "disease". The federal government estimates that by 2050 approximatley 48 million Americans will have type 2 diabetes if nothing changes in prevention and treatment between now and then. This will absolutely crush us financially.

How about cost? The American Diabetes Association estimates that in 2007, the cost of diabetes in the U.S. exceeded $174 billion. They take into account $116 billion in excess medical costs that are attributed to diabetes, and another $58 billion in reduced productivity. They also say that people with diabetes have about 2.3 times the healthcare costs as compared to others. All considered, about 1 in every 10 healthcare dollars are attributed to the care of diabetes. That is an astonishing cost considering that most cases are preventable, given their strong association to obesity, which is a lifestyle choice.

How about life expectancy? Depending on whose statistics you reference, diabetes is the fifth leading cause of death in the U.S. Most cases of type 2 diabetes can be avoided through simply changing habits. A study published in the *New England Journal of Medicine* made headlines, estimating that they expected the steady rise in life expectancy over the past two centuries to possibly come to an end. The manifestations of obesity as expressed in cardiovascular disease and diabetes will likely reduce the life expectancy of our children by about 5 years if things remain unchanged. In a separate analysis looking at the famed Framingham Heart Study, diabetic men and women died on average 7.5 and 8.2 years earlier respectively than those who did not have diabetes.

So whether you want to live longer, live healthier, or reduce your healthcare costs along the way, it is your choice whether or not to tackle your health. I will add my personal prediction to all of this as well. I have been saying for the past few years that I expect our U.S. life expectancy to begin a reversal in the near future. There have been great gains made in the cessation of smoking, which has had enormous benefit, most notably in the reduction of lung cancer. As we see those numbers get thrown into historical averages, they will begin to get overtaken by less appealing numbers. Cancer, cardiovascular disease, diabetes and other diseases will begin to ramp up as time passes. In 10 or maybe 20 years, you will see a significant reduction in our U.S. life expectancy numbers. We are living with polluted water, poor food, high stress, and sedentary life styles. Drugs may very well begin to reach the limits of their effectiveness, assuming they are effective in the first place. These are all choices we make. Whether or not you choose to exercise, supplement, drink clean water, eat healthy food, or reduce your levels of stress, it is a decision that has long-term consequences. So let's refocus on diabetes for a moment, and consider supplementation of vitamin D as an affordable consideration for your health.

The pancreas, or more specifically the beta cells of the pancreas, is the site of insulin production. As stated previously, the pancreas has vitamin D receptors, as well as the enzyme 1-alpha hydroxylase, which is necessary to make active D, the 1,25(OH)2D. We know that a vitamin D deficiency reduces insulin secretion in humans, plays a role in insulin resistance, and, conversely, an improvement in levels to regenerate beta-cell function and glucose tolerance. We also know that obesity itself, a huge contributor to type 2 diabetes, is associated with a vitamin D deficiency. Fatty acid synthase is an enzyme that converts calories into fat. Higher vitamin D and calcium levels inhibit this enzyme, while lower levels increase its production significantly. So, the more vitamin D you have floating around, the less likely you are to put on additional weight, the more likely you will produce higher levels of insulin, and the more likely your cells will respond to the insulin thereby taking up sugar from your blood, which is a good thing.

Not to be discounted in all of this is the impact of genetic variations across the board in making and using vitamin D. The most used, and probably best-identified gene regulating vitamin D is that of the vitamin D receptor (VDR). Although I believe this to have a role in some, the vast majority simply don't get enough intake of vitamin D. This vitamin D genetic flaw is probably best addressed here in the diabetes subsection, as we have sufficient data with which to elucidate this point. We know that mutations within this gene are associated with diabetes, Addison's, Graves, and Hashimotos disease. (5) In addition, compromises in this gene have also been associated with breast, colon, and prostate cancer, and, of course, bone mineral density. Its role is seemingly not only in affecting the beta cell function of the pancreas, but also as that of an anti-inflammatory modulator. In regards to type 1 or even type 2 diabetes, for that matter, the best course of action is that of prevention. It has been shown that in type 1 diabetes, if vitamin D is administered before the formation of the circulating antibodies to the beta cell, vitamin D can be expected to achieve a much higher level of success than if administered afterwards. In fact, if you do wait, and the antibodies do form, it has been shown that the successful administration of vitamin D would then also requires a T-cell immunosuppressant (6). Used preventatively, it has been shown that vitamin D intake has the capacity to prevent or significantly reduce the development of type 1 diabetes.

To illustrate this preventative medicine component, a very interesting study published in the *Lancet* in 2001, monitored over 10,000 infants born in 1966 in northern Finland for vitamin D intake, and years later for type 1 diabetes development through to 1997. Yes, that's 31 years later. It was found that those who as infants who took 2,000 IU/day or more of vitamin D *during their first year of life*, and presumably beyond, had almost a 78% less chance of developing type 1 diabetes than those who did not supplement. Those suspected of rickets in the first year of life, i.e., those with a vitamin D deficiency, showed three times the risk of developing type 1 diabetes. This tells us on both sides of the equation that vitamin D can play a significant role in diabetes prevention and/or causation. (7) It has also been shown that increased vitamin D intake during pregnancy significantly reduced beta cell autoimmunity in the corresponding offspring. Cod liver consumption during pregnancy and infancy has also been shown to reduce the occurrence of type 1 diabetes. How about type 2 diabetes? After all, some 90% of all diabetes cases out there are of the type 2 variety.

Type 2 diabetes is characterized by reduced insulin secretion and/or insulin resistance. Vitamin D has been shown to improve upon both of these parameters. Does that mean that vitamin D is the cure for diabetes? No. It is a tool available to you in this battle.

We know that vitamin D supplementation improves insulin secretion in response to an oral glucose load in those with mild type 2 diabetes, in healthy subjects, and in those with a vitamin D deficiency. We also know that when vitamin D levels are restored in those with a deficiency, glucose tolerance is improved. It has also been shown that women with type 2 diabetes show an improved insulin response with vitamin D supplementation. Further evidence shows us that vitamin D treatment for those with osteomalacia, which is a compromise in bone mineralization resultant from a vitamin D deficiency, improves insulin secretion and glucose tolerance. (8) Additionally, several studies show that diabetics have poorer glycemic control in the winter, which is a connection not hard to make to vitamin D.

It must be noted that all trials do not support the connection. This shouldn't be surprising, since this is true for most everything in medicine, which is why the public is so often confused as to what is, and what is not healthy. However, most case control studies show that patients with type 2 diabetes or glucose intolerance have been found to have lower serum D concentrations than those without diabetes.

If you look at the preponderance of data, there is a correlation between diabetes, both type 1 and type 2, and vitamin D. Sure, there are studies small and large, short duration and long, varying on gender, disease state, ethnicity, and other components of trial design that seem to point in different directions. However, if you look at the complete picture of all of the data, and apply some common sense based on what we know vitamin D does in the body on a cellular level, you can come to the same conclusion. Also, when you consider broad epidemiology best expressed in studies looking at sun exposure via latitude, you can find more support for this conclusion.

Cancer

The evidence for vitamin D and cancer prevention and/or treatment is strong theoretically, good epidemiologically, and mixed clinically. Why is it mixed in clinical trials? If you were to analyze the colorectal trials, the evidence is quite strong. Not only is it supported in the treatment of colon cancer, but there is a proven strong association between low vitamin D levels and increased cancer risk. Of the 30 studies analyzed in a 2006 review on colon cancer, the risk of developing colon cancer or the mortality from colon cancer was significantly improved in 20 of them when higher vitamin D status was taken into account. (9) Five of the remaining ten showed a benefit as well, but were statistically less moving, thus not deemed as a "significant" benefit. If you were to look at breast cancer, the results are promising, but not as strong. Of the 13 studies analyzed, 9 reported a favorable association of vitamin D or sunlight with cancer risk. Prostate cancer was also considered in over 26 studies. In half there was a favorable significant benefit in regards to vitamin D. As you can see, the data is mixed once again. Here are a couple of thoughts on the matter.

It is the active form of D that is seemingly responsible for the anti-cancer benefits. These benefits boil down to an improvement in the cells becoming what they were intended to become (differentiating), and the inhibition of cancerous proliferation. Remember that active D is controlled fairly strictly in serum, and theoretically most anticancer benefit is derived from the tissue taking in the 25(OH)D and converting it via the enzyme to the active form from within.

In the case of prostate cancer, it has been found that while normal prostate cells possess the 1-alpha-hydroxylase enzyme, cancerous prostate cells have this capability enormously reduced, and consequently will not respond to supplementation. (10) Said another way, you can take all the vitamin D supplementation you want, but the prostate can't convert it well to the form it needs to fight off cancer when you already have cancer. As you can guess, this is a perfect example of preventative medicine. Assuming this is the predominate factor in the potential role of vitamin D in prostate cancer, then one would be wise to keep his D levels higher in the hopes of preventing the cancer.

In another study, which included 19,000 men, those with a 25(OH)D level below 16ng/ml had a 70% higher rate of prostate cancer than those above 16. (11) That's a significant difference. It seems odd that there can be one trial that shows such significant results, and yet another that may show none. One of the major contributors to this confusion is study design. To illustrate study design flaw, and the ultimate confusion as to what's best for your health, we'll look at a poorly constructed breast cancer study.

In the Women's Health Initiative (WHI) trial, there was an arm evaluating the development or lack thereof of breast cancer. 36,282 women were randomly assigned to receive daily doses of 1,000 mg of calcium and 400 IU of vitamin D or placebo for an average of seven years. There were overlapping groups within this subset of the trial. There were other variables such as dietary modification, and hormone therapy. As a result, 69% of the women in this trial were in the dietary modification group, 54% were a part of the hormone therapy group, and 14% were a part of both subgroups. In addition, personal use of vitamin D and calcium were permitted in both the supplementation and placebo arms of this trial. The researchers allowed for up to 1,000 mg of calcium and 1,000 IU/day of vitamin D above and beyond what they may or may not have been taking. This means the voluntary vitamin D levels were 2.5 times higher than the official amount of 400 IU outlined in the trial, which seems absurd to me.

What did they find? They found that those in the calcium and vitamin D arm did not have a reduction in breast cancer. I can't say that I am surprised. One of the many flaws was that a dose of 400 IU is too low to support efficacy. The BEST results I can find in the literature for 400 IU is a bump in D values into the mid-20s, which takes more than a year to accomplish. Other data shows us that an approximate 50% reduction in the occurance of breast cancer calls for D values in the fifties. Research seems to show for the prevention of breast cancer, optimal vitamin D levels should be maintained for a lifetime, whereas this trial used postmenopausal women, a late start.

My point is that for almost every trial that makes a claim, I can find another trial that will not substantiate that claim. So, when I tell you that the data is mixed for breast or prostate cancer, there are many factors at play. Some trials are simply constructed better than others. These many variables contribute to your confusion in virtually all facets of your health.

A researcher published in a 2007 paper that an estimated U.S. savings on all cancer costs could be $16-25 billion by simply supplying America with 1,000 IU per day of vitamin D. (12) This just considers cancer, and not a wide variety of others conditions that could be helped. It may be just an estimate, but a fraction of that $16-25 billion wouldn't be shabby. What if HMOs issued vitamin D supplementation to their members of 1,000 IU, 2,000 IU, or more a day? How would that help their bottom line?

In a meta-analysis, which is a review of existing clinical trials, it was found that there was a 50% lower risk of developing colorectal cancer at a serum D level of greater than 33, as compared with a value less than or equal to 12. Interestingly, at each quintile the risk went down proportionately with the levels of D between the two points given, or in other words, there was a precise risk/vitamin D curve, so to speak. (13)

A trial published in 2007 was looking at bone fracture incidence and cancer in 1,179 women over the age of 55 over a span of 4 years. They were given a placebo, calcium, or calcium plus vitamin D at 1,100IU per day. The women at entry were absent of known cancers, which means they may have had some at onset without their knowledge. There was a 77% reduction in all cancers in the calcium/D arm as compared to the placebo arm at year four. If you want to talk serum levels, they stated that for every 10 ng/ml increase in serum D, there was a corresponding 35% reduction in risk. Let me reiterate for you, a 77% reduced risk of cancer at four years out! (14)

One set of researchers analyzed the available data on vitamin D and cancer. What they found was quite extraordinary. They estimated that 50% of colon cancer incidence in North America could be prevented by keeping Americans at a minimum serum D value of 34. That 50% reduction would require an intake across the board of only 2,000 IU per day.(15) This conclusion was probably in part based on an earlier analysis in which most of these researchers were involved. In their review of five clinical trials on colorectal cancer, they showed a 50% lower risk for the cancer when at levels equal to or greater than 33 as compared to levels less than or equal to 12. (16) For reference, the National Cancer Institute (NCI) estimated that in 2008 about 150,000 new colorectal cancers would be diagnosed.

Those same researchers also took a look at breast cancer. They projected a possible 50% reduction in breast cancer incidence through the achievement and maintenance of a serum D level of 52 or greater. To achieve this level, they said, would require a universal 3,500 IU per day intake. Given that the NCI estimates 182,000 new cases of breast cancer in 2008, preventing 91,000 new cases would be very welcome news.

The Ludwigshafen Risk and Cardiovascular Health Study conducted in Germany published more compelling data in May of 2008. They took vitamin D levels from 3,299 patients, and followed up with the patients for about 7.75 years. 95 of the original 3,299 had died from cancer from their baseline to the end of follow-up. When the researchers controlled for other factors, they found that those who had the highest vitamin D levels had a 55% lower risk of dying from all cancers.

Cardiovascular Disease

There are many facets to cardiovascular disease (CVD). You're probably familiar with blood lipids, high blood pressure, stroke, heart attacks, angina, and congestive heart failure. You're probably less familiar with vascular inflammation and arterial calcification. There is a whole milleu of cause and effect associations within the vasculature. The end result may be death or incapacitation through heart failure or stroke. Vitamin D therapy or deficiency has been shown in many clinical trials to play a role in hypertension, left ventricular hypertrophy, congestive heart failure, vascular inflammation, heart attacks, stroke, atherosclerosis, and triglycerides. As you can see, vitamin D has been shown to likely help with whatever your current diagnosed cardiovascular condition happens to be. I will only highlight conditions around blood pressure and parathyroid hormone for you since a review of all the data is far too much for our agenda here.

The effects of a vitamin D deficiency can be seen in numerous studies to affect blood pressure. Chronic high blood pressure is not particularly good for your heart and arteries as you well know, initiating damage and inflammation. Whether in therapy or deficiency, vitamin D plays a significant role in two mechanisms behind blood pressure. Have you heard of rennin? It's an enzyme that is part of a cascade of events that causes an increase in fluid retention, referred to as the RAAS. This resorption of sodium at the kidney increases water in the serum, which in the compromised may increase blood pressure. Vitamin D therapy has been shown to inhibit this system, whereas a D deficiency has been shown to increase the activity of this system. That's pretty clear-cut, and it has been shown repeatedly. On a macro level, other studies have shown that the up-regulation of the RAAS results in an increased risk of developing high blood pressure, vascular calcification, left ventricular hypertrophy (heart enlargement), and an overall increased risk of CVD. We also know that when we breed mice to have no vitamin D receptor, their RAAS is up-regulated, and they go on to develop many of the same conditions.

Mechanism two, works via the parathyroid gland. A vitamin D deficiency results in less calcium in the blood. Reading this, the parathyroid gland sends out its hormone, PTH, to move calcium from bone to the blood. A chronic D deficiency results in a constant release of PTH, which is technically referred to as secondary hyperparathyroidism. We know from other studies that increased PTH results in increased blood pressure, inflammation within the vasculature, and a negative impact on the muscles of the arteries and heart. We also know that if you supply PTH to a normal patient, you can cause hypertension.

In a similar condition, known as primary hyperparathyroidism, the end result is the same. You have a chronic elevation in your serum PTH, just for a different reason. You still get all of the same nasty impacts of PTH on the cardiovascular system in regards to blood pressure. The way to resolve the high serum PTH in this condition is to surgically remove the parathyroid gland causing the problem. You have four of these glands, although usually only one is problematic. At least one study has shown a 40% lower risk of developing a heart attack or stroke in patients who had the problematic gland removed, and hence a reduction in PTH, as compared to the control group. (17) Let's move away from the more technical details, and get into some data with which you will better identify.

A German study measured the baseline vitamin D levels in 3,258 adults who were undergoing elective cardiac catheterization. They followed up with these patients for an average of 7.7 years. They found that the subjects in the lowest quartile of serum D had twice the risk of death, especially from cardiovascular disease, as compared to those in the highest quartile. (18)

Published in 2008, our next study looked at the association between vitamin D status and coronary heart disease (CHD). 18,225 men aged 40-75 were all free of diagnosed CVD at the start. During their 10-year follow-up, 454 men developed either a nonfatal heart attack or fatal CHD. Vitamin D deficiency was classified as those with a value of 15 or less, whereas those who were deemed sufficient had values of 30 or above. It was found that the deficient group had twice the risk of a heart attack compared to those who were D sufficient. (19)

In a trial with women over the age of 70, the calcium plus vitamin D group experienced a 9.3% decrease in systolic blood pressure, and a 5.4% decrease in heart rate as compared to the calcium only group. The amounts taken were 1,200mg of calcium and 800IU of vitamin D. The trial only lasted for only eight weeks. (20) In another blood pressure trial from 2007, 1,811 men and women were examined for the relationship between vitamin D and hypertension. *The risk of hypertension at four years out was over six times greater for the lower D group than the higher.* (21) The groups were defined as less than 15ng/ml for the lower end, and greater than 30ng/ml for the higher end. To reach a D value greater than 30 is not hard to accomplish at all with supplementation. In women, the risk of hypertension was almost three times as high when looking at the same parameters. These along with several other studies show a beneficial relationship between your vitamin D status and your blood pressure.

Peripheral artery disease (PAD) is atherosclerosis that is not of the coronary (heart) or carotid (neck) arteries. In a study published in 2008, researchers analyzed data from 4,839 participants. They found that those on the lowest end, having D levels less than 18 ng/ml, were more than two times likely to have PAD then those at the higher end. (22) This study is supported by other studies showing that vitamin D has a beneficial effect on the vasculature. In a similar study, researchers looked at the relationship between calcification of the coronary artery and vitamin D. Calcification is the deposition of calcium, in this instance into the plaque of the coronary artery. As you can imagine, plaque with calcium does not lend itself well to the good functioning of your arteries. These researchers found that there was a strong correlation between higher active 1,25-vitamin D levels and lower calcification. (23)

In yet another trial, 1,739 participants from the Framingham Offspring Study were enrolled to study the relationship between vitamin D and a first cardiovascular event. These subjects were followed up for an average of 5.4 years. Over this time, 120 of them developed a first cardiovascular event, such as a stroke or heart attack. They showed that for those with a vitamin D level of less than 15 ng/mL, the risk of having a first CVD event was about two times that of those over 15. (24) Fifteen is a really low vitamin D level. It would have been interesting to compare the low D group to a group above 30. The problem was that so many of these patients were D deficient or insufficient, this couldn't statistically have been shown.

Osteoporosis

You would think that with all of the calcium supplementation, dairy consumption, and general public awareness over the years in the United States, we would have eradicated osteoporosis and osteopenia (basically its predecessor). Think again. In 2004, more than 10 million people in the U.S. were diagnosed with osteoporosis. (25) In 2005, the cost for treating the approximately 2 million bone fractures resulting from osteoporosis was almost $16.9 billion. (26) That's a lot of money.

We can divide the term osteoporosis into two basic definitions, as if you and your bones really care. Primary osteoporosis occurs with bone loss as people age. I'm not a huge fan of this definition. It implies that it is inevitable. The fact is that people with appropriate lifestyles do not, by and large, develop osteoporosis. On the contrary, they get by fine on calcium intakes far lower than ours here in the states. To reiterate, osteoporosis to a large degree boils down to what you do, and what you choose not to do. If you'd like to consume a high protein and high sugar diet, smoke, avoid vegetables, drink soda, use excessive salt, and not exercise, then be my guest. We'll be counting you in the data along with millions of other Americans in the future. That $16.9 billion figure will only balloon higher. If you're relying on drugs to save you, I wish you well.

Secondary osteoporosis is caused by medical conditions, such as those of malabsorption, and by medications. Yes, medications. The very drugs you may be taking for one condition, may very well be causing another. We all know this to be true. One of the biggest reasons patients come over to natural medicine is because they want to do away with their drug because of side effects, and exchange it for a natural product, which has none, or at least in theory. The principle offender in this category are the glucocorticoids, but suspicion and maybe even fact, is strong for stomach acid blockers as well. You may know the glucocorticoids better as cortisone, prednisone, hydrocortisone, dexamethasone, methylprednisolone. When taken orally they can cause osteoporosis over the long haul. Even their package inserts state that osteoporosis is among the long-term side effects from its use, among a number of other joyous maladies. So, what is long-term use?

In a review article published in the journal *IMCJ* in 2008, Drs. Neustadt and Pieczenik quote numerous studies looking at bone health and steroids. Two studies claim that systemic corticosteroid use, such as that of oral prednisone, for more than six months has been found to increase the risk of osteoporosis. They go on to quote that even very small doses at less than 2.5mg/d (prednisone ranges from 1-50mg) for over approximately six months are associated with a 20-200% increased risk of vertebral fractures. Yet another study found that for each 10mg increase, there was an additional 62% risk in bone fracture. Lastly, another of their references states that the risk for fractures decreases after stopping the medications, showing a clear relationship. I could go on with other references, but the point is clear: long-term use of these drugs significantly contributes to the likelihood of the development of osteoporosis, as evidenced by even their package insert.

Now let's get to some data. In a British trial, 2,686 men and women over the age of 65 were given 100,000 IU of vitamin D orally once every four months for five years. I don't think this dosing schedule is ideal, but that's what they did. I think administration should mimic nature as close as possible, hence the daily dosing. In any event, after the five years, 147 of the folks had fractures in common osteoporotic sites, which were the hip, wrist/forearm, or vertebrae. There was a 33% reduction in first time osteoporotic site fracture in the vitamin D arm, as compared to the placebo. In addition, there was a 12% reduction in overall mortality. Adverse events were not seen. (27) Said another way, the risk of someone fracturing a bone in a location that is commonly associated with osteoporosis was only 2/3 the risk of those who did not take the vitamin D supplementation. This is even more interesting when you consider the age at which therapy was begun, the dosing schedule chosen, and the fact that critical additional bone building components such as vitamin K, magnesium, and calcium were not co-administered. The 12% reduction in death over that time span is a nice bonus as well.

Here's a study from the *New England Journal of Medicine* from 1992. 3,270 women were placed into two groups. One group was to receive 1.2g of calcium plus 800 IU of vitamin D and the other group a placebo. They did this for each day over 18 months, and a number of parameters were measured, to include femoral bone density, hip, and non-vertebral bone fractures. The average age was 84, and they were seemingly controlled well for other factors that may confound the results. The researchers showed that among the 1,765 women who completed the study, there were 43% fewer hip, and 32% fewer non-vertebral fractures in the D plus calcium arm. I would say that's significant. Also, of interest to note, the bone density of the femur for those on therapy increased by 2.7%, and for those on placebo, a decrease in 4.6% was seen. (28) This shows that women with an average age of 84 can still increase bone mineral density on natural medicine, and when considering the cost of bone fractures in the elderly, the cost savings is potentially enormous.

Another study took a look at both men and women. It is true that women are at the greatest risk for the development of osteoporosis, but about 5% of men over 50 will develop osteoporosis, and about a third will develop osteopenia. At the end of this 3 year study, 318 subjects completed the trial to the satisfaction of the researchers. Once again, a significant effect on bone mineralization was seen in the treatment arm that was taking 500mg of calcium and 700IU of vitamin D. This benefit was not seen in the placebo arm. Yet again, fractures were analyzed as well. The incidence of a first fracture in the treatment arm was 5.9% of the subjects as compared to 12.9% fracture incidence in the placebo arm. (29) So here is another trial that contradicts a long held belief that bone mass cannot be restored once lost, but the loss can just be slowed. Also, consider that the vitamin D level was not all that high, and other important factors, such as vitamin K, weren't utilized. Of course, there are some trials that do not support just vitamin D with calcium for bone mineralization, but we already covered these issues in bone health.

Musculoskeletal Pain/Fibromyalgia

Studies suggest that an amazing 9-20% of adults in the United States experience chronic pain. Of these, 89% have some degree of long-term or short-term disability. Additionally, it is estimated that their chronic pain costs us about $50 billion a year. (30).

What is Fibromyalgia? If you know, then please inform the rest of us. It's a catch-all basket when your provider doesn't know what to diagnose. Well, guess what? Natural medicine attracts these very same patients, those given an unclear diagnosis, where help seems to be elusive. Fibromyalgia (FM) only differs from Chronic Fatigue Synndrome (CFS) in one aspect. The primary diagnostic criteria in FM is musculoskeletal pain, while the primary diagnostic criteria in CFS is fatigue. All other symptoms are the same. Is it possible someone has been misdiagnosed?

CFS/FM could be one or more of the following conditions; lyme disease, other bacterial/viral/parasitic pathogens, adrenal fatigue, thyroid disorder, systemic candida, a food allergy, or one or more nutritional deficiencies, such as a vitamin D deficiency. This list is not meant to be all-inclusive, but probably covers most cases. I realize it is simplistic, but also relevant. For more information on FM/CFS read Jacob Teitelbaum's book, *From Fatigued to Fantastic*, or James Wilson's book, *Adrenal Fatigue: The 21ˢᵗ Century Stress Syndrome*.

Yes, I mentioned a vitamin D deficiency. Did your provider take a vitamin D level? Did he or she order the right test? Have you heard of osteomalacia? Osteomalacia is basically the adult form of rickets, which is in most cases caused by a vitamin D deficiency. It is similar to osteoporosis, but varies a bit since it is more of an inadequate mineralization than a simple demineralization. In any event, I think the two can certainly share space. What are the symptoms of osteomalacia? Well, they are fatigue, bone pain, and muscle weakness. Do these symptoms sound familiar? What if 10% of FM/CFS cases were mostly or entirely due to a vitamin D deficiency, how much money could be saved in our healthcare system? How much pain and suffering could be alleviated? How many people could go back to work and contribute? Again, it is a bit simplistic, but also relevant. The best part is it's really inexpensive to find out. So, take into consideration the following trials.

In an amazing trial done in 2000, five patients who were confined to wheelchairs for reasons of age and disease states were administered vitamin D therapy. Their confinement was due to weakness and fatigue from their condition. Treatment with vitamin D resolved body aches and pains, and, get this, all five became mobile within six weeks. (31) I'm pretty sure vitamin D costs less than the wheelchair, the pain medications, the physician care, and more. Let's not forget that there is a significant quality of life component here, and those who are younger can return to the work force as well.

Here is more fantastic proof for those of you suffering from musculoskeletal pain. You may have even been diagnosed with fibromyalgia. This illustrates for you that a deficiency in vitamin D is clearly linked to this kind of pain. Whether this is the case for you or not is up to you to discover. I would certainly think a vitamin D test is warranted, at the very least. This study was done in Minnesota. As you may gather, it could be a challenge for someone to get enough vitamin D living at that latitude, working many hours a week, and spending much of the remainder of their spare time indoors. These researchers looked at 150 patients between 2000 and 2002 who had presented with persistent, nonspecific musculoskeletal pain to the community university health care center. They were well represented by age, gender, and race. Of those who were of darker skin, 100% had deficient levels of vitamin D. A deficiency was defined as a count of less than 20. Of all patients, which included the remaining lighter skin patients, 93% had deficient levels. Believe it or not, five patients had D levels that were undetectable. (32) Now I'm not sure about you, but that demonstrates to me a pretty clear link between a vitamin D deficiency and pain. This is not to say that I guarantee resolution to all of you who get your levels into the optimal range, but for the cost it's certainly worth a try.

I'll give you one more interesting study to consider. This one comes from Saudi Arabia. I'm sure your initial thought is to question why anyone in the Middle East would have an issue getting adequate sunshine. If you consider cultural reasons, and consequently the clothes worn, then you might have insight into the cause. The authors state in their paper, published in 2003, that lower back pain is a well-recognized presentation of a vitamin D deficiency, and more specifically osteomalacia. Of course, they ruled out other possible causes of chronic lower back pain, such as a mechanical cause. From the 360 patients in the study, 83% were found to have low vitamin D levels. If that' not convincing enough, 95% reported a disappearance of low back pain after vitamin D therapy. (33)

In supplements, you will see vitamin D in two different forms. D2, also known as ergocalciferol comes from irradiated plants sterols or yeasts. D3 comes from irradiated lanolin. In a study published in the *Alternative Medicine Review*, it was found that D2 had possibly only 1/10th the potency of D3. In 2006, the *American Journal of Clinical Nutrition* went so far as to state that due to its inferiority, "Ergocalciferol should not be regarded as a nutrient suitable for supplementation or fortification." The results from other comparison studies are mixed. So, when you look at the label on your bottle, it is key to note the form of vitamin D, and with it, the corresponding dose.

You could use the aforementioned studies as guidance in choosing your appropriate dose. For those who are otherwise healthy, and looking for a dose for optimal health, then a couple of considerations should be made. First, what is your 25(OH)D level, and what is the time of the year? If you're above a D value of 32, and heading into the summer, and you happen to be a beach lover, then I'd consider lower doses, if any. If, however, you're at something less than 32 and heading into the winter in the northern 2/3 of the country, then it would be prudent to consider anywhere from 1,000 IU to 5,000 IU per day. Given that it is estimated that you can produce anywhere from 10,000IU to 20,000 IU per day from whole-body sun exposure, then these recommendations would seem quite conservative. In reality, it is whatever combination of sun, diet, and supplementation that keeps you roughly in the range of 30-65.

If you are obese, due to the fact that adipose (fat) tissue has been shown to sequestor vitamin D, you might want to consider a higher dose. Additionally, if you suffer from some disease causing malabsorption, such as Crohn's or Celiac, then consider the same. If you are of dark skin, then consider higher doses as well. One study comparing white women to African-American, found that the African-American women had ten times the incidence of low vitamin D as defined by that particular study. (34) On that note, another trial found that 800 IU or even 2,000 IU was not enough when specifically looking at optimizing the dose for African-American women. They recommended a dose of 2,800 IU for those starting above a reading of 18, and 4,000 IU for those starting at less than 18. (35). Also, as mentioned in the opening, should you have any compromise in liver or kidney function, please factor accordingly.

On one more note, there are variabilities between individuals, which adds to the confusion. Some of us can take less supplemental vitamin D and our 25-D values will shoot up quickly, whereas in others, it takes much more to increase by the same values. It may have to do with genetic variability in the liver enzymes that convert the cholecalciferol into 25-vitamin D. Likewise, as mentioned previously, we have genetic variability in our vitamin D receptors. So in theory, someone with low vitamin D levels and a homozygous flaw on their D receptor is at significantly higher risk for the cancers and other above conditions, than are others. Likewise, if you have zero flaws on the VDR, then you may very well need much less D than most others, and, in fact, there may be disadvantages in attaining some higher levels, which at this stage in the research seem beneficial.

The current U.S. guidelines, as set forth by the NIH are as follows: Age zero to 50 is 200 IU per day; 51-70 is 400 IU per day; and 71+ is 600 IU per day. These are not an RDA or DV, but an AI, which is estimated to ensure adequacy. Many experts consider these guidelines way too low. For example, the Canadian Pediatric Society recommends pregnant and lactating women consider taking 2,000 IU especially during the winter. In 2008, the American Academy of Pediatrics issued recommended intakes for vitamin D based on evidence from more recent clinical trials and the history of safe use of 400 IU per day of vitamin D in pediatric and adolescent populations. In November of 2008, a group of 18 scientists from the University of California suggested in a "call to action" the RDI/AI be upped to 2,000 IU per day. AAP recommends that exclusively and partially breastfed infants receive supplements of 400 IU per day of vitamin D shortly after birth and continue to receive these supplements until they are weaned and consume at least one liter per day of vitamin D-fortified formula (400 IU per liter) or whole milk (98 IU per cup). Of course, as you can gather, I flat out do not endorse the consumption of milk, or even formula over breast milk. Even though breast milk is a poor source of vitamin D, at about 25 IU per liter, it is loaded with numerous other health benefits. They also go on to say that infants, children and adolescents who do not obtain 400 IU per day through vitamin D-fortified milk and foods should take a 400 IU vitamin D supplement daily. There are liquid forms available for those with swallowing issues.

"At what cost?" you ask. To possibly help alleviate or resolve the health issues above there must be a high cost. What do you pay now? Or maybe better asked, "What could you pay in the future if you avoid preventative natural medicine?" If you shoot for 5,000 IU per day, then a 90 day supply will cost you about $19. Daily, this works out to 21 cents a day. This seems affordable to me.

Now let's discuss toxicity, or sensitivity. If you happen to be a practitioner or an otherwise savvy reader, you may be asking yourself about vitamin D toxicity. What is vitamin D toxicity? Well, you'll recall that vitamin D is a fat soluble "vitamin", and therefore has the potential to build up to toxic doses due to a longer half-life in the body. This is true. Hypervitaminosis D (high blood active D levels) itself is not a problem. The problem lies in the hypercalcemia (high blood calcium levels) caused by high D. The symptoms of high blood calcium, which is a possible result of prolonged high 1,25D, are fever, vomiting, constipation, fatigue, abdominal pain, anorexia, and, ultimately, kidney dysfunction. From a lab standpoint, although it does not have an exact definition, it can be defined as having calcium blood values of greater than 14 mg/dl, while the reference range is 8.7-10.4 mg/dl, and an elevated

25(OH)D level above 150 ng/ml. Active 1,25D would likely be elevated as well.

The literature does not contain evidence of toxicity for adults consuming 10,000 IU per day of vitamin D. However, this is in regards to acute toxicity, not chronic. There are only a handful of cases of toxicity, and most are accidental. Faulty industrial production (buy from someone reputable), labeling errors (same), and patient dosing errors account for the bulk. Ergocalciferol at high dose may have some toxicity.

There are a few basic things to do prior to partaking in vitamin D replacement therapy. We need to begin by asking some basic questions. Do I have pre-existing hypercalcemia? What would cause that? Primary hyperparathyroidism can. So, if you've been diagnosed with primary hyperparathyroidism due to a tumor on your parathyroid gland then I would certainly seek out medical advice. If you have sarcoidosis, a lymphoma, or tuberculosis then do the same. These latter three disease states produce unregulated active 1,25D, seemingly from activated macrophages. However, these conditions are rare. The vast majority of Americans can benefit from proper vitamin D therapy.

In fact, I am going to quote an entire paragraph from a renown vitamin D researcher. He can speak with more authority than I to the safety of reasonable vitamin D therapy. The author is Reinhold Vieth, and his review article was published in the *American Journal of Clinical Nutrition* in 1999. Vieth states:

"Throughout my preparation of this review, I was amazed at the lack of evidence supporting statements about the toxicity of moderate doses of vitamin D. Consistently, literature citations to support them have been either inappropriate or without substance. The statement in the 1987 council report for the American Medical Association states that 'dosages of 10,000 IU per day for several months have resulted in marked disturbances in calcium metabolism ...and, in some cases death.' Two references were cited to substantiate this. One was a review article about vitamins in general, which gave no evidence for and cited no other reference to its claim of toxicity at vitamin D doses as low as 10,000 IU per day. The other paper cited in the report dealt with 10 patients with

349

vitamin D toxicity reported in 1948, for whom the vitamin D dose was actually 150,000-600,000 IU per day, and all patients recovered. If there is published evidence of toxicity in adults from an intake of 10,000 IU per day, and that is verified by the 25(OH)D concentration, I have yet to find it."

He did make mention of an adverse event in infants reported in 1938. Their linear bone growth was seemingly suppressed when given 1,800-6,300 IU of vitamin D per day. If you'll recall, in the Finnish study from the section on diabetes, the dose given to infants was 2,000 IU per day, with very interesting results correlating a vitamin D deficiency with type 1 diabetes development. Again, I am merely supplying you with information. It is your call whether or not to give your infant vitamin D or not. Keep this conflicting data in the back of your mind for now.

Lastly, consider that it has been shown in no fewer than four studies that sun exposure results in the production of at least 10,000 IU of vitamin D. What type of sun exposure are we discussing here? Were these people frying in Crisco in the Caribbean for 18 hours a day? How about if you're white, and it's the summer time, somewhere around 20 minutes of full body exposure? The darker your skin, the longer it takes for the formed D to max out in your skin. Someone with very dark skin would be looking at somewhere around 2 hours.

Now that you're excited to get started on your vitamin D therapy, hold back. As wonderful as vitamin D may be, you should be aware of more information. As discussed in the book, nutrients don't operate in a vacuum within our bodies. There can be consequences for "overdoing" one thing as compared to another. With the wonders of vitamin D in mind, I introduce you to a chapter on vitamin A, and information of which virtually no provider is remotely aware.

Chapter 13   Vitamin A

We have for ourselves a natural medicine industry that is running to vitamin D and, by and large, running away from vitamin A. This is yet another example of this flawed mono-nutrient fixation we have, where single nutrients are viewed as "the answer", while others are dismissed. We should embrace vitamin A, along with the many other nutrients available to us. I cover vitamin A because so little is known about it, and yet it offers so much potential in natural medicine.

Most practitioners and many manufacturers are shunning vitamin A based on a handful of studies. There are primarily two categories of studies that scare people. There are those that show relatively moderate doses of vitamin A increase the risk of bone fracture, and that pregnant women have a higher risk of birth defects on higher levels of vitamin A as compared to those on lower doses. So let's take a look at a few trials to better understand the concerns in taking vitamin A.

From October of 1984 to June of 1987, 339 babies with birth defects were born from a much larger group of monitored pregnancies. When looking just at cranial-neural-crest defects, the women who consumed more than 15,000 IUs of preformed (active) vitamin A from diet and supplements had a 3.5 times higher risk as compared to those who consumed 5,000 IUs or less. (1) As this study got a lot of press, practitioners have this notion of vitamin A and birth defects cemented into the back of their heads, which is not necessarily a good thing for the general health of the overall population.

One dietary recall study looked at the vitamin A content of the foods of women with recent hip fractures as compared to other age-matched women. The researchers found twice the risk for those who had 7,500 IU or more of active vitamin A as compared to less than 2,500 IU per day. (2) In another dietary intake survey, the women who were estimated to have consumed more than 15,000 IU per day of active vitamin A from both food and dietary supplements had about 1.5 times the risk for hip fracture as compared to the women in the lowest fifth in terms of vitamin A consumption. (3)

The last piece of information to be included here in this limited view on vitamin A is that a vitamin A deficiency results in night blindness, and unless you have night blindness, you are not vitamin A deficient. There you have it. In general terms, this is what the vast majority of providers know, and thus they steer clear of recommending vitamin A supplementation for both legal ramifications, and a general lack of knowledge. So let's take a deeper look into this lesser known nutrient, and arm you with knowledge so that you can make informed decisions as the primary advocate in your healthcare.

Background

Vitamin A, at the very least, has roles in eye health, the skin, immune strength and regulation, fertility, bone health, red blood cell production, adrenal and thyroid regulation, mucus membranes to include the airways and gastrointestinal tract, embryonic development, growth, and gestational health. If you pair this up against many of our chronic degenerative conditions from IBD, hypothyroidism, adrenal fatigue, asthma, infection, autoimmune disease, infertility, iron deficiency anemia, bone health, and birth defects, you might notice a strong overlap between the two. For example, in the case of growth/fetal development, the German Nutrition Society recommends a 40% increase in vitamin A intake for pregnant women and a 90% increase for breastfeeding women. (4)

In 2004, it was determined from an international body that vitamin A supplementation is among the best strategies to improve global health in developing countries. According to one set of researchers, "Periodic high-dose vitamin A supplementation is one of the most cost-effective interventions to reduce child mortality, and has prevented an estimated 1 million child deaths from 1998 to 2001." (5) These same researchers took a look at the health of children in Indonesia who missed the twice a year 200,000 IU therapy, as compared to those who received it. They found that the children who did not receive the preventative vitamin A medicine within the last 6 months were at greater risk for underweight, stunting, wasting, anemia, and had higher rates of diarrhea and fever as compared to the children who received the therapy. (6) For those of you with IBD, they also state that diarrheal disease increases the risk of vitamin A deficiency.

The Merck manual, which is a physicians prescriptive and care guide, states, "Vitamin A treatment is recommended for all children with measles, and the dose to be given once a day for two days is as follows.

200,000 IU for older than 1 year
100,000 IU for 6 months to 11 months
50,000 IU for less than 6 months of age

I am by no means advocating such high doses for the general public, but I do advocate a consistent lower naturally occurring vitamin A blend at therapeutic doses based on need, balanced with vitamins D and K, not excluding the many other nutritional interplays within the body, more notably some of the B vitamins. Notice the inclusion of a naturally occurring vitamin A blend. In my review of the data on vitamin A, the potential for trouble arises when single more "synthetic" forms of high dosed vitamin A are administered, without any heed for other nutritional factors.

Our average dietary intake does not include liver, shellfish, and egg yolks which are the richest sources of active vitamin A. Liver tastes like hell, shellfish are probably contaminated with heavy metals, and although eggs yolks are one of the healthiest foods known to man, they are discouraged through a no-fat/no cholesterol campaign. However, vitamin A deficiencies during pregnancy lead to multiple birth defects, to include the face, heart, lungs, kidneys, bones, and eyes. Mortality is high in these newborns, as is susceptibility to infection. For the rest of us, vitamin A is depleted in times of infection, stress, sickness, lactation, and intense exercise. For the current epidemic of hypothyroidism, it should be noted that the thyroid gland requires more vitamin A than any other gland. (7)

We do get vitamin A supplemented through various foods, such as breakfast cereals, but the benefits of these isolated metabolites are debatable. Vitamin A from liver isn't just one specific molecule, but comes in a variety of forms. One form, for example, is that of the retinyl esters, which can come as palmitate, stearate, oleate, palmitoleate, or linoleate. The active form of vitamin A is retinoic acid, which has been shown to cause birth defects administered in synthetically high doses. The forms and pathways are outside the scope of this chapter, but common sense tells us that if we take too much of any one thing, without consideration for other factors, the results may not be good ones. For many generations, cod liver oil has been given to our youth and expecting mothers for its vitamin A content, as well as for its vitamin D and omega-3 fatty acids. We live in times where we increasingly abandon the practices passed down over centuries, learned the hard way, to marketing and convenience.

The world of vitamin A is a bit dense, and confusing. Researcher E.V. McCollum is credited with the discovery of vitamin A, although a case could be argued for others. In any event, he found that when cows were fed a carotenoid deficient diet, they failed to thrive, became blind, and gave birth to dead calves. Over one hundred years later, we are beginning to abandon this complex and poorly understood vitamin.

Carotenoid Conversion

This chapter is focused on dietary and supplemental active vitamin A. However, as you are likely aware, vitamin A can be synthesized in the body from carotenoids within plant matter, the most familiar source being carrots. Other yellow, orange, and even green leafy fruits and vegetables, such as sweet potatoes, spinach, and papaya, all contain appreciable amounts of carotenoids. The main consideration is whether or not the body is able to make enough vitamin A from these food sources for ideal health. If not, then dietary/supplemental vitamin A may be necessary, especially in certain conditions to maximize ones nutrient status.

You will frequently hear many "experts" claim that you can get all the vitamin A you need from carotenoid conversion. This message goes hand in hand with the message of avoiding active vitamin A. In the short term, it is most likely true that most people can get by just fine on carotenoids as a primary or exclusive source of vitamin A. However, for optimal health, for pregnancy and child development, and for a host of medical conditions, active vitamin A is preferable, if not flat out required.

If you think you're supplying yourself with enough carotenoids, then you may want to reconsider. The body has to absorb and convert dietary carotenoids into active vitamin A as needed. The steps of absorption and conversion leave a great deal of variability. The type of carotenoid source, the way the food is prepared, the fat content of the meal, stomach acidity, and many other nutritional factors affect absorption, and ultimately conversion to vitamin A. For example, the absorption from raw carrots is virtually non-existent, whereas the absorption from carrot juice is up to 60%. (8) The studies show a wide range from a factor of 4:1 all the way up to a factor of 28:1. In other words, you have to consume anywhere from 4 to 28 units of carotenoids to get one unit of vitamin A.

Here's what a study looks like that determines these things. In Boston, 14 subjects under strict dietary controls were given active vitamin A, and organically labeled carrots and spinach. The amount of retinol (vitamin A) and carotenoids in the blood was measured. It was found that in this healthy, well-nourished adult group, where pureed carrots and spinach were given with fat, that the conversion for carrots was about 15:1 whereas the conversion for spinach was about 21:1. (9) The point is, as one set of researchers puts it, "Foods containing preformed vitamin A (carotenoids) need to be consumed in atypically large amounts in order to meet the vitamin A requirements." (10)

This previous lab experiment was done with healthy adults. What about many others? Pregnant women, children, and people with certain conditions should all most certainly consider their vitamin A status. In addition, as the topic of genes keeps coming up, according to one researcher, "It should be remembered that human subjects may have different abilities to convert provitamin A carotenoids to vitamin A. These differences in conversion efficiency may be due to the genetic variability in beta-carotene metabolism of individual human subjects. Therefore, provitamin A carotenoids might not be a good vitamin A source for those subjects of the poor converter phenotype." (11) The only caveat here is that we simply don't know who these people are at this moment in time.

So let's take a look at a number of instances where vitamin A intake may very well be warranted. As you read through the rest of this chapter, keep a couple of items in mind. The only realistic source of vitamin A is from liver, although shellfish and egg yolks are a reasonable source as well. As our Paleolithic ancestors evolved over millennia, they excelled at the whole "free range" game. This would include the muscle meat we eat today, but the brains, marrow, liver, and other organs as well. I know it sounds repulsive, but it's as close to the truth as we can verify. Likewise, consider that our current standard American fare does not include liver, as we all know it's quite distasteful to put it kindly. Lastly, reconsider a few of the afformentioned properties of vitamin A, immune strength and regulation, mucus membrane integrity to include the airways and gastrointestinal tract, growth, and embryonic development. If you pair this up against IBD, asthma, infection, autoimmune disease, and birth defects, I would strongly argue that we are running relative vitamin A deficiencies in this country in the absence of rampant night blindness.

Infection

In the 1920s, researcher Ed Mellanby and associates found increased rates of infections, to include bronchopheumonia, were more prevalent in the vitamin A deficient induced dogs and rats as compared to controls. Upon examination, the deficiency of vitamin A appears to produce a breakdown in mucosal surfaces in the lungs, and elsewhere, allowing infections to occur. (12) In the 1930s, three trials were conducted looking at worker absenteeism resulting from respiratory illness, to include the common cold. In these three trials, absenteeism was reduced about 40-66% for those given a cod liver oil treatment, which is a premier source of vitamin A. (13)

Puerpural fever is a bacterial infection among women who have just given birth, and was a major challenge prior to hand-washing, sterilization, and antibiotics. In an effort to treat the condition with its approximate 5% mortality, the afformentioned Mellanby used cod liver oil as treatment, and reduced the death rate in a small group from a whopping 92% down to 29%. (14) When he used cod liver oil prophylactically, he saw a successful reduction in the most serious cases from 4.7% down to 1.1%. (15) Given this data, and much more, an old advertisement for Squibb, a pharmaceutical company, read:

"Whooping cough, measles, mumps, chicken pox, and scarlet fever may do greater harm than most mothers think…the children will have lighter cases, they recover quicker, and are less likely to be left with some permanent injury, if they build up good general resistance in advance to fight them…(is to give them) "resistance building" vitamin A. Vitamin A is the important factor which increases their fighting power in time of illness." (16)

Yes, this is the same Squibb that merged with Bristol-Myers in 1989 to form Bristol-Myers Squibb. As antibiotics became the standard of care, the emphasis clearly moved away from the non-patentable cod liver oil.

If you recall your history, during World War II, the Germans bombed England from the air. In an obvious move, the British moved their people below ground into subways and bunkers for safety. Arising from the concerns of respiratory and diarrheal diseases in these cramped quarters, the British Ministry of Food provided cod liver oil to children under five, and pregnant and breastfeeding women. (17) This would make sense as its immune-enhancing qualities should be given to those at most risk, and its growth-enhancing qualities given to those growing the most. It made sense then, but I doubt we'd do it today. This provides a nice segue into the fear of vitamin A-induced birth defects. The British seemed to not have an issue with it, so why do we?

Teratogenicity and Breast-feeding

Teratogenticity is a fancy way of saying birth defect potential. It's curious that vitamin A has been shown to cause birth defects in both deficiency and at high doses. This is also true in regards to bone health. So what are we missing from this data?

There are four things to consider in this equation. The first is that the vast majority of the data that shows teratogenicity in high dose vitamin A comes from animals exposed to insanely high doses, well above any range we'd consider. Second, the form of vitamin A must be taken into consideration. Vitamin A from naturally occurring sources occurs as a blend of various forms of the vitamin, and once ingested, the body properly stores and converts it as needed. Third, it has been very well established that vitamin A plays a major role in cell division, growth, and healthy development of the fetus, while the ability of carotenoids to support all the above is in question. Lastly, the balance with vitamin D must also be factored into this equation. We know that excess intakes of vitamin A can cause a "relative deficiency" in vitamin D, and likewise excessive intakes of vitamin D can do the same to vitamin A status. More on this in the next subsection.

Let's take another look at the study that launched this concern. In their 1995 study, the authors discuss how previous data has shown a potential link between high dose vitamin A and birth defects in animals and humans, and presumably this is why the study was conducted. They referenced two previous human studies to support their argument. However, one of these studies concluded that their findings were not statistically significant. (18) In other words, because no dose information was available, and small subject numbers were used, the results aren't worth referencing. I'm thinking dose information is an important consideration.

In the second human trial they mention, the risk of birth defect was low up to 40,000 IU per day, and rose to 2.7 times the risk after 40,000 IU, with most of the risk occurring in the first two months of pregnancy. (19) If we steer clear of 40,000 IU per day in general, high doses in pregnant women in their first trimester, and take other nutrients such as vitamin D into consideration, then we can still use vitamin A therapy.

They also referenced data referring to the use of isotrentinoin, which is a single vitamin A form, 13-cis-retinoic acid. Isotrentinoin was approved by the FDA in 1982 for the treatment of severe acne. By many accounts, the teratogenicity of this form of vitamin A in humans is clearly established. (20) You will not see this form in supplements. This was a specific metabolite of vitamin A manufactured for a specific treatment.

This reinforces the point that the form of vitamin A given must be considered. A naturally occurring blend of vitamin A from a liver source is a very different product than the single concentrated form used in the acne product. In 2005, researchers attempted to evaluate the blood levels of several vitamin A metabolites by increasing doses in 36 non-pregnant female subjects. Vitamin A palmitate up to 30,000 IU per day was given over the course of 21 days. They did not see any serum levels of any vitamin A metabolites at any dose that posed a concern. In their conclusion, they state, "Repeated oral doses of up to 30,000 IU of vitamin A in addition to dietary vitamin A were without safety concern." (21)

In fact, the metabolite of concern, retinoic acid, showed serum concentrations at the highest dose and duration comparable to those retinoic acid levels in another study where 160 pregnant women all gave birth to healthy babies. The average retinoic acid blood value for these pregnant women was only 4.7 nmol/liter. In contrast, therapeutic acne treatment with the retinoic acid acne product resulted in maximal blood concentrations of this metabolite of approximately 208 nmol/liter. (22) In other words, the concentration of this one vitamin A metabolite in the blood was more than 44 times greater in the acne group as compared to women taking high dose vitamin A in a different form. Let's look at this study.

In this European study from 1999, the researchers found no malformations among 120 infants exposed to more than 50,000 IU per day, and concluded, "The studied sample did not provide evidence for an increased risk of major malformations associated with high vitamin A intake..." (23) As other researchers noted from this study, when looking at those crucial first two months of pregnancy, "The study provided no evidence for an elevated risk of malformations with intakes of 10,000-30,000 IU per day during the first 9 weeks of pregnancy." (24)

In yet another study, researchers looked at vitamin A metabolites in various human and primate studies at various doses as compared to the normal vitamin A metabolite range seen in pregnancy. After considering all of the serum data, they concluded that "..a dose of 30,000 IU per day should also be considered as non-teratogenic in man." (25)

In a review of the literature looking at vitamin A, carotenoids, pregnancy, and breastfeeding, researchers came to the following conclusion in regards to vitamin A and teratogenicity, "The actual teratogenic substance is not vitamin A (retinol), but its metabolite retinoic acid, which does not occur in foods, but will only be synthesized from retinol in the body. Since the synthesis of retinoic acid from retinol is strictly controlled, even excessive retinol intakes will not result in supra-physiological levels of retinoic acid. Thus the warning against liver consumption is not based on scientific evidence, and may have caused the low consumption of liver to decrease even further, especially among young women." (26)

The goal here is to simply show support for reasonable naturally blended vitamin A consumption around the time of conception, either planned or not. A female patient should not be scared out of taking vitamin A to help treat a pre-existing condition, for general health, or for maternal/fetal needs based on one study out of many others not hyped by the press. Following delivery, vitamin A needs are just as critical, if not more so.

Obviously, pregnancy is a state of rapid growth, and requires many nutrients to support that growth for both mother and baby. As with other nutrients, the need for vitamin A increases during pregnancy and while breastfeeding. Especially during the last 2/3 of pregnancy, vitamin A is needed for fetal lung development and maturation, with many more needs likely to be verified.

Upon birth, the liver stores of the baby are so low, perhaps lasting for only a couple days, most newborns could be considered marginally deficient in vitamin A. (27) Should the mother have been marginally deficient herself during pregnancy, the A status of the newborn is even more compromised, the newborn may have a lower birth weight, and is likely at higher risk for other complications. As nature works, the colostrums of mother's milk has extremely high concentrations of vitamin A. However, during lactation, the mother must keep up her intake of vitamin A for both herself and the newborn, as dietary vitamin A intake has been shown to strongly affect breastmilk vitamin A content. (28)

Vitamin A in Bone Health

Vitamin A causes osteoporosis! I guess we should all stop eating foods that contain vitamin A? What nonsense! We do know that vitamin A deficiency leads to bone defects. But once again, you are the confused consumer wondering what to do given all of these conflicting authorities. Like anyone else, you're trying to live as healthy as you can, and maybe even do the same for your family. Too often, wacky statements about nutrition hit the media via the internet, television, or some other medium. Authors who are not immersed in all of the data make partially accurate statements that may have significant ramifications. I believe as a nation we've "out-thought" ourselves and lost common sense along the way. Before you avoid vitamin A based on concerns over your bones, consider these next two subsections.

A 2002 trial published in *JAMA*, implicating relatively moderate doses of dietary and supplemental vitamin A as a risk factor in bone health, has swayed a lot of minds. To reiterate the main point, of the 603 hip fractures analyzed from 1980 to 1998, those subjects in the highest fifth of vitamin A intake had 1.5 times the risk, as compared to those in the lowest fifth. (29) The highest fifth consumed only about 9,000 IU or more per day, which isn't a staggering number. So how can one study create such a stir, and contribute towards an even lower rate of vitamin A consumption than we already have?

We must first consider that this study is not alone in its observations. There are several other human dietary assessment studies that lead to similar conclusions, to include two Swedish studies with increased risk in intakes as low as about 4,500 IU per day. (30,31) 4,500 IU is a low vitamin A intake, and so something is amiss from this data. In contradiction, there are many more studies that have found no association between bone health and vitamin A intake. Beyond this, there are just as many studies that have shown a beneficial effect of vitamin A on bone health. So as you can see, the data is all over the place. Let's look at a few of the studies.

In a 2005 study in Britain, vitamin A intake was evaluated in 312 women over 75 years old who had experienced a bone fracture, and compared them to 934 control subjects. They used serum vitamin A markers as predictors of fracture, and followed these women for an average of 3.7 years. The researchers found that there was a tendency for increased serum retinol to <u>predict benefit</u> rather than harm in terms of bone mineral density, and that <u>multivitamin or cod liver oil</u>

supplementation was associated with a significantly lower risk of any fracture. (32)

A 2002 study gave 40 men 25,000 IU of vitamin A and compared their blood bone metabolism markers to 40 men who had been given a placebo. The researchers found no effect of 6 weeks of the vitamin A supplementation on bone remodeling markers. (33) Granted the study was only 6 weeks, but the dose was much higher than those shown in a few studies to have a negative outcome. Also, serum metabolites are likely are far more accurate measures than the dietary questionnaires used in almost every study, both pro, indifferent, and con, which are fraught with error.

One study suggested that dietary vitamin A worsened bone loss as determined by food evaluation and bone density of the femur. However, the researchers made an interesting comment. The negative outcomes on bone health were not seen when subjects consumed vitamin A supplements, mostly from cod liver oil. They go on to postulate that it could be the vitamin D content in the fish oil that is responsible for the observation. (34)

This brings us to one of the most recent works on the matter from 2009. 75,747 women from the Women's Health Initiative Observational Study were examined via dietary assessment as compared to hip and total fractures. They found that the only association between vitamin A and total fractures was in women with low vitamin D intakes. (35) They also went back and reviewed the work of the hip fracture study from 2002 Nurses' Health Study that fueled the vitamin A concerns. These researchers found that the vitamin D intake in the 2002 study was lower than that in the 2009 study, as well as another neutral study, both of which found no risk association in taking vitamin A.

As you can gather, there seems to be a role between vitamins A and D, an interaction that has by and large not been accounted for in these dietary analysis trials. There is a strong indication that for those who take higher doses of vitamin A in the presence of low vitamin D status, a primary effect can be bone degradation. In contrast, higher doses of vitamin D supplementation in the presence of low vitamin A status can result in primarily calcification of soft tissue. It is a balance of these two vitamins working in concert with one another that yields ideal health. In this model of mono-nutrient fixations, with the current trend on dosing up vitamin D while discouraging vitamin A, we're asking for trouble. A possible long-term consequence is soft tissue calcification of the heart, the kidneys, and other organs. I don't "push" one or the other, but a balance, as best as we can determine from the data. To confuse the matter even more, vitamin K, as discussed in the chapters on bone health and vascular health, is a key player in this relationship. These three fat-soluble vitamins, two of which are more like hormones, act in concert to regulate calcium, gene expression, and more throughout the body.

Think about the primary diseases of mankind today. This ridiculous spike in "autoimmune" diseases makes no sense. I put autoimmune in quotes, because we can't all of a sudden in human evolution have such a sharp increase in these diseases. There is something biochemical going on in the body. More in truth, it's probably several somethings, two of which are possibly vitamins A and D. Both vitamins have been shown to modulate the autoimmune response. Likewise, we Americans consume or synthesize, on average, very little of these two vitamins. We don't get much sunlight, and when we do, we lather up the sunblock. We don't consume foods high in A or D either.

Think about another condition that consumes our health, time, and money. Vascular disease is the number one killer in America. There are several reasons behind this disease, but vascular calcification is integral in this equation. Vitamin D has shown both positive and negative impacts on vascular calcification in studies. Vitamins A and K have shown positive effects on soft tissue calcification. It is these three vitamins working in concert, vitamins largely absent from our synthetic way of life, that contribute to health and longevity. Vitamin A plays a role in thyroid health, Vitamins A, D and possibly K play a role in cancer prevention. This list goes on. These are three crucial vitamins largely absent from the standard American diet. You can try to address your biochemical shortcomings with a drug, or you can try to address them by supplying the raw ingredients determined to be in need by the body. For each person, the needs are individual, but this is a part of in-depth natural/integrative medicine.

To better understand this connection between vitamins A, D, and K, I will have to highlight a number of trials as I have done so many times before. I present you with this data so that you can see for yourself what's going on out there in research, and from this you can begin to formulate your own opinions, rather than listen to a conventional practitioner who has no training in these matters, or some ad campaign looking to separate you from your money.

The next subsection will help to explain why there is so much confusion behind the use of vitamin A, and how it works with vitamins D and K. However, there is no concensus on this topic, and in fact, much debate. I don't offer up definitive answers to your health needs. In this honest approach, I present the data, much of which you are unfamiliar with, and you alone or in partnership with a qualified practitioner in natural medicine can try to find your best solution. The solutions are yours. As we have seen many times over, genetic variability plays a significant role in determining your nutritional needs. Some things like the avoidance of dairy is a fairly universal good practice, but others are less obvious.

I get turned off by doctors who speak in definitives. "There's nothing that can be done for your condition," is one that's heard. "Natural medicine doesn't work," is another. When you hear definitive statements from blow-hards who love to listen to their own voices, I would consider other options. There have been far too many people who've had their conditions resolved through an alternative to conventional medicine to prove these statements absolutely false, which is a definitive statement!

Interplay Between Vitamins A, D, and K

The human body is an amazingly complex marvel of evolution. The field of medicine has for the most part made many great strides over the centuries in its attempts to better our condition. The modern medical establishment is wonderful in the care of acute trauma, acute pain, acute infection, and more. For a patient with a broken bone, the x-ray is clear, the needs are clear, the standards of care are clear, and debate is low or non-existent. In conditions of chronic degenerative disease, such as auto-immune diseases, cardiovascular disease (to include stroke), cancer, and many more, the pathway is less clear, the biochemistry of the body is more complex, and in this grey area, drugs flourish as they many times treat symptoms, but don't get to the underlying cause. Underlying causes can be exceedingly hard to find. It can take many visits to a qualified practitioner of integrative/natural medicine to uncover these hidden burdens. They may be parasites, a high toxic burden, infection, or a nutritional deficiency to name a few. It is here where we will address the topic of nutritional deficiency with the complicated interactions between these three fat-soluble vitamins. I exclude vitamin E, not because there is no data to show that it has no role here, but to reduce mental overload.

There are numerous animal and human studies that have looked at the roles of vitamins A, D and K in relation to one another. Although the vast majority of the data shows that vitamin A and D are seemingly antagonistic, other data shows that they work together. In many trials, the negative effects of ridiculously high doses of vitamin A were ameliorated by giving vitamin D, and likewise, vitamin A helped to reduce or eliminate the effects of excessive doses of vitamin D. The simple fact is that the two vitamins work together in a variety of ways that we don't completely understand, and we don't know the appropriate ratio at which to administer them. This ratio varies from one person to another. For example, if you work outside in warmer climates, your body will theoretically synthesize the correct amounts of vitamin D needed, which is preferable to using supplements. Vitamins A and K obviously need to be ingested, but in what quantities?

On the surface, the vitamins would appear to counteract one another, and in some instances they probably do, but if one is in a state of deficiency while the other is in a state of excess, the effects of the dominant player will win out. For example, it has been shown that excessive intakes of vitamin D can cause soft tissue calcification of the heart and kidneys, whereas excessive vitamin A does not have this effect. Excessive vitamin A has been shown to result in other symptoms, most notably bone problems, which can be "treated" with vitamin D. Gla proteins are carboxylated by vitamin K, but too much vitamin D makes too many Gla proteins in the presence of low vitamin K.

We've already seen that vitamin K activates what's called Gla proteins, such as the osteocalcin in bone health, and MGP in vascular health. We've also seen that vitamin D is made from a cholesterol precursor in the skin, or ingested, and is converted to the 25(OH)D form in the liver, and converted to the active 1,25(OH)D form in the kidneys and at a cellular level. The active form acts on the vitamin D receptor (VDR), which is a plug-in port on a cell membrane for vitamin D. Likewise, vitamin A is converted from retinol to retinaldehyde, and then to all-trans retinoic acid. Like vitamin D, retinoic acid binds to several types of retinoic acid receptors (RARs). Data has shown that these two vitamins do not always act alone, and in some cases, they work together for a more potent outcome. They go on to form a heterodimer, which is a fancy way of saying the two vitamins are co-joined into one unit. It does this in thyroid and steroid hormone function as well.

It is this partnering synergy that may make them even more potent than either is alone. One of the better examples comes from a 2006 study done in Europe. Looking at cancer cells, the researchers found that vitamin D alone was unable to improve levels, whereas when it was combined with vitamin A, they found a strong synergistic effect. (36) This may be why some data shows vitamins A or D alone to be beneficial in some cancer trials, but not in others.

One research paper estimates that as much as 70-80% of the gene expression induced by vitamin D requires a vitamin A-derived molecule (RXR) in order to function. (37) In other words, vitamin D can't enter into the cell and tell the command center, the nucleus, to make various proteins, such as enzymes and hormones, without the help of vitamin A. So, if you're taking high doses of vitamin D, but are under stress, have underlying infection, have inflammation of mucus membranes, and have a low vitamin A intake, then you may be running "relative" deficiencies of vitamin A, and thus you may not be able to make enough thyroid hormone, or form the necessary A-dependent heterodimer at the thyroid receptor to induce thyroid hormone functions for optimal health.

As it would be unethical to give humans mammoth doses of either vitamins A or D, it has been done in many animal studies. With that said, there is a great deal of data to show that vitamins A and D require each other, counteract each other, and "use up" each other.

One of the better studies looked at varied doses of vitamin D, and its relation to vitamin A in broiler chicks. In essence, they found that high doses of vitamin A interfered with low or marginal levels of vitamin D, causing the familiar decrease in bone mineral content, body weight, and rickets. When vitamin D levels were increased, the toxicity of vitamin A was overcome. Likewise, high vitamin A intake prevented the toxic effects of high dietary vitamin D. (38)

In an in vitro study, osteoblast (bone building) cells were incubated with vitamins A and D alone, both of which increased the synthesis of osteocalcin, but when the two vitamins were combined, "a remarkable synergistic effect between the hormonal forms of vitamin A and D on the synthesis of this bone specific protein was observed." (39)

A 1974 study looked at vitamin D intake and heart attack, and found a correlation between the two. (40) They also found that those with the higher heart attack rates also had a higher history of kidney stones. They note that this was also seen in a 1973 study. Also referenced was a paper that suggested a relative vitamin A deficiency may cause coronary heart disease.

In an interesting Indian study, it was found that those subjects who had vitamin D levels above 89 ng/ml (which is within range of some recommendations) had greater than 3 times the risk for heart disease. Here, 143 men were compared to control subjects, from the ages of 45-65. Not only was sunlight in high supply, but the dietary levels of vitamin D in the form of D2 were quite significant. The researchers theorized that vascular calcification may occur with levels "beyond the normal range." (41) Remember that D2 seems to be less safe than D3.

Another set of researchers closely links the two conditions of osteoporosis and cardiovascular disease, as both have imbalances in calcium regulation. They mention how excess vitamin D induces both bone loss and cardiovascular health in both humans and animals.

Importantly, magnesium deficiency and high dietary cholesterol may play a role. (42)

Consider that primarily in animal models, the doses of either vitamin given were exceptionally high. Through this usage of short-term supraphysiological levels, the researchers are trying to interpret what elevations or imbalances over the long term may do in humans. We are not going to consume 1 million IU of vitamin D, or equally excessive doses of vitamin A. However, over time, if one vitamin is continually higher than the other, the gradual and unseen process of bone demineralization or soft tissue calcification can occur and lead to morbidity and mortality.

I am not trying to scare anyone out of using vitamin D, and I am not endorsing uncontrolled use of vitamin A. There is a balance, which is an elusive target. There are other researchers, some of whom were quoted in the vitamin D chapter, who have looked at this equation. (43) One of their concerns around using cod liver oil is that in current processing techniques, notably deodorization, much of the vitamin D has been stripped out, thus unable to compliment or counter the effects of the vitamin A still in the fish oil. Here again, in the process of large scale manufacturing to appeal to the masses in taste, the quality of the product has been compromised.

This extensive list of vitamin D proponents recommends that children obtain serum vitamin D levels greater than 50 ng/dl. They also feel there should be several times greater intake of vitamin D than vitamin A, looking something like 2,000 IU of D for a 50 pound child in the absence of significant sun exposure, with roughly 350 IU of vitamin A. (44) The level of vitamin D may be relatively accurate, but I believe the level of vitamin A recommended is too low for a growing child, or most anyone, for that matter.

Contrarily, the folks at the Weston Price Foundation, a group who for better or worse passionately adheres to the principles noted in Dr. Price's book, have a very different view. One of their authors, Christopher Masterjohn, who is very knowledgable on the interaction between all the fat-soluble vitamins, notes the naturally occurring ratios of vitamins A and

D in the liver oils eaten by healthy tribes. They recommend a ratio more along the lines of 10 parts vitamin A to one part vitamin D. He supplies extensive data in at least two articles, "Vitamin A on Trial: Does Vitamin A Cause Osteoporosis?" and "From seafood to Sunshine: A New Understanding of Vitamin D Safety."

To be perfectly honest, no one has the answer, and the answers put forth are highly variable. For example, Weston Price had no way to measure serum vitamin D levels, and thus we don't know how much the diet needed to supply, given extensive sun exposure. It is likely that we need on average more vitamin D as we avoid the sun, work indoors, and are fully clothed much of the year, particularly of concern in the northern states. Meanwhile, given our poor diets, high levels of stress, gut dysbiosis, and poor dietary sources, vitamin A is certainly worth considering. Curiously, both have been proven to have a role in bone health, vascular health, autoimmune disease, cancer, and more. These two vitamins seem to mostly work together, and your individual needs may vary, but a closer ratio is probably in order. Of course, if you have adequate sun exposure, the equation changes, as your body is able to self regulate the vitamin D, which is better than us trying to "out-think" it.

These two vitamins don't operate in a vacuum. Many nutrients work together, to include vitamin K. Is vitamin K the new calcium, the new vitamin D, the new "it" nutrient? I hope not. Although there seems to be no overdose toxicity, we usually find out these things later in time. Vitamin K deserves notice and balance along with the other nutrients, and is lacking in the American diet. How many people eat kale or fermented soy? Not many. So let's wrap up this section with some vitamin K data.

Decades of research show that very high doses of vitamin D cause soft tissue calcification, doses you and I would not take. Vitamin K has proven benefits in preventing soft tissue calcification. We know that vitamin D causes an increase in matrix Gla protein (MGP) and osteocalcin, the two vitamin K dependent proteins. Yet you'd think with this extra MGP in the cells of the vasculature, it would help keep out calcifications. Yet, there seems to be some type of "relative deficiency" in vitamin K with excess vitamin D. Thus, the MGP attracts calcium, but it is not used properly, as the MGP is inactive.

This was seen in a rat study. These researchers gave warfarin with vitamin D to rats, and quickly caused extensive arterial calcification. (45) Warfarin, as you may know, is a widely prescribed blood thinner. It works by counteracting the coagulation aspects of vitamin K. So in this study, you have a scenario with high vitamin D and a vitamin K antagonist in a rat model, illustrating what can happen to patients on warfarin, with extra vitamin D, and no vitamin A (which reduces MGP expression) and K. These rats were shown to have excessive amounts of inactive MGP in the calcified arteries, which makes sense given the anti-vitamin K activity.

Yes, this has been shown in humans too. 45 aortic valves were analyzed after routine cardiac replacement, and those who were taking oral anticoagulant drugs were compared to those who weren't. The researchers found more than twice the calcification of the anticoagulant treated valves, as compared to the others, and even low dose treatment for short periods of time showed a significant increase in calcification. (46)

Proof of the effects of vitamin K were shown in a study, which is a logical extension of the previous two. Warfarin-treated rats were given vitamins K1 and K2 to see if the vitamins countered the calcification effects of warfarin. K2 but not K1 countered the calcification in the arteries, further proof in support of conclusions in the bone health chapter. (47) If you recall, K1 had adequate activity in the liver for coagulation, and its efficacy outside the liver was questioned, whereas K2 had a longer duration in the blood, was seemingly more potent for these Gla proteins, and had the data to prove it. The warfarin doesn't just inhibit the clotting factors associated with vitamin K, but the activation of Gla proteins in general. It's kind of like taking antibiotics. They kill the bad bugs, but they also kill the good bugs in your gut.

It's also of interest to note that in rats the tissues with the highest concentrations of MGP are the heart, kidney, cartilage, and lung. It's hard to translate this to human data, but the evidence seems to be a match. At least the first three sites play extensive roles in human health. Additionally, vitamin K has also been shown to protect the kidneys from calcification (48)

Most practitioners in natural medicine will know that vitamin D increases absorption of calcium in the gut, and that it has a wide variety of fantastic benefits in the body as it acts at a nuclear level in hormones, cell division, and much more. What they often will not know is that vitamin D elevates marix Gla proteins, which seemingly increase the demand for vitamin K. It has been repeatedly shown that increasing these proteins, without adequate vitamin K, is not a good thing.

The relationship with vitamin A is even less known. The typical view is that vitamins A and D counteract one another, like osteoblasts and osteoclasts. The body is not that simple. Osteoblasts and osteoclasts regulate each other. There is a communication network built into the bone system, which balances the needs of the body with the needs of the bone. Remember, osteoclasts aren't evil. They are simply doing the job of returning calcium from the reseviour (the bone) into the blood to maintain that fine line of calcium balance. The body needs the calcium for one thing or another.

This balance of bone building and bone resorption between the osteoblasts and osteoclasts is exemplified well with the bis-phosponate drugs. They essentially turn off the osteoblasts, which would seem logical. Yet, the drugs seem to cause these odd fractures in a certain part of the femur. It would seem that the strength of this heavily burdened bone is compromised by interfering with the normal cycle of bone remodeling.

Likewise, vitamin A is required for bone health. It is quite possible that among other mechanisms, vitamin A allows for a slower, but more complete bone deposition, leading to more solid bone structure, which makes sense as research has shown too much vitamin D makes for weak bones. This better mineralization is the result of cross-talk between osteoblasts and osteoclasts driven by vitamins A and D, with support from vitamin K and a host of other nutrients.

Ideally, you'd strike a balance among these three, and all nutrients based on your individual needs. This can in part be determined through nutritional diagnostics available through many natural medicine practitioners. If you don't follow that path, just logically consider your condition and historical nutrition, and keep in mind moderation and balance.

Vitamin A in Mucosal Health

Asthma is a condition of the mucus membranes. In asthma, we look at our ability to breathe in the face of inflammation. As is well known without dispute, vitamin A is essential for these epithelial cells, which are integral in mucosal integrity. Likewise, the compromise in these cells from vitamin A deficiency disrupts this barrier to bacteria and normal function, creating a condition of inflammation. Sounds a bit like IBD.

In one study from the journal *Pediatric Allergy and Immunology*, researchers looked into the vitamin A status in children with asthma, and how it correlated with the disease. They observed that vitamin A deficiency was four times more common in children with asthma, with the levels being the lowest in those with the most severe disease. (49) They go on to state that due to the frequent inflammation, infection, and stress, the lower vitamin A serum levels are reflective of increased demand for vitamin A for these stressed mucosal cells. It must also be noted that only about 6% of the children in this trial had a clinical vitamin A deficiency, whereas a full 40% had low serum vitamin A levels. This is further proof that one does not have to present with a clinical diagnosis of deficiency to be deficient enough to cause health problems. For example, of an estimated 125 million preschool children with vitamin A deficiency, only about 6% show clinical evidence of severe deficiency. (50)

I want to stress this point, because its relevance to your health goes well beyond vitamin A. Modern conventional medicine is mostly about lab numbers, prescriptions, and the avoidance of risk/lawsuits. In the case of a relative vitamin A deficiency, if you did not present with night blindness, your average physician would exclude vitamin A as a metabolic need. Likewise, in the case of adrenal insufficiency, if you do not present with symptoms and labwork that shows full-blown Addison's disease, then you don't need adrenal support. In other words, you are either fully healthy, or near death, with no grey area in between. However, for those who have adrenal inadequacies, there is a very large grey area, and they need treatment and direction. This is a part of the art of medicine, which is now lost with our current systemic flaws in schooling, marketing, greed, lawsuits, managed care, and more.

In one more asthma study, children from Japan were analyzed under the same pretenses, that persistant inflammation and epithelial cellular damage depletes vitamin A. They added one more consideration as well. As vitamin A status can change with cases of infection, they decided to look at well-nourished children with minimal signs of an immune response. This could easily be your child or grandchild. They found that the vitamin A serum levels were 2/3 lower than those of healthy controls. (51) They concluded that there is a correlation between vitamin A deficiency and the asthmatic response.

In a similar light, we'll look at IBD. I stated within the IBD chapter that vitamin A is a crucial part of a much larger regimen to manage inflammatory bowel disease, and I deferred the data until here. Vitamin A plays more than one role in regards to GI health, but let's first look at some studies that show a correlation. Once again, you don't have to take my word; you can read the words of many researchers with multiple degrees who spend many hours researching but one aspect within all of natural medicine.

In a study published in 1983, 52 Crohn's patients with an average age of 39, were investigated for evidence of a vitamin A deficiency. According to their criteria, the researchers found that 21% (11 patients) had low plasma vitamin A, a far higher percentage than normal. Three of these 11 had impaired dark adaptation, night blindness, with an average blood level lower than the others, which was associated with extensive small bowel disease. The authors concluded, "This study has shown that vitamin A deficiency is a significant clinical problem in severe Crohn's disease. (52)

This study illustrates a couple things. One, the more severe the vitamin A deficiency, the more severe the Crohn's disease. I think this is a fairly strong correlation, albeit it with only 11 subjects. Second, once again you don't have to have night blindness to have a vitamin A deficiency that negatively impacts your health. They also noticed that fat absorption was a problem for some of the patients, which is relatively common in IBD. It's an unfortunate viscious cycle as vitamin A is a fat-soluble vitamin, and although it's in high demand, by its nature, it may be absorbed to a lesser degree.

In one study, rats were fed a vitamin A deficient diet, and then compared to others sufficient in vitamin A. (53) Their purpose in doing so was centered around the fact that vitamin A is essential for normal cell growth, differentiation, and maintenance of epithelial tissue. As epithelial tissue, even under normal conditions, has a high turnover rate, in vitamin A deficiency this tissue would be highly compromised. The villi are tiny finger-like projections within the GI tract, which exponentially increase the surface area to facilitate absorption. In their paper, the authors present stunning microscopic pictures of stunted and perturbed villi in the vitamin A deficient rats. The authors state that this observation has been seen in other rat, chicken, and mice studies. They go on to conclude that, "…vitamin A deficiency induces morphological (size and shape) and functional changes in the small intestinal mucosa and…demonstrates the important role of vitamin A in the integrity and functionality of the intestinal epithelium…"

Another study evaluating nutritional status in IBD looked at 23 patients admitted to the hospital for attacks of IBD. They were compared to 89 healthy controls. Among the many other nutritional deficiencies seen, there was at least a 40% risk for developing low vitamin A status. (54). In another trial looking at vitamin status in Crohn's, the fat soluble vitamins A and E were significantly decreased when compared to healthy controls, and there were a variety of other vitamin deficiencies as well. (55)

At Children's Hospital in Boston, 97 patients with IBD were compared to 23 controls. Although none of the control children had low serum vitamin A levels, 14% of the IBD patients did. (56) This rate of 14% is much higher than the less than 5% prevalence they uncovered in the general population. Although none of the subjects had any overt symptoms of deficiency, they theorized that they were at risk for deficiency.

Based on information similar to that above and more, some researchers tried to treat 86 Crohn's patients with 50,000 IU of vitamin A twice a day for an average of 14 months. (57) My first response is to the dose. We're looking at 100,000 IU a day for more than a year. This seems in total contradiction to the warnings we're getting about vitamin A, and I agree. This dose is excessive. They found no benefit of vitamin A in this trial, but they also saw no negative effect from such a large dose and duration.

To understand why this trial failed, you have to understand a bit more about vitamin A and IBD. They did not address any of the other issues of allergens, pathogens, genetic flaws, and inflammation as per the chapter on IBD. They had way too much vitamin A intake as compared to vitamin D in particular. Like many trials, they were trying to use a single agent to fix all the problems. We are not single-nutrient mammals. Vitamin A at more reasonable doses is a part of a larger regimen. Second, vitamin A is not your average vitamin. Like vitamin D, it has many roles at the nucleus of the cell. It basically tells different cells what proteins to make. If you don't have all the other nutrients to support the commands of vitamin A then it doesn't matter how much you administer, as your potential for success is highly compromised.

For example, if you were to build a house, vitamin A is a bit like the foreman. He can yell at the carpenters (the cell ribosomes) all day long to build, build, build. Yet, if you don't have any wood, nails, or other raw materials you can't build anything. Think of the proteins and fats you eat as the raw materials. Think of the other vitamins and minerals as the tools. You need all players to build a house, yet we keep throwing one or two items at a health problem. The fact is, we know enough about vitamin A to advocate its use. From animal, in vitro, and human data, we can say where and why it helps.

Vitamin A helps IBD, mostly on an immunological and epithelial level. We know from decades of research that vitamin A plays a key role in both of these manners. We know that in cases of infection, such as pneumonia, we can excrete up to 50% of the RDA of vitamin A per day in our urine. (58) We know that IBD has a component of infection to it, whether it be bacterial or fungal in nature. So with the pathogen chewing up more vitamin A, the inflammation of IBD putting greater demands on vitamin A by destroying the lining of the GI tract, and with the reduced absorption of vitamin A, there appears to be a clear need to supplement.

The atypical conversion of carotenoids to vitamin A must be noted as well. The primary site in the body to convert dietary carotenoids to active vitamin A occurs within the intestinal mucosa with the help of other factors, such as bile salts. This is not typical for vitamin activation. This ability of intestinal mucosa to convert "on the spot" is indicative of the importance of vitamin A within the intestinal mucosa. Similarly, some studies have shown that people with IBD are up to five times more likely to develop colon cancer. Given that vitamin A also plays a large role in cell division, and those with IBD have been shown to be deficient, the lack of local vitamin A may incapacitate the body from properly controlling cell growth, particularly under such inflammatory conditions.

Vitamin A not only plays a direct anti-pathogenic role from the immune perspective, but also helps the body to differentiate between friend and foe, which is not only of huge importance in IBD, but in any "autoimmune" condition. How vitamin A does this is extremely complicated biochemistry, which is still being unraveled.

Many studies point to the key role vitamin A plays in immune regulation, in particular within the GI tract. (59-67) The data gets extremely complex, so we'll only discuss a few generalities, and mention a few new key players.

The first new player is IgA. IgA is an antibody. It plays a critical role in mucosal immunity. More IgA is produced in mucosal linings than all other types of antibody combined. (68) By no coincidence, it is also high in the colostrum of breast milk. FoxP3+ T cells are a major subset of regulatory immune cells. They not only play a role in pathogenic resistance, but seem to play a broader role in self-tolerance, or recognition of which cells are "bad" and which are "good." The impact here is massive, as we're discussing "autoimmune" conditions. In other words, the autoimmune condition attacks your own cells as your immune system has lost the ability to distinguish between friend and foe. This general on the battlefield helps direct the battle to minimize friendly fire, and directs efforts toward the true enemy. The use of FoxP3+ T cells in animal models has led to significant reductions in conditions we call "autoimmune," such as diabetes, MS, asthma, IBD, thyroiditis, and renal disease. (69) Dendritic cells are also a part of the immune system, originating from bone marrow. They are present in parts of the body exposed to the outside environment, the skin and membranes of the GI and respiratory tracts. Their primary role is to process, identify, and, if need be, activate and present pathogens to other components of the immune system. They are a bit like RECON in the battle against pathogens. The last contributor to this equation is NF-KB. We've seen this player before. It has a key role in the pro-inflammatory immune response.

Much of the hard-core biochemical research has to be in animal and in-vitro models. It would be unethical to induce vitamin A deficiency, chemically induce IBD, and otherwise chop up humans to get this data, although it could be argued that it's unethical in animals as well. In any event, we have an immense amount of data, some of which we'll now review.

A rat model looked at the induction of colitis (IBD) on three groups, a vitamin A deficient, a vitamin A sufficient, and a vitamin A supplemented group. (70) What the researchers found most interesting were the morphological and inflammatory changes in the vitamin A deficient rats <u>without colitis</u>. The shortened villi, infiltration of immune cells, and activation of NF-KB was not seen in those on vitamin A. The intestinal changes were similar to those seen in the vitamin A sufficient rats where colitis was induced. The study showed that vitamin A deficiency induced inflammation and other negative intestinal changes, that the colitis was worse in the deficient group, and that vitamin A supplementation improved these outcomes, in part by inhibiting the pro-inflammatory cascade kicked off by NF-KB.

In a very recent review article from 2009, the authors' concluding remarks, although a bit dense, are so well put, I had to include them in their entirety for your review.

"A functional immune system is essential for efficient protection of the organism against invasive pathogens as well as invasive transformed autologous (think cancer cells) cells. Aberrant immune responses directed towards non-self harmless agents or normal endogenous cells can lead to severe pathology and autoimmunity. Many regulatory mechanisms are in place and in particular FoxP3+ regulatory T cells are indispensible to prevent excessive and self-destructive immune responses. The intestine, which forms the largest entry surface for invading pathogens but also contains a vast load of harmless antigens derived from colonizing commensal (think probiotics) bacteria and absorbed nutrients, imposes a unique challenge for the immune system. In particular, the ability to mount a highly efficient protective immune response needs to coincide with the steady state prerequisite of tolerance towards innocuous agents. An improper balance between inflammatory and suppressive immunity can jeopardize mucosal homeostasis (balance) and destroy the integrity of the mucosal barrier (think IBD). The intake of vitamin A as part of the food absorption by the intestine and the ability of the vitamin A metabolite, retinoic acid, to drive the differentiation of the induced FoxP3+ regulatory T cells and to suppress the differentiation of the pro-inflammatory effector cells, provides an expedient mechanism to secure tolerance when protective immune responses are not advantageous. The plasticity of the system and the ability of innate and pro-inflammatory signals to override the RA controlled immune suppression provides the mucosal immune system with a key control to allow for protective immunity in the face of steady state immune tolerance." (71)

In another review looking at IgA, the authors noted that IgA is the most abundant immunoglobulin (antibody) produced in the body, that about 80% of the cells which secrete IgA are in the gut mucosa, that mice lacking or having impaired IgA are more susceptible to intestinal toxins and pathogens, and rats with depleted vitamin A have decreased IgA. (72) This confirms what has long been observed in humans, particularly in the third world, that a vitamin A deficiency is associated with an impaired intestinal immune response.

An interesting in vitro model from 2008 looked at the activity of vitamin A metabolites to affect the pro-inflammatory NF-KB as it relates to asthma. They looked at a pro-inflammatory cytokine (immune signaling protein) named TSLP. The TSLP is up-regulated in inflamed airway epithelial cells, such as with asthma. Through various tests, they state in many ways that vitamin A inhibits NF-KB directly, and that this NF-KB inhibition modulated TSLP expression. In other words, you should strongly consider taking vitamin A if you have asthma. They conclude that, "…these data suggest that the use of RXR agonists (vitamin A) may be useful as a therapeutic modality in treating allergy." (73)

Another rat study looked into vitamin A and its effects on dendritic cells, the immune RECON force. As supporting background information, the authors stated that dendritic cells are the most powerful antigen-presenting cells, and are critical players in intestinal immune defense. (74) Although these dendritic cells reside in the entire intestinal mucosa, they have a concentration in the terminal ileum, the end of the small intestine, which by "coincidence" is the primary site of Crohn's disease. These immune cells guard against pathogens, and previous research has shown that vitamin A has direct effects on these cells. Although more precise mechanisms have yet to be identified, the authors state that, "…vitamin A may be able to maintain mucosal homeostasis and strengthen humoral immunity to invasive antigens and that vitamin A may be potent in reducing intestinal inflammation and restoring impaired antibody responses in a vitamin A deficient situation."

In a mouse study looking at vitamin A status and FoxP3+ T cells in a Crohn's model, the authors concluded, "Our results identify novel pathways of inducing highly suppressive FoxP3+ regulatory T cells that can effectively control inflammation. The results have significant ramifications in treating inflammatory bowel disease." (75) Statements like this aren't common from researchers, especially from institutional ones, as these were from the Purdue Cancer Center. The premise for their research is that these FoxP3+ T cells have been shown to be highly effective in suppression of intestinal inflammation, and that one of the most notable clinical symptoms of someone with a mutation in their FoxP3 gene is enteritis (inflammation of the small intestine). They further justify their research by saying that vitamin A and its metabolites are required for proper immunity to pathogens by promoting IgA and its role in FoxP3+ T cell activity. Taken all together, this is "big news." Well, I have more big news for you.

In a review of vitamin A metabolism, the authors note a few very important factors, which have significant ramifications. (76) They first inform the reader that in situations of high demand for vitamin A, such as inflammation and disease, the supply of vitamin A storage from the liver to the rest of the body can be slow, due to the processes involved in packaging up vitamin A for delivery. This can cause localized deficiencies. They make this point in regards to chronic obstructive pulmonary disease (COPD) from smokers. COPD is found almost exclusively in smokers. They state that although smokers with COPD do not have systemic vitamin A deficiencies, a local deficiency in the lung occurs due to the toxic, oxidative, high cellular turnover rate, and that this local deficiency will finally lead to cancer. The risk for COPD increases with decreasing vitamin A serum levels, and this risk is strongly decreased with the intake of vitamin A in a dose-dependent manner.

They also comment on how a vitamin A deficiency leads to night blindness, and eventual blindness, but long before these clinical signs appear, an increased incidence in respiratory tract infections becomes evident. This paper encompasses many of the facets of this chapter. The concept that a patient may have local deficiencies in any given mucosal area which may not present with the classical symptoms associated with vitamin A deficiency, to include blood levels and night blindness, despite being very ill. Lastly, vitamin A therapy can turn this process around before it's too late.

Suffice it to say, vitamin A is a very complex vitamin. Its complexity contributes to its misunderstanding, or lack of understanding. The fact that it has so many metabolites, that these metabolites work in very complex ways at the nuclear level, and that they kick off so many processes, which are equally mysterious, is its burden to bear. Given its grave importance within the body, and its lack of content in the standard American diet, combined with an ever increasing list of diseases that seem to have some links to a vitamin A deficiency, then doesn't it stand to reason to incorporate it more into our daily routine?

We're not talking about 30,000 IU per day here. Depending on your condition, your other nutrient intake, and your dietary intake, levels of no more than 10,000 IU per day over an extended period of time would appear to be both efficacious and quite safe, according to the extensive data presented here.

Chapter 14   Probiotics

In natural medicine there are some products you take on faith, some that are garbage, and some that have quick therapeutic impacts. Antioxidants for example, have supportive clinical data, but you can't tell me that you can "feel" a difference. A well-manufactured probiotic is one of those special tools we have in the arsenal, and they work. If you have a GI issue, then you will notice whether they are working in a relatively short period, usually within a week or two.

You may be surprised, but probiotics are a valuable tool for many more conditions than those of the gastrointestinal tract. As you will see in the supporting data, they have immune enhancing, urogenital, dermatological, cancer, and other benefits beyond the GI tract. Probiotics are one of those "no-brainer" supplements that should be a part of your daily or weekly regimen. Unless you've been breast-fed, had no antibiotics, a perfect diet, no stress, perfect genes, and no chlorinated water, then you may not need them.

This whole probiotic concept was officially recognized back in 1907. Nobel prize winner Professor Elie Metchnikoff theorized in his book, **The Prolongation of Life**, that certain cultures that consumed fermented milk products derived an immunological benefit from the good bacteria, which explained their health and longevity. Of course fermented foods go back well before the days of Metchnikoff, but he was the first to theorize the health benefits of regular consumption, and the positive effects these newly described microbes could play in regulating pathogenic bacteria.

Over 100 years later, we are still debating the issue. Here we are, awash in a nation of illness, obesity, and skyrocketing healthcare costs, and conventional medicine dismisses the extraordinary work of researchers decades and centuries ago for the pursuit of profitable and patentable drugs and devices. In some cases, the answer is not some expensive drug, but as simple as "You are what you eat, and digest." In this chapter, and throughout this book, I hope you will have come to an appreciation that we truly are what we eat. The impact of a poor diet is not relegated only to the GI tract. The effects can range across the entire spectrum of illnesses in the body. Cancer, dermatological issues, rheumatoid arthritis, type 1 and type 1 diabetes, heart disease, and many other conditions can be traced in one way or another to your digestive tract. Probiotics are not quite the magic bullet to your health, but they play an integral role.

The clinical data is coming out fast and furious on probiotics. There is so much published data that I won't even have to reference any animal or test tube trials. We'll cover human data, on living people, to illustrate the value to you. Not all data is supportive, and there are several explanations for this. Some clinical trials, especially older ones use very small numbers of probiotics. We have come to learn that certain general minimums are required for effect. Second, some probiotic products are not made well; therefore, many of the beneficial bacteria are dead upon administration, or die in the stomach. This is your biggest obstacle in finding a good probiotic, as they are the most difficult thing to manufacture in natural medicine. Although some very limited data suggests dead probiotics can be of value, (1) the vast majority of the data, to include that of Professor Metchnikoff, suggests that live probiotics are of therapeutic value. Additionally, some studies used a single species or strain in various pathologies, while as research has progressed, we have found that some species work better for certain conditions. Lastly, probiotics are but one aspect of a disease state. If you have IBD, then in addition to probiotics, the next best step would be to remove any existing food allergens and coat your GI tract with mucopolysaccharides to halt inflammation.

In the newborn, the GI tract is a sterile environment. Some of the micoflora that initially inhabit the GI tract come from ingested fluid during delivery. However, following delivery, breast-feeding plays an integral role in establishing a healthy colonization of the GI tract. Lactobacilli and bifidobacteria are the main beneficial bacteria found in breast milk. In a revealing study, researchers found that 1 month old breastfed infants have about 10 times more beneficial bifidobacteria in their stool as do bottle fed infants. (2) This sets up a healthy GI tract to resist pathogenic organisms, solidify GI integrity, and enhance immune function.

The value of probiotics has not gone unnoticed to large multinational corporations, such as Dannon. Their product, bifidobacterium animalis DN-173 010 (aka bifidus regularis), is available in their product-line. They are not alone. There is much work being done behind the scenes to selectively breed, and consequently own, better and stronger strains of probiotics. It's much like selectively breeding flowers or vegetables. Over time, you propogate the ones that do best, however you define best. Once you've bred a strain that's new, you own it. Then you run clinical trials to see if it actually works in the real world. A few successful trials later, and you have a marketable product. So if large well-financed companies see the value in all of this expense and work, then isn't it quite possible that probiotics just might work?

When you're in the store buying a probiotic, several different things on the label will jump out at you. First, there are many genera of probiotics for sale. The two most common and clinically proven are of the lactobacilli genus and the bifidobacteria genus. Within these genera, there are many species. Names such as lactobacillus acidophilus, plantarum, rhamnosus, and bifidobacterium bifidum, longum, and lactis are frequently found on the labels. If there are any little alpha-numerical designations after the name, that is the strain designation. So how do you know which one is right for you?

You will sometimes see a single bacterium in a product, such as lactobacillus acidophilus. You will then see some reflection of how many of these guys are supposed to be alive inside the product. The clearest way to represent this is by stating the CFU, or colony forming units. So if a product has 1 billion CFU, then there should be about 1 billion live lactobacillus acidophilus bugs in the product at the time of sale.

You will more often see a blend of bacteria. In other words, lactobacillus acidophilus, plantarum, and reuteri can all be combined together with species from bifidobacterium, such as longum, breve, lactis, and more. What you are looking for are a few things. First, you'll probably want a blended product. This will enable you to affect both the small intestine and the large intestine, as well as address a wide variety of health benefits. Recall that I stated earlier that some species and strains within the genera have different benefits that vary according to your condition.

Use the clinical data referenced later in this chapter as a guide to your needs.

Along with the genera, species, and strains, you'll want to play close attention to the CFU count in the product. What is stated on the label is not necessarily what's alive inside the packaging, and what will make it alive to your lower GI tract. Also, the total count needed is up for debate, but minimal counts somewhere around 1-5 billion CFU have been proven efficacious. If your product has a count less than 1 billion CFU, I'd rethink things. Also, if the product states a CFU count "at time of manufacture," I would also have concerns. What I ultimately want to know is the amount that makes it through the acid in my stomach. A CFU at time of manufacture tells me that the maker of the product is unsure of, or has no confidence in, the number of live bacteria in the real world use. After manufacturing, the product will spend time on the shelf of the manufacturer, likely a distributor, in transit, a retailer, and ultimately on your shelf. If the company does expiration testing, and states the count at time of expiration, then you can have more confidence.

If this wasn't enough, there is the issue of stomach survivability. The HCL in your stomach is there for a number of reasons, which is why taking H2 blockers and PPIs for GERD and heartburn for years is not such a good idea. One of the roles of HCL is to kill potential pathogens, such as molds and bacteria. However, the stomach doesn't know the difference between good and bad bacteria, just like antibiotics. So it can kill the product on which you just spent good money. During breast-feeding, the combination of the calcium in the milk to buffer the acidity of the stomach, with the lower HCL output in an infant, allows these good bugs to survive the gastric environment. In the adult, manufacturers take extra measures to ensure survivability of the probiotics.

Don't be fooled by labels and claims. As we've seen, there are many products with wonderful claims that don't contain what the label says. There is more than one way to ensure survivability of probiotics. The issue is to find a product that has the bugs you need, where the CFU count is appropriate, they are alive in the box, and survive past the stomach. There are a number of fine products out there, and there are a number of questionable products available for sale as well. For you, the average consumer just trying to get better, you don't want to have to roll the dice several times to see if you come up a winner. This is one reason why many of those who dip their toes into natural medicine walk away feeling as if it doesn't work. Well if your drug didn't have an active ingredient in it, or at the right dose, then that wouldn't work either.

For example, in one **ConsumerLab.com** analysis, they pulled 13 probiotic products off the shelf for sale in the U.S. and/or Canada. Only two passed the testing which was measuring the number of bacteria that were alive and viable at time of the testing as compared to the label claim. The actual CFU count as compared to the label claim in some of these products was as low as 7%, 10%, and 13%. Keep in mind that **ConsumerLab.com** was just trying to culture the probiotics from the packaging. No consideration was given to stomach acids, which is why in some cases a simulated gastric environment is used to replicate the acid exposure in the stomach to see if anything survives.

On a similar note, the folks at Bastyr University, with funding from the NIH and the Washington State Department of Health, looked at probiotics and their label claims. They purchased 84 products for sale, and tested for viability and identification, not for count. They found that although 88% of the samples had viable bacteria, only 8% of the products were both viable and had no additional bugs that "snuck in". In other words, they found 71% of the product tested included at least one extra organism. You may think you're getting more for your money, but 10% of the products tested had more than one potentially pathogenic organism, which could pose a health risk. They didn't count the CFU, and they didn't perform a gastric environment test.

This is one reason why it may be best to seek out a qualified practitioner in natural medicine. In theory, they have already tried a number of different products, and have settled on one or two with which they have had the most success. This natural medicine business is a complex one, as I'm sure you have come to appreciate.

Should you want to avoid the supplemental route, and try a yogurt that contains probiotics, then have at it. I would caution you to re-read the chapter on dairy before doing so. Although there are products in the marketplace that have clinical data to support their use, there are others that don't test out so well. With studies in Australia, Britain, and the U.S., many brands show a marked drop in viable probiotics, with some having none. (3) There are a number of factors that can affect the viability of probiotics in yogurt products, which include: acids, oxygen, strains used, sugars, growth promoters and inhibitors, temperature, competition and more. (4) Even when there are some bacteria still present, authors question the validity of any beneficial label claims, as the CFU remaining has questionable efficacy.

I often get questions regarding when a probiotic should be taken, such as with a meal, at bedtime, etc. Opinions vary, but my recommendation is first thing in the morning. You are ensured of an empty stomach, and so it will pass through quickly. The acidity upon awakening is less so than during the day on an empty stomach. I don't recommend taking it with food as the food will remain in the stomach for hours, albeit at a higher pH, but the duration of exposure is longer. In addition, the bile salts and pancreatic enzymes released with food digestion also play a factor in probiotic survivial in the gut. None of these issues are present when you first wake up.

Some products will contain "prebiotics," which are essentially fuel for bacteria. There are both pros and cons for their use. As prebiotics, such as inulin, provide fuel for probiotics, they have also been found to feed pathogenic bacteria as well. I don't see any need for prebiotics, assuming you have a healthy diet with fiber for the bacteria to feed upon. I will not reference any data on prebiotics.

Urogenital Effects

We'll begin with the vagina, as that's where our first encounter with probiotics occurs in life. In vaginal ecology, we're covering the same types of pathogens as would be seen in the gut, such as pathogenic bacteria and yeast. So the potential conditions that can be treated include vulvovaginal candidiasis (yeast infections), bacterial vaginosis, and urinary tract infections. These conditions are the results of an imbalance, just like in the gut, between the good bugs and the bad bugs. Antibiotics are often used for bacterial vaginitis, but as you will recall, they kill off all bacteria, both good and bad. Bacterial vaginitis is characterized by changes in the flora of the vagina, with reductions in lactobacilli and increases in bacteria you don't particularly want there. The flora in the vagina is dominated by lactobacilli bacteria in healthy women, and this is recognized as a protective measure from pathogens. (5)

Like other conditions, the research shows certain species and even strains work better than others. In the vagina, the differences likely revolve around the ability to kill candida and bacteria, and adhere to the lining of the vagina and cervix. For example, one trial involved 106 women diagnosed with bacterial vaginosis. They were treated with Flagyl 500mg twice a day for 7 days, and received oral probiotics or placebo for 30 days. The probiotics used were a lactobacillus rhamnosus strain and a lactobacillus reuteri strain. At follow-up, 88% within the probiotic group were cured as compared to 40% in the antibiotic-only group. (7) Of those who weren't cured, the outcomes in the probiotic arm were better. Lastly, high counts of lactobacillus species were found in the vagina in almost all probiotic subjects, but only in half of the non-probiotic subjects. Yes, oral intakes of probiotics can work their way into the vagina.

In 2001, several researchers showed for the first time that oral probiotic lactobacilli can be delivered within the body to the vagina via oral intake. They used 10 women with a history of recurrent yeast infections, bacterial vaginosis, and urinary tract infections and gave them strains from lactobacillus rhamnosus and fermentum suspended in skim milk twice a day for 14 days. They recovered and identified the strains from the vagina verifying viability and delivery. Of note, 6 of the 10 cases were resolved in one week. (7)

In a candidiasis study, 55 women were treated with a single dosing of fluconazole, and then given a placebo or a probiotic product with lactobacilli rhamnosus and reuteri strains for the next 4 weeks. About 4 times as many subjects in the placebo group cultured for yeast, while very few of the probiotic group did. (8)

Cancer

There is a fair amount of evidence for considering the use of probiotics in cancer prevention strategies. Like any other data, there is no definitive conclusion on benefit and mechanism of action. It is theorized that there are possibly several mechanisms behind the use of probiotics in cancer prevention, most notably colon cancer. These mechanisms include: a change in intestinal pH, binding to or inhibition of the release of carcinogens, short chain fatty acid production, immune system support, and an anti-pathogenic-bacterial role.

Colorectal cancer is the third most common form of cancer, has unflattering survival rates, and doesn't seem to be decreasing given the vast sums of money spent on pharmaceuticals. Colorectal cancer is an important issue for both men and women; thus it's something we can all appreciate.

With cancer, prevention is especially the best option. With researchers always divided, what constitutes prevention? High fat diets, low fiber diets, and diets with chemicals such as nitrates have all been shown to promote cancer development. Probiotics have been associated with lower rates of cancer, but more studies are needed.

Let's look at just one aspect to try to understand the broader picture. The GI tract hosts a complicated series of events. Its health is affected demonstrably by the things we put down our throat. Likewise, our overall health is clearly impacted by the health, or lack thereof within the GI tract. Just one consideration is a detoxification pathway that can affect several cancers. Glucuronidation is a detoxification pathway in the liver that binds up a toxin to glucuronic acid, which has consistent data in its support. Toxins like drugs, food additives, and hormones are metabolized in this pathway. What the liver has done is to bind up a toxin with a chaperone, excrete it through the bile, and hopefully it will leave the body and land in the toilet. There are several considerations to be made, one of which is the bacteria present in the gut.

Some pathogenic bacteria have the ability to cleave, or separate the toxin from the chaperone through enzymes. Once on its own the toxin is capable of being reabsorbed. As you can imagine, this isn't a great idea. Especially when you consider that the average American diet is loaded with toxins, and it's likely that many livers are already overburdened. A diet high in animal fat may be unhealthy, but you also have to consider that animals concentrate their toxins in their fat just as we do. These cattle are fed in feed lots, on feed laced with pesticides, herbicides, and more that wind up in their fat, as do the drugs these animals are administered. As the top member in the food chain, you have to be able to detoxify these chemicals for your health.

Some strains of probiotics have been shown to decrease the enzymatic activity, beta-glucuronidase, of these pathogenic bacteria, thus leaving the detox-complex intact for excretion. Probiotics positively impact other potentially harmful enzymes as well, to include nitroreductase and azoreductase. As for the other mechanisms, we already know that probiotics have the ability to kill off pathogenic bacteria by a couple possible mechanisms. As we will soon see, they also have the ability to boost the overall immune system. It's likely that any anticancer benefit seen would be from several aspects.

In looking at colon cancer, a Japanese study found that the incidence of cancer was lowest when the colonic population of bifidobacteria (probiotic) was the highest, and when the bacteria clostridium perfringens was the lowest. (9) Clostridium perfringens is one of the most common causes of food infections, and is the leading cause of gangrene.

In regards to breast cancer, a French study with 1,010 breast cancer cases compared to 1,950 healthy control subjects found that yogurt consumption, or the probiotics in the yogurt more specifically, had a protective benefit. (10) In addition, the risks of breast cancer increased with cheese consumption (a concentrated dairy source), and the level of fat in the milk. A Dutch study found much the same thing. They compared 133 breast cancer subjects to 289 controls in regards to fermented milk consumption, and stated, "Our results suggest that a high consumption of fermented milk products may have a protective effect on the risk of breast cancer." (11) These two fermented dairy trials essentially mimic what Metchnikoff observed. Of course, you can get probiotics in a pill, and avoid the dairy, which would seem to be the best of both worlds.

The benefits for breast cancer are likely from two primary mechanisms. As probiotics decrease the enzymes able to free up toxins for reabsorption, the implications are for more than the colon. In addition to the many other toxins, one of the compounds excreted through beta-glucuronidase is an estrogen metabolite. For breast cancer, an estrogen-dependent tissue, excreting excess estrogen would be ideal. This is just one of many ways probiotics are of value. Another likely mechanism is from overall immune enhancement. It's likely that an elevated healthy immune response can reduce cancer incidence. So let's look at the immunity connection.

Immunity

There are a number of animal and test-tube data to support several theorized reasons for probiotics in immune health. Without going into the complicated world of the immune system, it would seem more valuable to highlight some great clinical data. In the end, you as a patient don't necessarily care about T-cells, gut-associated lymphoid tissue, IgA, and phagocytes. Your main concern is that if you spend your hard-earned money on a probiotic product, will there be measurable benefits?

A recent trial from 2009, published in the mainstream journal, *Pediatrics*, illustrates the power of probiotics on the immune system. In 326 children aged 3-5 years, a lactobacillus acidophilus strain, a combination of lactobacillus acidophilus plus bifidobacterium animalis strains, or placebo were given for 6 months to see if they reduced cold and flu-like symptoms. The single acidophilus probiotic reduced fever incidence by 53%, coughing by 41%, and runny nose by 28% as compared to placebo. The dual probiotic administration resulted in an even more impressive reduction in incidence of fever by 73%, coughing by 62%, and runny nose by 59%. Antibiotic use was reduced by 68% with the single strain, and by a whopping 84% in the dual strain. As you would expect, these kids missed about a third fewer days of school. (12)

In a similar trial published in the same journal, three M.D.s studied probiotics for the prevention of infection. Encompassing 14 child-care centers in Israel, 201 children aged 4-10 months were given either placebo, a bifidobacterium lactis strain, or a lactobacillus reuteri strain over the course of 12 weeks. Although the bifido lactis group on average did better than placebo, the reuteri group did exceptionally well. Episodes of fever, days of fever, episodes of diarrhea, days with diarrhea, clinic visits, absence from daycare, and antibiotic prescriptions were all significantly reduced. (13) Unlike in the previous trial, respiratory illnesses were no different from placebo and probiotic groups. Again, you have to consider the differences in strains used, as research shows different strains appear to have different benefits within the body. This is an excellent argument to buy a diversified probiotic product with multiple strains.

In one more immune health trial, we'll now look at adults. This trial out of Sweden compared 94 subjects receiving lactobacillus reuteri to 87 getting a placebo over 80 days in a workplace environment. The study demonstrated that a daily intake of probiotics was able to reduce the workers gastrointestinal and respiratory tract diseases by 60%! (14)

Dermatitis

Eczema is a general term for skin conditions that include one or more of the following: swelling, itching, blistering, flaking, crusting, redness, dryness, oozing, and bleeding of the skin. Contact dermatitis can arise from an allergic response to poison ivy, for example, or from an irritant, such as the many chemicals in our clothing, furniture, bed sheets, etc. Atopic dermatitis is a subset of eczema, typically in children, and seemingly with a genetic predisposition. Atopic is defined as a genetic predisposition for an allergic reaction, which could present as a respiratory outcome, such as asthma, or a dermatologic one, such as dermatitis.

Dermatitis can arise from direct contact, but not necessarily. It can also be "in the blood," and thus come from something else, such as food. In fact, it is recommended that for infants with atopic dermatitis, they be breast-fed and the introduction of complex proteins such as wheat, dairy, and soy be postponed. This brings us to probiotics. As we've learned, food can cause a wide array of issues, not just isolated to the GI tract. In the chapter on dairy, I showed how ear infections, dermatitis, eczema, and asthma could all be traced to dairy consumption. Clearly, in order to reduce the inflammation for your child, you should address several aspects of their care, first and foremost being the diet.

As clinical trials will typically only look at one variable at a time, we'll look at probiotics and their role in skin inflammation. As with IBD, probiotics are not THE answer, but a part of the answer. This is why the data is not conclusive. The theorized benefits behind the use of probiotics for skin applications revolve around the GI tract and the immune system. More specifically, within the GI tract it is thought that probiotics help with the mucosal barrier. If you recall, we covered gut permeability in IBD, but a refresher will help. In a compromised, inflamed GI tract, the integrity of the cells that line the tract is compromised. Instead of being a single organ with tight junctions with their neighbors, candida, NSAIDs, inflammation, and genetic flaws can compromise this wall from only letting in little food particles to accidently letting in larger full proteins, which skip into the blood. The immune system attacks these proteins, as the only full proteins that should be in the blood are the ones made by the body. A continuous ramped-up inflammation in attack mode on these various proteins may result in some conditions we've seen such as type 1 diabetes, rheumatoid arthritis, or skin inflammation.

Probiotics are thought to help retain the barrier in the gut by several mechanisms, as well as modulate the immune response, much like vitamin A. With this in mind, researchers out of Germany looked at intestinal barrier function in children with atopic dermatitis. In 41 children with severe atopic dermatitis, a lactobacillus rhamnosus and reuteri strain were given versus placebo for 6 weeks. The probiotics resulted in a significant decrease in severity of eczema and GI symptoms as compared to placebo, and improved the lactulose to mannitol ratio. (15) So what's a lactulose to mannitol ratio? It's an interesting test. You drink two sugar molecules, which the body can't metabolize. After collection of urine, the lab determines the amount of these two sugars you excreted, which means the amount you absorbed through your GI tract. The more lactulose, which is the larger molecule, the more permeable your gut is between your cells, allowing in larger proteins and toxins kicking off inflammation and immune reactivity. The more mannitol absorbed, the more your cells may allow small antigens to cross. The lab comes up with a ratio, which is presumed to be ideal.

So in this study, when the authors state an improvement in this test, they are saying that probiotics are able to stabilize the intestinal barrier, which allows in fewer proteins and the like into the blood, resulting in less immune response and inflammation, resulting in a significant decrease in skin inflammation.

In another trial, a lactobacillus rhamnosus strain and a bifidobacterium animalis strain were given to pregnant women and their newborns to 2 years of life. The infants who had received the rhamnosus strain, but not the animalis strain, had half the rate of eczema at 2 years. (16) In a very similar study, 62 mother-infant pairs were given probiotics during pregnancy and lactation. For the probiotic-exposed infants, the risk of developing eczema in the first two years of life was only 15% as compared to the 47% risk for those who were on placebo. (17) In addition, a genetic link back to the mothers proved to be a clear risk factor.

This trial shows us a couple things. First, a mother can pass on probiotics administered orally either in utero, in breast milk, or both. Second, genetic links keep coming up throughout this book. We all have genetic compromises. The trick is to know what they are, and work with them through natural medicine. Recall that half of natural medicine is your diet. So whether your genes push you towards rheumatoid arthritis, asthma, dermatitis, Crohn's, ulcerative colitis, high homocysteine, or any of the other myriad issues addressed in this book, it's up to you to work with those flaws, and manage your care accordingly.

Not all studies are as supportive for probiotics. Another German study found no benefit in administering L. rhamnosus to infants suffering from atopic dermatitis. (18) And in a review of 13 trials looking at atopic dermatitis control with probiotics, the authors illustrated weak support for probiotics, but held L. rhamnosus above all others for performance. (19)

What should be made of the data? First, either marked benefit was seen, or none. Notice there were no negative effects in using probiotics. Second, once again it appears the type of probiotic, in this case rhamnosus, has more beneficial effects. Third, the condition is multifactorial with foods being a prime suspect. Also, supplements to modulate the immune response and inflammation such as vitamin A, fish oil, and quercetin may be of added value. Last, there may have been variability in the quantity of probiotic count administered and viability of the bacteria. You will only know after you've tried a multifaceted approach.

Diarrhea

Although not as much of an issue here in the states as in developing nations, infectious diarrhea is still a concern. The very young, the very old, and the compromised patients are at greatest risk, but if you've ever had food poisoning or a stomach bug, it's no fun for anyone. The pathogen can be E coli, Shigella, Clostridium difficile, or rotavirus. As if these weren't enough to try to avoid, antibiotics can also cause diarrhea. As we know, antibiotics kill all bacteria, both good and bad. Depending on who you reference, Clostridium difficile is responsible for 15-50% of all cases of diarrhea associated with antibiotic use. (20, 21) So if C difficile is a bacteria, and antibiotics kill all bacteria, then how does antibiotic use cause diarrhea induced by C difficile?

As we know, some pathogenic bacteria have become resistant to antibiotics. C difficile in recent years has developed a new and very powerful strain. This new strain, associated with increased morbidity and mortality, is getting much attention. In 2004 and 2005, the CDC emphasized that the risk of C. difficile-associated diarrhea has increased, to include not only antibiotic use, but surgery, healthcare setting exposure, serious underlying illnesses to include immune-compromised, and aging. (22) In addition, patients on PPIs (proton pump inhibitors for GERD) and heart transplant patients are also at an elevated risk. In fact, C difficile is now more common in the general population as well. This viscious tissue destroying bug is able to colonize the gut better because the antibiotics disrupted your normal intestinal flora, the good bacteria. (23)

Even if C difficile is not the culprit, the rates of antibiotic-induced diarrhea reach as high as 62% of patients. (24) As antibiotics clearly disrupt and kill the normal flora of the gut, studies have been conducted using probiotics to re-inoculate the gut following antibiotic therapy, and as a preventative measure while on antibiotics. If you take probiotics while on antibiotics, the question remains: "Is the antibiotic killing off the good guys?" There are varied opinions on this, and it will depend on the practitioner.

As is always the case, the data for diarrhea treatment and prevention is mixed in support of probiotics. Logically, it makes a lot of sense to use them, and you'd expect consistent results. Of course, the same variables remain, that of CFU count, viability, and strain chosen for the bug in question.

For example, one study used a lousy 60 million probiotic cells of L rhamnosus to treat diarrhea from rotavirus in 684 patients, half of whom were controls. (25) They found no difference between the two groups in terms of diarrhea frequency or duration, vomiting, or length of hospital stay. I'm not surprised, as 60 million is a lot less than billions of bacteria. What I am surprised by is that the same authors in the same year used the same paultry 60 million count to treat persistent diarrhea caused by E coli, Shigella, or C difficile, and they halved the duration of diarrhea, and significantly reduced hospital stay as compared to placebo. (26) Although supported by this last trial, using 60 million is asking for failure. As the research has rapidly progressed in the field of probiotics, you will now usually see minimums of 1 billion. Even 1 billion is considered more of a maintanence dose, whereas something on the order of 5 billion+ is considered therapeutic.

Another trial used L rhamnosus to treat infectious diarrhea because the authors noted that it has previously demonstrated the most consistent effect in reducing the duration of diarrhea. These researchers found the L rhamnosus strains to be effective for rotavirus specifically. (27) There have been many reviews of probiotics and diarrhea undertaken, and the conclusions vary from supporting their use, to requiring more data. One review, which did not support the use of probiotics in pediatric antibiotic-associated diarrhea, stated that the dose (CFU) and strains used may be responsible for the mixed results. They went on to imply that a count of 5 billion CFU or more per day, for certain strains to include L rhamnosus, would show stronger evidence. (28)

In a recent study, strains of L casei, L bulgaricus, and Streptococcus thermophilus were used in 135 hospital patients with an average age of 74. The objective of the study was to see if this probiotic drink could reduce or prevent diarrhea associated with antibiotic use, to include C difficile. (29) These researchers out of a London Hospital, published in the prestigious *British Medical Journal*, found that only 12% of the probiotic group developed diarrhea, as compared to 34% in the placebo group. Notice these strains are different than the one advocated previously. Interestingly, they noted in reference to skeptical reviewers, "This is a major advance on previous meta-analyses (reviews) which called for further definitive trials and expressed considerable doubt as to the efficacy in preventing C difficile associated diarrhea." In their conclusion they noted that probiotics have the potential to decrease morbidity, healthcare costs, and mortality if used routinely in patients over 50. Why start at 50?

I know this is all confusing, and contradictory, but a good probiotic product does work. It may very well depend on the strain, and it certainly depends on the CFU count and viability as well. You can use the data to seek out a product that has strains specific to your needs, or you can buy something with multiple strains, for broad-spectrum support. The sad fact is that in this relatively unregulated industry, it's hard to tell the good products from the useless ones.

IBS

Depending on whom you reference, IBS affects 3-25% of the population. (30-32) There are several types of IBS: diarrhea predominant, constipation predominant, alternating between the two, and undefined. (33) For all intents and purposes, the average IBS patient doesn't care how some egghead defines it, they just want relief from diarrhea, constipation, bloating, pain, heartburn, gas, and systemic effects such as fatigue, headaches, and more. Classically, IBS is alternating constipation and diarrhea. There are a number of theories as to why IBS occurs, but I'll focus on bacteria, with just a couple of caveats.

First, I'd like to say that it's not in your head. Many practitioners and some researchers want to lump IBS in with psychological issues. With that said, there is definitely a connection between the brain and the gut. Serotonin, the "feel good neurotransmitter," for example, is even more abundant in the gut than it is in the brain. In fact, SSRI's are given to IBS patients in this vein, but as you can guess, if they were successful, many

Americans wouldn't still be searching for answers. So there's more to IBS than "It's in your head." In fact, if you've been ill for some time, and gut permeability messes with your immune system, your sleep, pain, fatigue, and most anything else you can imagine, I think anyone would be a little psychologically off. I can't tell you how many patients have heard from a doctor that the condition is in their head, or they are lying, or something to that effect. As if the patient has nothing better to do with their time and money. The gall and arrogance of these doctors who have no empathy. If you hear "it's in your head" enough times from enough "authority figures," then you begin to believe it's true. Because IBS has no consistent biological marker or unifying framework, the symptom-based approach lets the unskilled doctor off the hook by putting the blame on your mental status.

Wouldn't it be nice to hear: "I honestly don't know why you are having these symptoms, but it's not in your head, your symptoms are real, this is the body's way of communicating to you, and so I'll do my best to help you. It may take some time and some effort on your behalf, but we'll do our best to get to the bottom of it." That would be a nice change from the accusatory doubt-riddled comments preceding the SSRI or benzodiazapene prescription.

My second caveat is the role of food allergies. Throughout this book I believe I have demonstrated their potential role in your overall health, and the difficulties in identifying them short of going on a hypo-allergenic diet for a long period of time. Make no mistake, your IBS could be an allergy to the proteins in dairy or wheat. The pain, binding, bloating, run-down feeling can be from a food that we're all better off not consuming, but you for whatever reason are more susceptible than the rest of us. With all that said, we'll now refocus on a relatively new concept.

In IBS, there is an interesting theory about bacterial infiltration and imbalance known as small intestinal bacterial overgrowth (SIBO). In the ideal GI tract, there are many times more bacteria in the colon or large intestine than in the small intestine. As you work your way upstream from the rectum, the amounts of bacteria diminish the closer you get to the stomach, with either a sterile environment or dramatically reduced bacterial counts in the first section or two of the small intestine.

Therefore, when you eat starches/carbohydrates (ie simple or complex sugars) any fermentation should occur in the colon, which has an escape route nearby for the gas. However, if you have more bacteria and the wrong kind of bacteria too far upstream in the small intestine, then you can get fermentation there, but the anal escape route isn't exactly right around the corner. This leads to bloating and the binding pain associated with it.

For example, in a study with 202 IBS patients, SIBO was determined by a breath test. The theory here is that bacteria that are further up in the GI tract than they ought to be produce certain gases, in this case hydrogen, which can be measured upon exhaling. They found that 78% of the 202 patients had abnormal hydrogen. When 47 of these SIBO patients were given antibiotics, 25 had eradication of SIBO as determined by the breath test. (34)

This is similar to clinical experience. Usually an IBS patient feels better during antibiotic therapy. It can be assumed that the prolific bad bacteria in the small intestine have been mostly killed off by antibiotics, but so have the good guys. But this is a temporary fix. After discontinuation of the antibiotics, the gut will repopulate dependent on what survived and your diet and exposure. Also keep in mind that antibiotics don't kill yeast. So while the good and bad bacteria are dying, space has been freed up for candida, hence all the books and talk on candida and yeast.

So why are these bad bugs creeping up the GI tract, and in large numbers? The healthy body has several mechanisms in place to control this. One is breast-feeding, which gets your GI tract off on the right foot. These good bugs do a great many things for your entire body. However, the body never budgeted for antibiotics. We didn't exactly evolve with them. Since their discovery and use, they have been mostly excellent tools for our health. However, with their current overuse, we suffer needlessly, and create some nasty resistant pathogens as well. As breast-feeding isn't an option for most of us, I know there's a joke in here somewhere, probiotics are the next best thing to re-innoculate the gut.

The body produces HCL in the stomach to kill bacteria, break down proteins, and activate nutrients. However, we treat heartburn with drugs that block acid secretion, and in turn increase our risks for several conditions, one of which is SIBO. (35) HCL production declines with age as well. In fact, one of the most significant risk factors for developing IBS is an acute bacterial infection, such as Salmonella or Campylobacter. (36,37) The HCL in the stomach would help to kill off much of these invaders, and a strong GI tract and immune system with vitamins like A especially, should help defend the body well. Also, bile and pancreatic enzymes are antibacterial, and help to keep the upper small intestine clean. However, our pancreas is overworked with the "dead foods" we constantly eat, and many Americans have had their gall bladders removed, which affects the absorption of vitamins A, D, E and K, as well as helps to control pathogens from feeding off of newly ingested foods.

If this wasn't all bad enough, the pathogenic bacteria can move outside of the gut, through a process called translocation. (38) It's basically gut permeability for bacteria. These nasty bacteria tear apart the GI tract through various toxins they create, and the GI tract responds with inflammation. The net result is the ability of these bacteria to get into the rest of your body and wreak havoc. A potentially important consequence of this translocation is immune activation, which was verified in a study. (39) The immune system, or some other mechanism, may in turn cause problems with the musculoskeletal system, as seen in fibromyalgia. In fact, in one fibromyalgia study, 100% of the patients had an abnormal breath test indicating SIBO. (40)

The therapeutic goal is to reduce the overall bacterial burden in the small intestine, convert from bad to good as much as possible, and do the same in the colon. As we know, probiotics have a wide variety of benefits in this regard. They support the physical mucosal barrier between the gut and the body, they compete for nutrients with the bad guys, they have antibacterial properties, and they positively affect the immune response in the gut. These are all enormous benefits in IBS and IBD. Unlike antibiotics, they also kill yeast. In one review, lactobacillus plantarum seemed to show the most consistent benefit for IBS. (41) Trials with other probiotics, such as l rhamnosus and bifido strains, have also shown to be of use, depending on your individual needs and response.

It's interesting and refreshing to note that one duo of researchers addressed the issue of probiotic quality. They noted that given the lack of regulation of commercial probiotic products, it's important to have a product with the strains and concentrations claimed, and to not have any contamination with potentially pathogenic bacteria. (42)

In one study, the severity of IBS was cut in half in just 14 days on probiotics, whereas it was only reduced by 8% with placebo. (43) In another study, bifidobacteria longum reduced constipation in 27% of the patients who were compliant with the regimen, with only 11% improvement in those who weren't compliant. (44) Interestingly, those who were on laxatives experienced a worsening of constipation. In a constipation study with children, probiotics given for 4 weeks to 45 kids with chronic constipation under the age of 10 showed better results than placebo, and equal results to the laxative magnesium oxide, but with much less abdominal pain. (45) In yet another study with children, an L rhamnosus strain improved IBS treatment success to 33%, compared to 5% for the placebo group. (46)

Without going into the heavy science babble about the immune system, the enteric nervous system, in vitro and animal studies, and more, I think you have an appreciation for the effects imbalances in the gut can have on the rest of the body. This is why one of the main driving tenets in naturopathic medicine is to start with the gut. We truly are what we eat, or more precisely what we eat, digest, and the digestive environment within. As we have looked here primarily at the small intestine, we'll now look primarily at the large intestine, with the more severe cousin to IBS.

IBD

The clinical data supporting probiotics is very mixed in the treatment of IBD. There are some trials that are very supportive. For example, L rhamnosus was as effective as a drug to prevent a relapse in ulcerative colitis out to 12 months. (47) For 10 Crohn's patients for whom drug therapy had failed, six had complete remission, with one having a partial response to probiotics measured out to 13 months. (48) In yet another trial, children with newly diagnosed ulcerative colitis had much higher success rates with a combination of probiotics and drugs, as compared to drugs alone. 93% had remission in the probiotic group compared to only 36% in the other, and 21% in the probiotic group relapsed within a year, whereas 73% did in the drug-only group. (49)

However, for every supportive trial, there is a trial with no beneficial results. As you can imagine by now, there are many factors to consider. When discussing food allergies, we get into this "chicken or the egg" conversation. For those who've had their guts torn up by celiac, you can imagine how the constant inflammation and tissue destruction could result in a compromised GI lining, letting in larger proteins, and resulting in additional food allergies. Likewise, it is well recognized that pathogenic organisms tear apart the epithelial lining of the GI tract, also creating permeability, and consequent food allergies. In the end, you'll have to avoid any foods that cause you inflammation. This concept was not addressed in these trials.

In addition, as seen with the rest of the data on probiotics, success may be dependent on the probiotic chosen, and the count and viability of the product. As we've seen, extensive clinical data has shown that beneficial bacteria (probiotics) improve the mucosal lining of the gut, positively impact the immune response, and are antibacterial and antifungal. Now compare that to a quote from one of the better review articles on IBD. "IBD...results from continuous enteric microbial antigenic stimulation of pathogenic T cell responses in individuals with genetic defects in mucosal barrier function, innate bacterial killing, or immunoregulation. Altered microbial composition, defective clearance of bacteria and enhanced mucosal uptake in Crohn's disease and ulcerative colitis increase immune stimulation. CD and UC preferentially occur in areas of highest intestinal bacteria concentrations and fecal flow sustains inflammation of CD." (50) Translated, IBD occurs in people with genetic flaws for which probiotics lines up perfectly as a treatment option.

Many of the more recent published opinions are in agreement on these flaws and many of the underlying factors. (51-55) Instead of listing more trials, we'll review the most recent data on IBD, and you can apply some reason, and determine if this is something you would like to try.

IBD is a nasty condition, with subsequent diarrhea, weight loss, nutritional deficiencies, ulceration, perforation, and possible surgery and colostomy bags. There is hope. Although "incurable", it can be managed. We've had an entire chapter on IBD, so we'll just briefly discuss findings pertaining to bacteria in the gut.

It has been shown that the introduction of an acute infection from some kind of pathogenic bacteria can set off a series of events leading to IBD. In one study involving thousands of U.S. soldiers, single episodes of an infectious gastroenteritis significantly increased the risk of developing IBD. (56) In either case, the disease is self-limiting. In other words, you don't suffer from food poisoning for the rest of your life. However, most people will go on to maintain a "normal" GI tract from then on. Then there are those who have genetic flaws in mucus lining, antimicrobial killing, and immune regulation in the gut. It could very well take one or two hits to this sensitive person to disrupt the balance in the gut, which given our diets, antibiotics, and lack of breast-feeding, probably wasn't a terribly good balance in the first place.

It is in these people that a shift in balance of bacterial occupants in quantity and quality occurs. The initial offending bacteria may be gone, or in the case of MAP, it may still be present. This is why research has not been able to consistently identify one particular bacterium as the cause of IBD. It simply requires an insult to the fragile system to dysregulate it. Once that happens, flaws in bacterial killing, mucus production, and immune regulation lead to persistent inflammation. The end result is diarrhea, tissue destruction, and the many other unpleasant features of IBD.

To make matters a bit more confusing, not all cases require an initial insult, or so it's thought. With these background genetic flaws, poor diets, antibiotics, and the like, a gradual shift has been noted in the occupants of the gut. There is data to show that the diversity of bacteria and types of bacteria shift. For example, in one fairly invasive trial, researchers went in and took biopsies from the sites of inflammation from patients with active IBD and compared them to controls. They found that the diversity (the number of different types of bacteria inhabiting the gut, which is in the hundreds) in Crohn's was half that of normal, and was only 30% of normal in UC. (57) In another study, other types of beneficial bacteria were significantly depleted in number. (58) If you recall from the IBD chapter, butyrate is a short chain fatty acid produced by certain beneficial bacteria, which is fuel for the epithelial cells that line the gut to produce mucus, among other things. Shifts in bacteria may result in the production of more hydrogen sulfide and other substances, which can injure these cells, and less of the fuel they need for sustenance.

Genetic flaws may support this gradual slide to a pathogenic state over time. In fact, it has been found that normal E coli strains, not of the food poisoning variety, have become more numerous and pathogenic in these susceptible individuals. (59,60) In the end, no pun intended, we're still staring down the same barrel. You have a situation of flaws in mucus, immune response, and bacterial killing, with subsequent diarrhea, inflammation, tissue destruction, malabsorption, and food/chemical allergies/sensitivities.

The focus of treatment has to be multifactorial. This is why any single solution, whether it be probiotics, a drug, curcumin, fish oil, or anything else, will only be partly successful and temporary. But this is how most clinical trials are run. Someone wants to see if their "baby" is the next magic bullet. It is a flaw in how we practice medicine and in how we design research protocols.

As you now know, the bad guys need to be killed, the lining of the gut needs to be refurbished, allergies and sensitivities need to be removed, inflammation needs to be reduced, and re-innoculation with probiotics needs to be undertaken to help compliment all of the three identifiable genetic flaws in IBD. This regimen in some capacity or another is likely a lifelong commitment, which for many turns out to be a superior alternative to drugs, surgery, and a wide array of horrible manifestations.

Chapter 15　Fish Oil

This chapter on fish oil is the last of four supplements discussed, and is certainly worth your consideration. I have tried to emphasize why all four are essentially required in our modern standard of living. Fish oil is probably the most known and most used of the four, and arguably the number one slot belongs to fish oil, at least among the fish oil sales people and companies. I believe it is a requirement, but not in the doses you may be using. In the same spirit as much of this book, I'll provide information, which you have likely not heard or read, along with balance, and a good dose of controversy.

What is fish oil, and why do we even need it? Like it or not, fat is a crucial component of our bodies, which is in contradiction to these many low-fat, no-fat diets we've been following. By the way, have you noticed that all these low-fat, no-fat products for sale haven't helped our obesity problem in this country? In fact, it has grown steadily worse. For example, about sixty percent of our brains are composed of fat, and every cell in our body has a lipid (fat) membrane. Fat as a solid, or its equivalent oil, a liquid, is essentially made of three fatty acids attached to a molecule of glycerol, hence the name triglyceride. It is these fatty acids that play a critical role in our health. There are a number of different fatty acids available in our diets. They vary in length, and in saturation or lack thereof. You will always see any natural fat source as a mixture of various fatty acids, with one or more predominating over the others. For example, butter is a fat. It is composed of eleven different fatty acids. Its most prevalent fatty acid, oleic acid, comprises about one third of its total constituency. This is the fatty acid you associate with the avocado, the olive, and the almond, to name a few. There are ten more fatty acids in butter alone.

Of all the fatty acids in our diet, we need to ingest two, which is why they are referred to as *essential fatty acids*. They both happen to be polyunsaturated fatty acids. You probably know this, since there are many savvy patients in this field, but we'll do a quick biochemistry review. The length of the fatty acid is dependent on the number of carbons. When two hydrogens are missing from adjacent carbons, a double bond is formed. A fatty acid may have no double bonds (saturated), one double bond (monounsaturated) or more than one double bond (polyunsaturated). The water-insoluble end is called the methyl end, which is a carbon attached to three hydrogens and ends the chain. The water-soluble end is called the acid end, which is two oxygens and one hydrogen. As you're probably muttering "who cares," these little variations play an enormous role in our health. That is why you hear from everyone, "Take fish oil." You know it's supposed to be good for you, but you don't know why.

There are two kinds of essential fatty acids, those of the omega-3 family, and those of the omega-6 family. We ingest way too much of the 6 variety, and not nearly enough of the 3, which is the point of this chapter. The base fatty acid, the starting block of the omega-3 family, is alpha-linolenic acid (LNA). It has 18 carbons, and the first double bond occurs at the third carbon from the methyl end, which is why it's called an omega-3 fatty acid. It has two more double bonds at the six and nine position. You mostly associate this source with flax, which itself is over 50% LNA by fatty acid ratio. From here, the body can manufacture other longer and more unsaturated fatty acids such as EPA and DHA. Here's the catch. Depending on whom you reference, who you are, and what you eat, the body has marginal to significant challenges converting LNA to EPA and DHA. For example, as one set of researchers states, "As only less than 5% of LNA is converted to EPA and DHA in the human organism, the dietary sources of these are also considered essential." (1) In other words, you'd be healthier consuming EPA and DHA from fish oil, than trying to convert LNA from a source such as flax, which is why the data on flax oil is not nearly as strong as it is for fish oil.

EPA and DHA are longer chain fatty acids the body needs, which can be made from LNA, or eaten in the diet. When you buy your bottle of fish oil, the very reason you're taking the product is for EPA and DHA, unless it's a liver oil for vitamins A and D. It is these highly unsaturated, loosely connected, oxygen-attracting fatty acids, EPA and DHA, which you want in your cell membranes for energy, detoxification, and a myriad of other health benefits.

So, how is fish oil going to reduce your healthcare expenses, how much do you need to take, and is all fish oil the same? All fish oil has

EPA and DHA at varying doses; most kinds are relatively free of toxins; but they do vary in their stability. Although the source of fish may vary, the goal is to provide you with the afforementioned EPA and DHA. The debate over cleanliness is really a non-issue. This is where one company says, "Our product is free of heavy metals and toxins." This is not where one fish oil can hang its hat versus another. The manufacturers all do a pretty good job of cleaning their oils. When I say "manufacturers" I'm referring to "fish oil suppliers." Relatively speaking, there are only a handful of fish oil suppliers to the market, but hundreds of different fish oil labels. In the summer of 2008, **ConsumerLab.com** released data on numerous fish oil supplements and a handful of fortified foods. They found that none of the products they chose were contaminated with heavy metals and toxins. I don't find this too surprising, since about two years earlier, I reviewed a number of fish oil products, and using their own data from independent labs found that every fish oil I researched was tested for the same heavy metals and toxins to the same levels of detectability, and showed the same results. This is a credit to the industry, especially when you consider that if you were to buy fish from a market, whether it were farm raised or wild, that fish would most certainly have higher toxicity.

The differences between fish oils reside in their stability, or conversely, their rancidity. You may have had the unpleasant experience of burping up nasty fish oil. Aside from buying a quality shelf-stable fish oil, you can help alleviate that problem a few ways. First, refrigerate your fish oil. I don't care how stable it is, or someone says it is, it's fish oil. These fatty acids oxidize extremely quickly, which means they spoil quickly. Two, take your fish oil with the first bites of a meal; don't take it at the end and set it on top of your meal because you'll be asking for trouble. Third, ensure you take a high gamma mixed tocopherol (vitamin E), even though the label will say it's added. Also, you probably don't need to take as much fish oil as you've been lead to believe, as you will read.

Stability is where fish oils part ways. Some are more stable than others. That rancid taste and/or smell are your primary sensory indicators signaling an oxidized oil. If you dare, bite into that softgel you've been buying, and if it tastes rancid, get a different product.

Rancidity can be tested, and it is. But here's the caveat: it's tested at the time of manufacture, which is not real world. The Council for Responsible Nutrition (CRN) is one association that helps to set standards for this industry. When it comes to the stability of fish oil they set standards based on laboratory markers. There are two such markers, a peroxide value (PV), and an anisidine value (AN). These are markers of oxidation. Combined, they form what's called a total oxidation number (TOTOX), which equals two times PV plus AN.

In their monograph they state that the proposed limits are for a PV of no more than 5 meq/kg, and an AN maximum of 20 meq/kg, with a maximum TOTOX of 26, which represents the most stringent quality standard for EPA and DHA. You will see many fish oil products state the PV, and even some will discuss AN, but keep in mind this is at time of manufacture. We know that these oils are unstable, because you've belched them back up. Some will cover the taste with enormous amounts of flavoring, lemon being the favorite. I'm sure you're well aware of the health benefits in taking fish oil, some of which we'll now cover. However, did you know that there can be "side effects" from rancid oils? <u>You can probably get more bang for your supplement buck by taking less fish oil, but a higher quality one.</u>

How did we get started on this fish oil kick anyhow? Our initial inkling of the benefits of cold water fish came from the Eskimos. The Eskimos, although consuming a high fat diet, suffer significantly less from cardiovascular disease, joint disease, skin, and other inflammatory illnesses as compared to their standard American diet (SAD) counterparts. Their marine based diet is rich in omega-3 fatty acids, so much so that it is approximately 20 times our levels here in the states. This allows for cell walls to become less rigid and thus respond better to the constant flux of incoming and outgoing cellular components. Whether it's suppleness of skin, fluidity of joints, responsiveness to insulin, elasticity of the vasculature, or whole organ support, it is crucial for your cells to have omega-3 fatty acids as a part of the cell wall. These Eskimos with their high protein and low fruit and vegetable diet aren't altogether models of health, but the inflammatory association was the impetus of massive amounts of research and money expenditures.

The reduced inflammation results from a shift in your inflammatory response. So what does this mean? One of the beneficial effects of EPA and DHA is that they provide the raw materials to your body to down regulate the inflammatory response to an insult. An insult can be a physical injury, an inhalant allergy, and much more. It's not so much that fish oil is anti-inflammatory, it is just less inflammatory than a response from omega-6 dominated pathways. So if you have a diet high in vegetable oils and animal proteins from farms that feed their animals corn, then you have "pre-loaded" your cells with lots of omega-6 fatty acids. Upon an insult to the body, these fatty acids form what's known as eicosanoids from the parent compound arachidonic acid. Certain prostaglandins, thromboxanes, and leukotrienes (all eicosanoids) can impair the immune system, promote clotting, promote inflammation, and constrict the arteries. We don't want to eliminate all omega-6 fatty acids from the diet, just as we don't need to eliminate all saturated fatty acids either. We just need to ingest healthy ones and in reasonably healthy ratios. It is the incorporation of these oils into your cell membranes, with the accompanying shift in inflammation pathways, that makes fish oil so beneficial.

Numerous highlights in the research will make my point that these fatty acids are crucial to your good health. Preferably you'd get them from eating fresh vegetables and nuts, and fresh fish and wild game. I repeat, ideally you would ingest your omega-3 fatty acids from freshly caught fish, a recently fallen nut, or a just-killed wild animal. This is important, because polyunsaturated fatty acids do not do well over time. This speaks to rancidity, and possibly to toxicity to you. However, we no longer reside in that world. That was the world of our ancestors thousands of years ago with an abundance of food, and little human population. Now with over six billion people smothering our planet, our food comes from far away, processed, packaged, preserved, farmed, and exposed in a system that prides itself on efficiencies of scale. So what do we do? We make supplements in efficiencies of scale to counteract our nutritional diversion. Understand this: your need for these fatty acids is in your genes, and it's expressed in a multitude of subtle ways.

There is data to support the use of fish oil in a variety of conditions. We'll focus on four general areas that have high prevalence and cost. Of course fish oil has many other potential uses. Numerous patients present with eczema, psoriasis, or simple dry skin, all of which may benefit from its use. Omega-3 fatty acids may help with weight loss. Significant cancer data shows benefit in omega-3 fatty acids, and risks with saturated and omega-6 fatty acids when in excess. IBD, osteoporosis, asthma, brain health and more all have supportive data as well.

CVD

A recent trial out of Norway with 2,412 participants, where patients were followed for an average 57 months, essentially showed no benefit for the use of moderate to high doses of fish oil <u>when looking at coronary events</u>. The researchers did not find any benefit in taking more fish oil as compared to lower intakes. There was a slightly increased risk in those consuming less than about 1/3 gram of oil per day. (2) In translation, you don't have to consume tons of fish oil to reduce your chances of coronary events.

Is that true? Is this just an anomaly? Do I only have to take more than 1/3 gram per day? Hasn't fish oil been shown to have a vast array of beneficial properties in much larger doses when it comes to cardiovascular disease? Let's take a closer look at some of the data. Keep in mind that there are scores of papers on fish oil. Next to calcium, it may be one of the most studied natural ingredients.

In terms of CVD risk, fish oil has been shown to have a beneficial role in regards to HDL, arrhythmia control, vasodilation, plaque stability, triglycerides, platelet aggregation (how much blood cells stick to each other), inflammation, blood pressure, and more. As is the case with all other clinical trials, there is wide variability in how studies are constructed. There are many in vitro studies that look at activity outside the body, there are post-mortem studies looking at fatty acid profiles, there are epidemiological studies looking at whole populations, and many more. The real driving question is: "Do these individual beneficial components lead to better outcomes in CVD disease, and ultimately in mortality?"

One of the many variables is that of population. For example, if you are a Sicilian who eats cold water fish 2-3 times per week, then the benefit of adding 1-3 grams of fish oil may not be as pronounced as giving fish oil to someone from Arkansas getting by on corn fed pork and beef, no offense to Arkansas. If you're conducting a dietary recall study on a population, how accurate will their memory be of how often they ate fish, and what kind of fish it was. All fish is not the same. Warm water fish, for example, have much lower levels of EPA and DHA as compared to their cold water cousins.

Plus, you have to consider toxicity. Heavy metal toxicity has been linked to CVD. So if the researchers are using clean fish oil in a trial, and another trial uses fish caught off the shores of northern New Jersey, then you may have some confounding factors. With all that said, the aforementioned CVD benefits are reasonably universal.

So what was wrong with this Norway trial? These patients already had diagnosed coronary artery disease. They used a food frequency questionnaire. They covered both supplements and fish intake. There were a lot of patients, and they followed them for almost 5 years. Is this trial an anomaly? A bit, but not totally off base.

In a different trial, data from 20,551 male physicians aged 40-84 at baseline was collected as part of the Physician's Heath Study. Among other things, a food frequency questionnaire was used to determine fish intake. In this cut of the data at 11 years follow-up, there were 133 sudden cardiac deaths. It was found that for men who consumed fish at least once per week, the risk of sudden death was about half. (3) Fish consumption once per week likely provides less EPA/DHA than 1 gelcap of fish oil per day, dependent on quantity and fish type. Sudden cardiac death is a death that occurred within one hour of onset of symptoms. However, fish consumption was not associated with benefits in total heart attacks, nonsudden cardiac death (took more than one hour to die), or total CVD mortality in this study. To complicated things further, it did significantly improve overall mortality.

In an extension of this data at 17 years follow-up, previously collected and stored blood was analyzed for fatty acids in 94 men who had died. The researchers found that the risk of sudden cardiac death was much higher, up to 5 times, in those with the lowest amount of omega-3 fatty acids incorporated into their cells. (4) In other words, the more omega-3 fatty acids one consumes, the more you'll have incorporated into your cells. This makes sense, and basically supports the previous trial.

For 2,033 men who had recovered from a heart attack, three different dietary protocols were given, one of which was to increase fatty fish intake. The subjects who were advised to eat the extra fish had a 29% reduction in all deaths at 2 years out. (5) None of the dietary regimens positively affected deaths as a result of additional heart attacks. The daily consumption of EPA and DHA was approximately 900 mg. (6) Again, there was a benefit in total mortality, but less so for subsequent CVD.

The JELIS study out of Japan had 18,645 patients with high blood lipids, while over 3,500 had a previous vascular event. They were given either a statin drug, or a statin plus 1.8 grams of only EPA. The addition of the fish oil resulted in a 19% reduction of major coronary events as compared to the statin-only group. (7) They stated that, "Serum LDL cholesterol was not a significant factor in a reduction of risk for major coronary events." In this case, sudden cardiac death did not differ between groups.

In a re-cut of this data a year later, the authors focused on CVD risk factors other than LDL in those subjects *without a history of coronary artery disease*. These included high total cholesterol, obesity, high triglycerides, low HDL, diabetes, and hypertension. Those on fish oil had fewer of these risk factors, and the two markers where fish oil really helped were with high triglycerides and low HDL. The risk of coronary artery disease was more than halved for those with both low HDL (less than 40) and high triglycerides (equal to or more than 150). (8) They stated that, "High triglycerides and low HDL represents a particularly potent risk factor." Fish oil has been repeatedly shown to help in both of these parameters.

In an Italian study, 11,323 heart attack survivors received either 850 mg of EPA and DHA with 300mg of synthetic vitamin E, or the usual standard treatment. The researchers followed the patients for 3.5 years, and found marked improvements. The risk of cardiovascular death was 30% less, coronary death was 35% less, and the risk of sudden death was 45% less in the fish oil + vitamin E group. (9) This study is complicated by the fact that vitamin E was also used, which has proven heart health benefits of its own, especially in a more natural format, as opposed to the synthetic one given.

On one last trial, the omega-3 fatty acid levels were taken from the red blood cells of 334 patients who had died of sudden cardiac arrest, yet with no history of clinical heart disease, and compared to controls. When those with the lowest amount of omega-3 fatty acids were compared to those in the third quartile, there was a 70% reduction in the risk of sudden cardiac death. (10) In their conclusion, the researchers state, "Dietary intake of omega-3 polyunsaturated fatty acids from seafood is associated with a reduced risk of primary cardiac arrest."

Two main themes should jump out at you, with a few others in support. The first is that you really don't need to take a lot of fish oil to derive benefits from its use. Doses on the order of 1-2 grams per day would seem to do. Secondly, fish oil seems to have its greatest benefits in total mortality and sudden cardiac death, of course not shown in all trials. The mechanism behind the reduced risk in sudden cardiac death probably has something to do with the sensitivity in cellular signaling with increased membrane fluidity, possibly as seen in studies showing support for heart rate and arrhythmia control. In fact, one set of researchers states, "Experimental and clinical research should establish that the antiarrhythmic effect is the more natural candidate to support the efficacy of omega-3 fatty acids." (11) In other words, of all the reported beneficial changes fish oil has on cardiovascular risk factors such as clotting, vascular pliability, lipid changes, and more, it is seemingly the improvement in cellular signaling within the heart muscle that may be the greatest benefit.

Also of note, should you have low HDL and/or high triglycerides, then fish oil may be an excellent choice to add to your daily regimen. Another set of researchers establishes a dosing regimen that seems supported by the literature. They recommend for general preventative medicine in regards to CVD a daily dose of 300-600 mg of EPA/DHA, which is about 2 grams of regular unadulterated fish oil. If you have some history of cardio risks, then 900-1,200 mg per day of EPA/DHA should do, which is about 4 grams of total fish oil. For high triglyceride levels,

3,000-4,000 mg of EPA/DHA per day would be recommended, which is a lot of fish oil. (12)

I would just add some caveats to the above recommendations. Given that fish oil is highly unstable, as you will soon read, I would shy away from such high doses, and instead prefer dietary changes and exercise. Granted some fish oils are better made than others, but given the pro-oxidative effects of fish oil, I'm not convinced going above 2 grams per day is such a fantastic idea. Especially when you consider the overall data on mortality is great at doses closer to 1-2 grams per day. Plus, you also have to consider that many of these trials are not life-long trials. At high doses, fish oil may have detrimental pro-oxidative effects not shown in the limited scope of any given trial. This is similar to drug studies. Pharmaceutical trials are run for just enough time to show efficacy, and no frank side effects, but as we've learned the hard way, there can be, and often are, long-term issues, which don't pop up on the limited radar screen within the confines of a clinical trial.

Rheumatoid Arthritis

Rheumatoid arthritis (RA) is an inflammatory condition mostly affecting the joints of the hands, feet, wrists, ankles, and knees. About 2% of the population is affected, with women in greater numbers than men. Genetic factors appear to play some role, but twin studies infer that the disease is by no means purely genetic. (13) For our purposes, we'll assume that you or a loved one has been diagnosed with RA, and you're looking for natural help. This is not intended to serve as a diagnostic aid, but rather an honest assessment of whether fish oils are efficacious in the treatment of RA.

The pro-inflammatory oxidative affects of RA result in cartilage destruction. Pro-inflammatory compounds like the ones discussed in the chapter on IBD have been found in higher concentrations in the synovial fluid of RA patients. Consequently, drugs that inhibit TNF have shown promise as a method of treatment. So we know that it's a condition of inflammation with consequent tissue destruction. How do we treat it? We do so with anti-inflammatory pain medications such as aspirin, NSAIDS, and corticosteroids. These approaches only serve to address the symptoms and not the underlying cause. Long-term studies looking at the efficacy of conventional aggressive drug therapy show very unimpressive results. (14) Beyond that is the risk of side effects with the use of NSAIDs or corticosteroids. In fact, most experts and medical textbooks state that long-term use of corticosteroids to treat RA is not advised due to the side effects. (15) When it comes to NSAID use, I refer you to chapter one in this book and the statistics on internal bleeding and annual deaths. Making matters worse, NSAIDs seem to compound the very problem they are used to resolve. Research shows us that NSAIDs accelerate cartilage destruction and inhibit its synthesis. (16)

With a "chronic" condition that only has treatments that address the symptoms, you are ensured of its chronic status. Beyond this, the treatments themselves are toxic when used chronically. This is why so many people seek out a natural medicine provider. One of the supplements that will most commonly be "prescribed" to you by these practitioners will be fish oil, which brings us to our topic.

Fish oil is but one of several steps to take in addressing your RA needs. Fish oil is in effect not much different philosophically from the use of standard pain therapies in that the goal is to reduce inflammation. As you may discover in this book, many of our ills are traced to inflammation, which can in large part be traced to diet and other habits. RA is no exception. A high omega-6 diet with low omega-3 intake feeds the pro-inflammatory condition. Several studies show marked changes in inflammatory markers in the synovial fluid of RA patients when dietary shifts are undertaken. (17) In a typical example of this, I will highlight the following two trials.

In a 2000 study done in Spain, researchers measured the fatty acid profiles of 39 RA patients and compared it to 28 healthy controls. Remember, it is the fatty acids that serve as the reservoir of raw materials to produce either a series of pro-inflammatory compounds, or lesser inflammatory compounds. Changing a diet from a high omega-6 based one to one that has a healthful ratio of omega-3 fatty acids seemed to be the key. This study found that the synovial fluid of the RA subjects had significantly lower levels of EPA and LNA and lower levels of DHA, although not significant. (18) In another study, fish oil administration caused a 30% reduction in the pro-inflammatory eicosanoid LTB4, which is sourced from omega-6 fatty acids, as opposed to the much lesser inflammatory LTB5, which is sourced from omega-3s. (19)

However, the sole administration of fish oil does not solve the problem. It simply helps to change your inflammation from one that is more inflammatory, to a pathway that isn't as inflammatory. The underlying cause is still there for the inflammation, and that needs to be addressed. The fish oil can play a reasonable role in the management of RA, and hopefully other avenues in natural medicine will be able to identify the offender, and make the condition a manageable one, if not resolved.

The data for the use of fish oil in the treatment of RA is fair. There have been a number of studies looking at this connection. In your typical trial, fish oil would be matched up against some type of control. Corn oil has been used on a number of occasions. Coconut oil and olive oil have also been used in some of these trials. Several subjective measures, and even some labs are taken to determine efficacy. Labs are all well and good, but if only the lab number improves while your pain doesn't, then perhaps we're barking up the wrong tree.

Your typical subjective measures will ask questions of the subjects pertaining to morning stiffness, grip strength, swollen and tender joints, overall assessment, and the like. Harvard-based researchers conducted a meta-analysis of 10 studies that measured 8 parameters of disease activity in RA. These studies involved 368 subjects, and lasted for at least 3 months. This duration is important too, since it takes some time for the fatty acid profile in your body to change as you consume more omega-3s in relation to your omega-6s. This should serve to inform you that fish oil will not work right away, but take around 3 months or so to "kick in".

In their conclusion, they state, "Fish oil caused a highly significant decrease in the number of tender joints and a significant shortening of morning stiffness in RA patients." No significant changes were observed for the other parameters measured. (20) Having reviewed most of their referenced studies, and others, I find this conclusion to be reasonable.

Typically you'll find an improvement in one or two parameters, but not in all. In a couple of studies there was no improvement seen at all.

Here's a typical trial with typical results. 16 RA patients were enrolled in a trial and randomized to receive either a mostly EPA capsule or coconut oil placebo. In the preceeding 3 months, fatty acid supplementation was forbidden. The patients took one pill for 12 weeks, and then crossed over to the other pill. Drug therapy was continued. In the end, joint swelling and duration of morning stiffness were significantly improved, while the other subjective measures were not. In addition, LTB4 levels dropped, and LTB5 levels rose. (21)

A more recent study from 2006 illustrates the likely real-world benefit of fish oil in RA. In this Australian study, 31 RA patients, who were all taking drug treatments, were enrolled, and 18 were put on fish oil supplementation. After three years of treatment, those on fish oil reduced their NSAID use by 75%, whereas the decline in NSAID use was only 37% in the other group. (22) If you are unable to uncover or treat the underlying cause of your RA, maybe fish oil in combination with less pain medication may be able to reduce its severity to the point where drug side effects and costs are also reduced. For anyone who has taken drugs, you well know that they can be quite harsh, and if we can lower the dose, then why not.

I would be doing this section a disservice if I did not mention the role of the gut and other considerations in RA. The use of fish oil serves to aid the degree of inflammation, but does not resolve the underlying cause. Think of your RA as a campfire. You can pour gasoline on it, which are the omega-6 fatty acids, or you can add tree branches, which resemble omega-3 fatty acids. In either case the fire will burn, just with varying degrees of intensity. We need to put out the fire itself. Just as in IBD, if you do not remove the offender, which is likely to be a pathogen or allergen, then fish oil only serves to modulate the inflammation. Also as in IBD, gut integrity can play a role in the management of RA.

RA is yet another condition that plagues us here in "the west", but is not such an issue with others globally who consume a diet that is more in accordance with our genetic roots. It is this disparity that serves as the basis for the notion that diet plays a key role in RA. This should come as no surprise, given the close association of diet and virtually every other condition known to man.

Studies show that dietary changes can result in the complete remission of RA or significant improvement in the majority of patients. (23) Some of these trials instituted a modified fasting period followed by a vegetarian diet. Given that the most common offenders have been shown to be wheat, corn, dairy, beef, nightshades (tomato, potato, eggplant, and peppers) and food additives, a total vegetarian diet may not be entirely necessary, as well as somewhat impractical.

The mechanism behind this marked improvement is probably multi-factorial. The first would be an imbalance in the microbes in your gut, also known as dysbiosis. Trials have linked an unhealthy balance of gut microflora to RA and the improvement of this balance has been linked to an improvement in RA symptoms. (24) This imbalance between the good and bad bacteria in your GI tract, aka dysbiosis, can very well lead to gut permeability, which we covered in IBD. In review, larger food proteins are able to pass through the normally tight and well-controlled defenses of the GI tract. Once these proteins are in the blood, immune defenses assume they are pathogens and put together an assault they deem to be necessary to protect the body. Ideally, only amino acids, simple sugars, and mono and diglycerides are supposed to pass through the gut into the body. When gut pathogens or NSAID use tears holes in the GI tract, the opportunity for full proteins to pass through occurs.

Much like in IBD, proper digestion plays a key role in the treatment of RA. Think of RA as the IBD for those with a genetic compromise in their joints instead of their GI tract. If you recall, there were a few possible genetic flaws in those with true IBD. Even though the flaw was always there, it took an offender such as a high pathogenic load or a dysbiosis/gut permeability-induced allergen to kick things off. The genetic flaw serves to help perpetuate the issue. In RA, about 70% have a genetic marker that implies a susceptibility to RA. (25) Think of the other 30% as the IBS component of RA; in effect, they suffer from poor diet, pathogen, and antigen but lack the genetic flaw, so to speak.

Other digestive aids, such as HCL and enzymes, would be supported here in this issue of digestive support. They too will help break down complex proteins for more complete absorption. Fish oil is but one part of the total equation. To a degree, many of the benefits seen in the dietary modification trials in RA have been attributed to the shift in fatty acids in vivo necessary to make the eicosanoids. However, fish oil will do nothing to resolve dysbiosis, food allergens, and gut permeability. This is why it is necessary to see an experienced well-versed visionary type of provider in natural medicine. Adrenal and thymus health, plus antioxidant status are other considerations in the holistic approach to RA. In this vein, we need to treat the whole patient, not just the symptoms of pain and inflammation with the usual suspects, which only serves to perpetuate the condition and cause other issues.

Reproduction

Within reproduction, we'll cover pregnancy, postpartum depression, and the development of the child. The conception itself is not possible without both mom and dad being fertile and able to conceive. As you well know, fertility is big business. The costs, whether funneled through an HMO or paid directly by the would-be parents, are astronomical. I wish I could provide you with solid evidence in the use of fish oils as related to fertility. There is plenty of theoretical, biochemical, and anecdotal evidence, but appropriate studies for either male or female fertility are seemingly lacking. We have to operate, therefore, from what we do know from a biochemical viewpoint.

Several animal studies have indicated that supplementation with omega-3 fatty acids may improve fertility. Our domesticated animals face many of the same diseases we face as humans, given we are in control of their food supply, as we are for ourselves. With that said we must consider a couple of drawbacks in these studies. First, not all studies show a benefit. Second, as we are not animals, all animal data cannot be correlated to us. Third, some studies used animal sources of omega-3 fatty acids given to animals that are herbivores. Therefore, with a general lack of animal and human data, let's apply some common sense.

We know that our consumption of omega-3 fatty acids is about $1/20^{th}$ of what it should be based on evolutionary data. We also know that all polyunsaturated fatty acids (omega-6 included) play a pivotal role in reproduction, particularly in the production of semen. Beyond this, omega-3 fatty acids are used to help women with dysmenorrhea (painful menstruation), which is said to affect up to 50% of all women. It is the pro-inflammatory diet high in omega-6 fatty acids (vegetable oils) that leads to vasoconstriction in the uterus for these women. Some data suggest that the reduced blood flow to the uterus may negatively affect a women's fertility, and administration of fish oil may improve blood flow, thus improving the prospects of conception. (26) Lastly, we know that other dietary measures contribute to increased fertility, such as carnitine, zinc, vitamin A, vitamin D, and vitamin B12 for men. If supplementation with these other depleted nutrients helps in reproduction, then why couldn't it be true for something like omega-3s, which are widely underconsumed?

Fortunately, I am able to share data supporting the use of fish oil in pregnancy, depression, and the neurological development of children. The fact is, the mother's diet, both before and during pregnancy, plays an important role in the health of the mother as well as the infant. Curious cravings for pickles and ice cream don't do as much to serve health as do cravings for fish and other wholesome foods. Certainly EPA and DHA are not the only fatty acids needed by pregnant women, or for anyone else, for that matter. As with most everything else, moderation and balance are key. However, here in America we usually don't do either. As for moderation, we may feel if something is good, then more is better. As for balance, we've already established that our diet, on average, supplies far too many omega-6 fatty acids, and too few omega-3s. As the developing fetus solely relies on the mother for nutrition, it is obviously crucial that her nutrition be sound. However, given our toxic environment, our own government warns against the consumption of fish during pregnancy. This paves the way for a need for fish oil supplementation as an effective replacement.

During pregnancy the demand for essential fatty acids is quite high. This is necessary for the development of human brain tissue, among other needs. The final products of these essential fatty acids are arachindonic acid (AA) in the omega-6 family, and docosahaexanoic acid (DHA) in the omega-3 family. Both of these end products are of extreme importance in the development of neural tissue, which also includes vision. It is no wonder that one study, which looked at the total amounts of serum plasma fatty acids during pregnancy, found that all fatty acids were increased, but DHA was higher by an amazing 52%. (27) In other words, the mother's DHA reserves were mobilized to supply the fetus with much needed DHA. Consequently, if the mother doesn't have much DHA to give, the fetus may be compromised, as well as the mother, just in different ways.

Common thought and research tells us that the content of fatty acids plays an important role in the second and third trimesters. Although this is true, there is data to support its equal importance much earlier. It is argued that in the early stages following fertilization of the egg, maternal nutrition has its greatest role. It is theorized that the mother's nutritional status at that time strongly influences the composition and the function of the placenta. (28) Although there is much data in support of later supplementation, first trimester support is limited.

On the other end of the gestation spectrum, preterm births are thought to occur in about 10% of all human pregnancies, and this rate is associated with 70% of newborn deaths. (29) Curiously, it is the impact of cortisol on prostaglandins from omega-6 fatty acids that is generally accepted to play a key role. (30) Data from both sheep and rats show us that diets high in omega-6 fatty acids increase 2-series prostaglandins, which induce early labor, and diets high in omega-3 fatty acids increase gestational length and birth weight. Is this true for humans as well?

Studies show higher AA acid levels in the red blood cells of women who delivered prematurely. Remember that AA (arachidonic acid) is the 20-carbon end product of omega-6 fatty acid metabolism. In one such study, essential fatty acid status was measured in women and their newborns in preterm delivery and controls. It was found that the amount of AA in the blood was significantly increased in pre-term deliveries as compared to full term controls. (31) The authors went on to suggest that altered essential fatty acid intake and/or metabolism and increased maternal blood AA increases the risk for pre-term birth.

In another study, it was shown that in blood collected 2 days following delivery, women with higher omega-3 long chain fatty acids (EPA,DHA) had a significantly longer pregnancy duration. (32) In another trial, fish oil, olive oil, or no supplementation showed that pregnancies in the fish oil group as compared to the olive oil group were longer. Also of note, the biggest improvements were among those taking the fish oil who had a low fish intake at the start of the study. (33) Later additional support looked at women with high-risk pregnancies. One study showed that women with a previous pre-term delivery had their risk cut in half for a current pre-term delivery when on fish oil supplementation. (34)

In one study, 291 pregnant women showed that the administration of DHA could increase the duration of gestation. Chicken eggs with either 33 or 133mg of DHA were administered from about the 26th week of pregnancy until birth. It was found that the duration of gestation was significantly increased when DHA intake was increased during the last trimester. (35) It is of interest to note that the dose of DHA was quite low and the administration didn't occur until well into the pregnancy.

In a trial from 2002, the risk for a pre-term delivery for those who never consumed fish was 3.6 times higher than for those who consumed it the most. (36) The authors concluded that, "Low consumption of fish was a strong risk factor for preterm delivery and low birth weight." It is of interest to note that the estimated fish oil consumption was not that high for the highest group. Approximately 445mg of long chain omega-3 fatty acids were consumed per day by this low-risk group, which equated to about 2 grams of natural fish oil a day. The implication here is that it is both affordable and tolerable in terms of pill burden.

When I was a little kid, I remember my grandmother telling us, "Eating fish makes you smart." It is interesting that over the years so many of these sayings of unknown origins have been proven true in one sense or another from research in natural medicine. This is no different for fish. As stated earlier, the brain consists of significant sums of fats, and the DHA from fish oil plays a large role in the brain as well. With that said, if you are pregnant then your need for essential fatty acids is increased along with that of your developing child. Your DHA will be depleted during gestation, and during breast-feeding. It's in everyone's best interest that you make sure you both have the right nutrients.

During the last trimester, the size of the fetus' brain triples. It is this need for brain growth which goes all the way back to our beginnings and which takes a toll on the mother's levels of essential fatty acids. As you'd expect, women who have recently given birth show marked decreased levels of omega-3 fatty acids in their blood. It is these natural needs that have somehow been recognized by "ancient" cultures, which *discourage continuous pregnancies in quick succession.* These cultures have adopted learned behaviors over millennia that have been shown to produce the most robust children in body and mind. These natural laws have been lost to us, with possible consequences in fetal health and severe postpartum depression.

As is the case throughout this book, and in science in general, there is almost never an uncontested "fact" proven by the data. This is true for fish oils, as it is for antioxidants, vitamin D, and more. Once again, we have to apply logic, and look at the bulk of the good data. Although there is plenty of data to show DHA supplementation in certain doses leads to increased DHA levels in newborns and in breast milk, I can't state all data supports the use of DHA supplementation to ensure a full term delivery. Although the bulk of the data does support this conclusion, there are always conflicting data. You must realize that there are study design flaws in both pro and con data. For example, the dose of DHA used, and the time at which administration began, varied wildly between studies. The data is much stronger than for the omega-3 oil from plants, such as from flaxseed. This is just some data to support the notion that we are truly omnivores.

It's been estimated that the fetus requires 50-60 mg per day of long chain omega-3 fatty acids, mostly DHA, during the last trimester of pregnancy. In order to compensate for those needs, it has been consequently estimated that the maternal intake should be about 100mg/day. (37) Are you taking in about 100mg/day of DHA as an expecting mother? That's easily accomplished with one gelcap per day.

When it comes time to breastfeed, fish oil supplementation is still just as important. For example, DHA is not only important for brain development, but it is also needed for the eyes. In fact, some data suggests that DHA represents up to 50% of total fatty acids in the eyes. (38) Is it possible that so many of our children need glasses so soon in life in part due to our DHA deficient diet?

We know that infants who are breastfed have higher levels of DHA and lower AA in neurological tissue, as compared to infants receiving cow's milk based formulas. (39) We also know that breast-feeding proportionally increases the content of DHA in the infant while AA content remains stable. Other researchers have estimated that a nursing mother loses about 70-80 mg of DHA per day in addition to her natural losses. This is supported by several studies that show a roughly 30% decrease in blood DHA in breast-feeding mothers in the weeks following delivery. (40) Again, this loss can be made up with about 1 gram, or one gelcap a day.

In studies specifically looking at visual acuity, it has been shown that the source of the infant's nutrition can make a significant difference. In studies comparing human breast milk, a formula with marine omega-3 oil, and a formula devoid of DHA, visual tests at 57 weeks showed that those getting DHA had better vision. As further proof, those with the highest DHA present in their blood had the best visual acuity. (41) Further indications from this particular study support the use of fish oil more than something like flaxseed oil, which only supplies the basic precursor to EPA and DHA. This makes sense, as we've discussed the fact that the body has to convert LNA through several steps to DHA and this process is a slow one, with potential genetic variabilities in capacity.

In another study, which looked at mental development, 133 exclusively bottle-fed children were compared to 291 children who were never bottlefed. In this study, the researchers found that early breast-feeding was associated with better intelligence at 8 and 15 years of age, ranging from math, pictures, non-verbal, and sentence completion. (42) In further support of this theory, 855 newborns were enrolled in yet another mental development study. Breastfed infants had significantly higher scores at 2, 3, and 4 years of age. (43) It all makes sense, doesn't it? If the brain is widely composed of a fatty acid found in only a couple of sources, then shouldn't the brain develop better when flooded with the nutrient as compared to others who don't get quite as much?

In one of the larger and longer studies that looked at omega-3 fatty acids in intelligence, the results are weakly supportive. In this study out of Norway, pregnant women were recruited in week 18 of their pregnancy and given either cod liver oil or corn oil until three months after delivery. The cod liver oil contained huge amounts of DHA. At four years of age the children were given three different tests that measured problem solving, information processing, and the like, to measure intelligence. The children who had cod liver oil supplementation in-utero and into breast-feeding, scored significantly better on only one test than did the corn oil group. There was a tendency for higher scores for the other two tests, but the difference was not found to be significant. (44)

In their follow-up study three years later, when the kids were at 7 years of age, there were no differences seen between either group in any of the tests. (45) I believe there are a couple of flaws in the trial. The first consideration is that the study came from Norway, a coldwater fish consuming population. As we have seen from many trials, it doesn't seem to take much EPA/DHA to have an effect, on the order of 1-2 grams per day, sometimes less. Although the researchers administered two food questionnaires, the mothers were asked to continue their habitual diet during the study. The second consideration is that Norwegian guidelines for infant nutrition recommend that all infants receive 5 mL of cod liver oil daily from 4 weeks of age. This cuts short the study by 2 months, as it went three months post delivery. So the real question is if a mother has adequate EPA/DHA intake, does adding additional high doses result in any benefit? In the first half of the study, it might appear to be of benefit, but at 7 years, it didn't make a difference.

The real risk to the child would appear to be with women who have had chronically inadequate diets. If your eating habits consist of fast food and other junk, and the only fish you eat comes as breaded frozen flakes in the grocery store, then you ought to consider eating fish high in omega-3 fatty acids or supplementation. If you are a pure vegan, but have had a healthy diet consisting of plenty of LNA for years, and you spread out your pregnancies, then you may have lower risks than one would think. Given that some of these studies come from nations that consume fish as a staple, such as in Scandinavia, the differences between groups may be less than one that is truly controlled. Also, if you are part of the research group, and the theory is that fish oil is best for fetal development, wouldn't you sneak some in on the side even if you were in the placebo group?

We still have much to learn, and studies are unfortunately fraught with possible design errors due to human nature and other reasons. In all of the studies, either a benefit was seen, or no benefit was seen. Not one study I reviewed found fish oil to be detrimental for maternal/fetal/child health. Given our biochemical needs, the very low risk "side effects" in using a low dose stable and clean fish oil, and given the numerous potential benefits, it seems reasonable to me to include clean cold water fish in your diet at least 1-2 times a week, and/or supplement with 1 gram of fish oil per day.

The needs of the developing fetus, particulary for the developing brain, may deplete the expectant mother of her needed nutritional status. If you combine the fact that our standard American diet is very low in omega-3 fatty acids, and the needs of a developing fetus are high for these same nutrients, one could reasonably expect problems across the board at a national level. This has, in fact, been borne out by evidence. Based on intelligent reasoning, researchers have looked at the DHA status of women who have given birth to one child as compared to those who have given birth to two or more. It has been shown that these long chain polyunsaturated fatty acids are significantly lower in newborns of two or more in number, such as twins and triplets. (46) So what does this mean? It implies that there is a finite source of the complex essential fatty acids when the diet contains little to no EPA, and especially DHA. The finite source is the mother, and thus her stores are depleted for the sake of the child. In the end, both wind up with suboptimal DHA for health. As has been shown in more than one study, the amounts of these fatty acids in umbilical and maternal plasma are strongly correlated, which is to say that the more DHA the mother has, the more DHA the child will have. For this section, we'll focus on the mother in post-partum.

The issue is made even more complex when you consider the consumption of our standard diet in a woman who has had one pregnancy after another. Perhaps both mom and child were perfectly fine in the first birth, perhaps even for the second, but a woman's health risks increase as she has more children in quick succession. In addition, should you be breast-feeding, as one should, even more of these essential fatty acids and other nutrients are leaving your body for your rapidly developing child. As you can imagine, this can have a detrimental effect on the health of the mother. When it comes to depleted DHA, one consequence is that of depression.

As previously stated, the cells of our bodies incorporate fatty acids in their membranes. A deficiency in one type with an abundance of another will shift the composition of any cell membrane to something other than ideal. With a diet high in saturated fats and low in EPA and DHA, the membrane will be less fluid. It is this fluidity that helps to let molecules in and out of cells. Since the brain is so rich in fatty acids, and since proper nerve cell function is very dependent on proper fluidity, a "rigid" membrane may negatively impact mood and mental function. Studies have shown that the physical properties of brain cell membranes, including their fluidity, directly influence neurotransmitter synthesis, signal transmission, uptake of serotonin and other neurotransmitters, neurotransmitter binding, and the activity of the enzyme monoamine oxidase, which breaks down serotonin and other neurotransmitters. (47) All of this neurotransmitter talk should sound familiar to someone who has taken drugs for depression. Whether your drug is an SSRI (selective serotonin reuptake inhibitor) or an MAOI (monoamine oxidase inhibitor), they both work on neurotransmitters for depression.

I am not implying that fish oil is the answer to all depression. It may be a part of the solution for you. There are other natural remedies to consider, such as certain B vitamins, 5-HTP, or SAMe. I am implying that when it comes to post-partum depression, logic indicates that given obvious deficiencies and depletions, the use of omega-3 fatty acids for this type of depression makes the most sense. The CDC informed us in 2008 that in any 2-week period 5.4% of Americans aged 12 or older would be experiencing depression. If that is so, then why is it that post-partum depression affects 10-20% of mothers? Doesn't that seem a bit out of balance? Sure, there are new challenges with an infant, but there are also the rewards of staying at home to care for your new baby.

There is evidence to back this up as well. Epidemiologic studies show that societies with high fish consumption appear to have lower rates of depression. In one review of the literature, researchers looked at 10 qualifying studies using fish oil in cases of depression. Their recent review of the literature found that omega-3 fatty acids had a significant anti-depressant effect on those with clearly defined depression and bipolar disorder. (48) Keep in mind this was for general depression for men and women. The hypothesis presented here focuses on postpartum depression, where I submit the impressive finding would be even greater.

With that specifically in mind, we'll look at a trial that focused exclusively on omega-3 fatty acid supplementation and post-partum depression. In this recent study, subjects were randomized to receive .5 g/day, 1.4g/day, or 2.8 g/day of omega-3 fatty acids. The trial lasted 8 weeks. The researchers used two subjective scales to evaluate depression: the Edinburgh Postnatal Depression Scale (EPDS) and the Hamilton Rating Scale for Depression (HRSD). To further explain, we'll take the EPDS. The EPDS has been used in at least 23 countries, and has shown to be accurate. A maximum score of 30 is possible, which is most indicative of depression. Scores of 10 or more are indicative of possible depression. For these subjects, the average scores at the start of the study were 18.1 (EPDS) and 19.1 (HRSD). In all groups the average depression score was cut in half in just 8 weeks. (49) As you can see, not only did fish oil work great for postpartum depression, as one would expect, but it also worked in fairly quick order, and not much of a dose was needed to get a benefit, as those getting ½ gram per day did just as well.

Diabetes

For the purposes of this chapter, we're referring to type 2 diabetes or non-insulin dependent diabetes mellitus, (NIDDM), which affects about 90% of those who are diabetic. NIDDM is a disorder of macronutrient metabolism, most often associated with high blood sugar. Typically through diabetes, but not always, NIDDM is the result of either the pancreas not secreting enough insulin for the needs of the body, the peripheral cells becoming increasingly resistant (a dulled response) to insulin, or some combination thereof. Almost all cases of NIDDM can be resolved through appropriate diet and exercise, and that is essentially what we're covering when we discuss fish oil. It may be in pill form, but it obviously can be adequately and easily achieved in the diet, unlike some other supplements to attain therapeutic levels.

Since about 90% of NIDDM patients are obese, and given that proper exercise and nutrition can resolve most cases, then in a perfect world we can dramatically reduce our healthcare costs by simply doing the right things. Drugs, supplements, devices, lab work, and doctor's visits could be dramatically reduced. Unfortunately, many Americans can't or won't comply. Perhaps they don't have the time for the gym, they don't want to change, think it's too much work and expense, or are confused about what foods are actually good for you. The diet-exercise-obesity-diabetes connection has severe consequences, not just for our health, but for our costs as well.

NIDDM has its roots firmly set in our lifestyle, which is why it is so prevalent, and becoming even more so. In fact, diabetes, especially among our young is so pervasive that the life expectancy of children born today has recently been lowered due to the explosion of NIDDM among our children. Other cultures that eat whole foods and engage in regular physical exercise do not see anywhere close to our levels. NIDDM results primarily from a combination of our highly refined diet, and the abundance of animal products with saturated fatty acids. Exercise is certainly not to be dismissed, as not only does it burn off excess calories, but also sensitizes the muscle cells to insulin, thereby stressing the pancreas less.

Insulin resistance is the end result of a see-saw chronic cascade of events related to wild swings in insulin secretion and adrenal fatigue. We won't get into blood sugar tests, symptoms, or the like. For the sake of this discussion, we'll assume the diagnosis of diabetes has been given, test results are understood, and the reader is interested in supplemental measures to aid in the management of NIDDM. Fish oil is not your only supplemental option, as you may know. Other considerations include ginseng, chromium, gymnema sylvestre, and others, which have clinical data ranging from good to poor. We merely discuss fish oil here, along with probiotics, antioxidants, magnesium, vitamin A, vitamin D, and vitamin K, because there is strong data to support its almost universal use for many Americans.

Should we use fish oil in NIDDM? As you've seen thus far in this chapter, it has strong clinical support. Since NIDDM patients have 2-3 times the risk of dying from atherosclerosis, 3-4 times the risk of coronary heart disease, and 65-70% of all those who suffer a heart attack either have diabetes or are prediabetic, then fish oil is certainly a valid consideration beyond its NIDDM specific effects. (50-52)

In an ideal world, you wouldn't need to bother yourself with buying fish oil in a bottle. You'd do just as the Okinawans or Medditeraneans do, and consume fresh fish almost daily. Back here in reality, that is not always possible, given geographic constraints and the like. You may have mixed feelings on this, but find it interesting to know that it is likely that your fish oil in a bottle has fewer toxins and heavy metals than the fresh fish in the store. This is both a sad testament to the pollution of our planet, and a testimonial to the general quality of manufacturing when it comes to purity. Where the differences lie between fish oil products is in shelf stability, which is the primary caveat of the next section. So let's take a look at some data to establish a good foundation of knowledge for you in regards to using fish oils in the management of NIDDM.

Fish oil can improve NIDDM by several mechanisms. One, it has been shown to increase the body's sensitivity to insulin. Two, fish oil has been shown to increase lipid oxidation (the usage of fats for fuel) through its enhancement of what's referred to as the PPAR system, which is how fibrate drugs work. Lastly, fish oils help to reduce inflammation, which as we've seen earlier in the chapter on dietary choices, can play a key role in NIDDM. There are too many research articles on fish oil and diabetes to list here. To avoid putting you to sleep, I'll reference a handful of them to give you a flavor of what the data has shown.

Here is a typical trial in <u>healthy subjects</u>. This model is used to potentially extrapolate data to those with NIDDM. Five subjects were given 6 grams per day of fish oil, which is a lot, for three weeks. Sugar loads were ingested and blood parameters were measured. It was found that the fish oil essentially kept the normal and post-load blood sugar levels unchanged, but showed a 40% decrease in insulin. (53) So what does this mean? Evidently, it means that the fish oil made the cells more sensitive to insulin. The subjects needed less insulin to send home the same amount of blood sugar as before. The researchers also found that carbohydrate oxidation was reduced and lipid oxidation was increased by 35% after the sugar loads. In essence, the body shifted more to burning fat for fuel, and less to burning sugars.

So does this healthy subject data translate well into NIDDM patients? In one trial, 10 grams of fish oil were given to mild NIDDM subjects resulting in a fasting blood glucose increase of 14% during three weeks. (54) Serum insulin and insulin sensitivity were unchanged. These results aren't what you'd want. The improvements seen in healthy subjects weren't seen here, and blood sugar went up. Ten grams is a lot of fish oil, but not impossible for any patient to tolerate.

In another trial at half the dose, a significant increase in glycosylated hemoglobin was seen over 6 weeks (55) Glycosylated hemoglobin is a representation of the amount of sugar in the blood over time, the more sugar in the blood, the more that is "stuck" to proteins such as hemoglobin, above and beyond what's considered normal. There was no effect on blood sugar or HDL. Triglycerides were significantly reduced as well. All results, both pro and con, were lost after 6 weeks off the fish oil. From this trial, we can note a few things. One, the fish oil did not help with blood sugar control, but in fact marginally hindered it via glycosylated hemoglobin. Two, although the usual increase in HDL was not seen, significant improvement in triglycerides were, another CVD hallmark benefit. Lastly, it appears that to get any benefits from fish oil, unless you change diet and exercise, they will be lost not too long after discontinuation.

In a trial using a whopping 18 grams a day, fasting glucose rose 19% and the average glucose response to meals rose 24% in NIDDM patients. (56) These levels are seemingly absurd, and could not easily be obtained by eating fish for most of us, as you would need about 3.5 lbs of fish a day to get this much oil. It does bring up a couple items though. First, when taken to an extreme, the negative results were also extreme. As is not always the case, if some is good, more is better. Second, these levels are possibly close to what Eskimos had consumed. Don't forget that in these people, inflammation, CVD, and diabetes were a rarity. So the format of the trial is not too ridiculous. Could there be a difference between the fish the Eskimos consumed and this fish oil?

In a different twist, 15 patients with NIDDM were studied over alternating three-week periods in a metabolic ward. A metabolic ward offers the researchers the opportunity to control the foods ingested by the study groups. By alternating diets, all patients ingested both regimens, which helps to exclude inter-patient variability. A diet higher in saturated fat was compared to a diet higher in polyunsaturated fats (PUFA), notably omega-3 fatty acids. Interestingly, the blood glucose response to breakfast, daily blood glucose, and fasting blood glucose levels were all significantly worse in the polyunsaturated arm than in the saturated group. (57) The good news is that triglycerides were on average reduced a whopping 40% on the PUFA diet. This trial did not use supplements, but food. It was complicated by the fact that there was a high level of omega-6 fatty acids in the diet. The ratio of omega-6 to omega-3 in the diet was actually better in the saturated fat group. With its flaws, the authors question the value of PUFA diets in NIDDM management.

I mention these studies, and there are more, not to alarm you but to inform you. There are several studies that show no impact on blood sugar parameters with the use of fish oil. These studies tend to be at lower doses, in the 1-3 grams per day range, which is very affordable, and more in line with the theme of this chapter. To my knowledge there is only one study that shows a significant improvement in insulin sensitivity with the use of fish oil in NIDDM. (58) Even in this trial, fasting blood glucose was not improved, but the glucose clearance rate was.

Obesity and its consequent high blood fatty acid load combined with excess fat deposits in the liver and muscle hinder blood sugar metabolism. These excess cellular fatty acids impair the fluidity of the cell wall and alter the expression glucose transport in the muscle and liver. In essence, there's too much fat gumming up the cells, which decreases insulin's effectiveness. For normal patients who do not have pre-existing NIDDM, the cells quickly respond by burning more fats for fuel, which helps insulin to better do its thing. The anti-obesity effects of suppressing liver fat production and enhancement of fat burning has been shown in a number of studies (59) This is not to imply that fish oil is the next weight loss cure. Although studies show improvements in insulin sensitivity and fat burning when switching from saturated fats to polyunsaturated fats, the evidence for weight loss is limited at best.

In NIDDM you should be aware of the potential impacts of fish oil. This is not to imply that I do not recommend its use for those who have NIDDM. In fact, the CVD benefits seem to outweigh any risks from its use. The bulk of the data shows us that there is potentially a shift in the substrate used for fuel. In other words, your body starts to burn more fat for fuel, and consequently less sugar. For those who are healthy, it matters not. For those who have NIDDM, you should be aware of the fact that it may very well impact your blood sugar levels. This impact is mostly related to dose, with higher quantities ingested potentially impacting your levels more than lower quantities. In fact, <u>two recent review articles on this matter go so far as to imply that the use of fish oil fails to have its insulin sensitivity benefits once NIDDM is established</u>. (60,61)

Measuring insulin sensitivity isn't so cut and dry. A rise in blood sugar may just reflect an ongoing shift from burning sugar to fats. It doesn't necessarily take into account cellular sensitivity. There have been studies looking specifically at the impact of fish oil at the cellular level showing that there is an increase in sensitivity. It's all fairly confusing, which is why the researchers can't come up with a unifying guideline.

In review of this data, and more, the following conclusions are fair. Fish oil should be considered as a part of a diabetes regimen, not only for its cardiovascular benefits. Second, the dose need not be excessive, and probably *shouldn't be*. Total fish oil intakes of 1-3 grams per day appear to blend efficacy with caution. Lastly, the fish oil should be a shelf-stable un-oxidized oil. There are many oils out there on the market, and as is true with most everything else in life, there are varying degrees of quality. If you buy fish in a capsule as most do, then bite into it to see if your supplement is rancid. You wouldn't buy smelly fish at the fish market, right? Then why would you not sample the fish oil you're throwing down the hatch?

Oil Stability

To further drive home this concept, we'll review some data looking at the consequences of ingesting oxidized fish oil. Keep in mind that oxidized oils can come from more than just fish. Fish oil only gets attention because of its extreme instability. Americans ingest plenty of other oxidized oils in the course of a day, with the leading culprit coming from fried foods. Consider that oxidation (ie *from oxidized oils* and excess iron) is one of several aspects of aging and degeneration. Others discussed in this book to varying degrees are: the slowing of methylation, toxic load, hormonal decline, glycosilation (from *excess blood sugar as in diabetes*), nutritional deficiencies, genetic flaws, and inflammation. You'll hear that saturated fats are bad for you, which is partly true, although they are still required in the diet to a degree. You'll hear about fruits, fiber, and other food constituents. But the long-term side effects from our American diet touch on all the above aspects of degeneration. Food is both essential, and causes what would be considered aging. This is probably the primary reason why caloric restriction diets have consistently been shown to increase life span.

The fact is that life itself is pro-oxidant in nature. The oxygen we need to survive from minute to minute is a pro-oxidant. The food we eat spins off free radicals through its metabolism. There is no age-reversal supplement or gimick. You can only take actions to slow down the aging process. So when it comes to the foods you eat, you should choose options that are less age-accelerating. Hence the frustration with all the reports we see in the media. At some point you become absolutely frustrated because you're left with nothing to eat. There is so much research out there that everything can be blamed for one thing or another. You just have to make the best decisions for you and your family.

Believe it or not, fish oil is not exempt from negative press either. I'm not talking about PCBs and heavy metals. Although we are exposed to an onslaught of data supporting the use of fish oil in CVD, you will unlikely hear about the possible issues with the use of fish oil as a supplement.

That's what this book is all about, giving you the little known facts about matters of health only known to a handful of people. So let's take a closer look at the stability issues that surround fish oil.

I do believe that fresh clean wild caught fish plays an essential role in the ideal health of humans. Ideally the fish is caught, and then eaten in short order. Cold water fish has more of the omega-3 fatty acids EPA and DHA that we have come to cherish. These fatty acids have an array of physiological benefits, many of which have been discussed earlier in this chapter. Omega-3 fatty acids are "essential" as we cannot manufacture them from other dietary precursors, and without them we suffer morbidity and mortality. We don't even need them in large quantities. Free range game offers up a significantly higher ration of omega-3 fatty acids than the grain-fed livestock we're used to, but not in the quantity per serving seen in fish.

In the aim of providing better health and profits in our quasi-free market society, companies offer you an array of choices to meet your EPA and DHA dietary needs. As we've covered, lab testing shows that these companies bring forth clean products when it comes to heavy metals and toxins. The other issue of concern is the stability of the oil.

EPA and DHA are the most unstable oils there are. They are long chain fatty acids with numerous double bonds able to interact with heat, light, and air. This is the reason why an unclean fish market smells the way it does. A bad fishy smell is naturally unappealing. To you it's an issue of taste. To our genes, it's a way of saying, "No, that's not good for you." This is why manufacturers load up their oils with tons of lemon flavoring. There is mounting data to suggest that the ingestion of fish oil is pro-oxidative, thus depletes serum vitamin E, and goes on to cause other downstream problems. Like everything else, there is debate even in taking fish oil. Researchers do the best they can with our limits in testing and knowledge to bring forth "facts" to serve as guidelines to better health. However, these "truths" are often at odds, and we are left to try to distill knowledge to the best of our abilities from the conflicting data.

Take, for example, LDL cholesterol. We currently believe that it is the oxidation of LDL that is vitally integral in the clogging up of your arteries. This is one major reason why nutrients such as vitamin E have been used in studies in the role of antioxidants. A number of studies have shown large increases in markers of oxidized fatty acids in those who consume fish oils in trials. The consumption of this highly unstable partially-oxidized oil is theorized by some to lead to a potential increase in risk for diseases such as CVD in the long term.

Researcher Jin Hyang Song has authored papers with others on the effects of fish oils on lipid peroxidation in the body. Peroxides are the primary way that fish oils are measured for stability, although other methods are available, which leads to inter-study confusion. In one of his papers he states, "Although dietary supplementation with DHA oil has shown preventative value in relation to cardiovascular disease by a reduction in plasma triglyceride levels, and possibly by inhibiting platelet function by reducing arachidonic acid levels in tissue lipids, it may also be a health risk because it substantially increases lipid peroxidation." His conclusion is similar to mine, in that he recommends extra antioxidant use to gain the atherosclerotic benefits without the unintended side effects from ingesting processed fish oil. To take this several steps further, I recommend that the fish oil you consume be the most stable one available, the antioxidants you use to be properly dosed mixed tocopherols, the quantity of fish oil consumed be reasonable in nature, the oil refrigerated at all times, and that you reduce other dietary oils that may cause oxidative burdens.

In an interesting Norwegian trial, 300 subjects with recent acute heart attacks were recruited into the trial and given either concentrated fish oil or corn oil to the tune of about 4 grams per day. (62) The subjects began their oil supplementation between 4 and 6 weeks following the heart attack. Vitamin E was added to the capsules to protect against oxidation. The supplementation went on for at least one year per subject. So what do you think they found? One would assume that the recurrent heart attack rate would be lower in the fish oil group. Once you've had a heart attack, your chances for another go up quite significantly, and so that's one of the parameters the researchers measured. The good news was that they found a highly significant improvement in both triglycerides and HDL in the fish oil group as compared to the corn oil group. Curiously, the rate of recurrent heart attacks was essentially the same in both groups after one year of intervention. In those who did have a recurrent heart attack, the measures of lipid oxidation were similar. Think about it. The results were equal to 4 grams of CORN OIL. By every account I have read, corn oil is something to avoid. It did no better. Why? Oxidation.

Another point of interest was the level of oxidation in all the subjects compared to a matched sampling from the healthy general population. The 12-month increase in fatty acid oxidative markers went way up for both the fish and corn oil groups, and was much higher than the general population. The oxidative markers for fish oil were slightly higher than those for corn oil. So it may seem that excess oil ingestion in general from the polyunsaturated family will increase in vivo oxidative stress. Although the fact that omega-6 fatty acids (as found in corn oil) significantly contribute to lipid peroxidation as seen in trials, one would expect fish oil to confer much higher levels of oxidation. This suspicion is backed up by other research specifically looking at corn oil vs fish oil and resultant oxidation ex vivo (out of the body). There were marked differences seen in oxidation of fish oil as compared to corn oil, even when synthetic and natural antioxidants were added to the fish oil. (63)

So what gives with this trial? Wouldn't one reasonably expect fish oil to significantly improve the outcomes in post-heart attack patients as compared to lousy corn oil? If fish oil doesn't work here, then where would it work? Perhaps there is something going on inside the body that we don't yet completely understand. Perhaps all polyunsaturated oils will contribute to oxidation.

Much of the data showing detrimental pro-oxidative problems with fish oil comes from animal data, humans deplete in vitamin E, high doses of fish oil, rancid fish oil, or more than one of the above. I could go on quoting this data, but it is only partly relevant to what you'd be consuming as a supplement, but it does serve as a guideline. For example, in some of this data it has been shown that the administration of vitamin E significantly reduces markers of oxidation. (64). In one human trial with cod liver oil at high dose, MDA (a marker for oxidation) went way up, yet with a different fish oil product that was seemingly more stable, MDA excretion was not significantly altered.

439

Even as a pro-oxidant, fish oil has its theoretical uses. Studies have shown when used as a part of cancer therapy, the cancer is killed more easily either by the body or by therapy. The theory goes as the cancer becomes larger and as more of your diet incorporates omega-3 fatty acids, the cancer incorporates these highly oxidizable fatty acids into its own structure, and upon exposure to radiation, the cancer cell dies more easily as the cell membranes are more easily destroyed. Here is clinical proof of the instability of these fatty acids, and a different twist on their use. Don't forget, there's radiation coming from the sun as well. What does that do to the skin of people who consume excessive quantities of fish oil?

<u>A number of researchers advocate the administration of vitamin E along with fish oil due to the increased body requirements for the vitamin, as vitamin E acts as the primary antioxidant for oxidized fish oil</u>. It has also been shown that there is an apparent reduction in the absorption of vitamin E in the presence of fish oil (65). Why would so many researchers advocate the use of an antioxidant if there were no issues with fish oil causing oxidation in the body? Of course, the need for vitamin E will vary, as better fish oil products will require less as the product is less oxidized, whereas lesser products may require more.

This is particularly true for those who are diabetic, as research has shown that poorly controlled diabetics have significantly higher plasma peroxides than do healthy controls. (66) Additional research shows that extra vitamin E was necessary for *healthy* blood sugar control in men with high triglycerides. (67) Although this research was done on a stable fish oil, the dose was very high, which is in agreement with our previous findings. Interestingly, higher dosed vitamin E has been shown in studies to improve insulin action, which may help to counteract the possible sugar imbalances from fish oils.

So what are the conclusions on taking fish oil?

- It is most preferable to eat clean freshly caught local cold water fish about 1-3 times per week. It's not entirely necessary to go overboard with consumption as some of the longest lived peoples don't have fish every day.

- If you can't comply with number one, then ensure you're buying a stable fish oil product. If it's a flavored oil, it will be hard to tell by taste. If it's a gelcap, then bite into it and judge for yourself. Buy the most current dated bottles off the shelf. When you get home, either freeze or refrigerate. On days you eat fish, you won't need your fish oil, assuming the fish is cold water.

- Take fish oil with extra vitamin E. Ensure it's a mixed tocopherol, and not just dl-alpha tocopherol, which is a cheap synthetic version. Yes, the manufacturers add vitamin E to their product for stability, but data shows us that it is only partially effective. Synthetic antioxidants are even more effective, but you don't want to ingest those.

- Each product will rave about its stability, but keep in mind that this is at the time of manufacture. There is ample shelf and transportation time for your fish oil to oxidize away. Remember the products that failed analysis in the chapter on supplement quality, despite claiming great quality. Buyer beware.

- Consume your fish oil in reasonable doses. More than 4-5 grams a day is probably ill advised. Cardiovascular benefits have been seen at lower doses. If you are diabetic, the dose and usage of vitamin E is even more important.

- There are boosted products and there are "natural" products. When a manufacturer boosts a fish oil, they are increasing the amount of EPA and DHA in the oil per serving size. A manufacturer will separate (hydrolyze) the fatty acids off of the glycerol backbone, and then re-esterify more of the EPA and DHA in place of the saturated fatty acids and monounsaturated fatty acids. You love it because you get more EPA and DHA per serving/dollar, and as far as you know, you want the most EPA and DHA you can get. But does this extra manufacturing degrade the quality of the oil? Any supporting epidemiological evidence for fish oil, such as that of the Eskimos, was from natural dietary fish oil, not from a boosted product.

- Reduce your exposure to all oxidized oils. If you're currently ingesting cheap rancid fish oil, you eat a lot of fried fast food, and when cooking you cook at higher temperatures with the usual processed vegetable oils, then you're asking for trouble. Insults to the body here and there are normal and compensated for, but chronic marked insults are a recipe for disease.

- If you're thinking of taking flax oil instead, which is alpha linolenic acid (LNA), the vegetable precursor of EPA and DHA, you may want to rethink it. I'm not saying it's not healthy; it's just also oxidized. It's better to buy packaged whole flax seed, and grind on the spot with a coffee grinder. Also, the clinical data for LNA is not as impressive as the data for fish oil.

- Free-range meats and eggs are a better source of omega-3 fatty acids than the animal products you're used to. Fat composition is just one of a number of differences between the products, and the extra effort and expense in raising these products are reflected in the price.

Your conventional MD's are beginning to buy into this natural medicine "thing". Many now recommend fish oil and vitamin D, and some even recommend probiotics and CoQ for patients on statins. As more people get better through natural medicine, as more clinical data emerges to its use, and as the word spreads, natural medicine will become even bigger. Your doctor will probably have limited information in recommending a product, and none pertaining to quality. In fact, you will probably know more than most conventional providers. Natural medicine is now big business. In these massive economies of scale, quality and integrity are lost at times to profitability. Read, learn, question others, and use common sense for your own sake. Don't be another lemming in "the system".

Chapter 16   My Story

I too have worn the shoes of a sick and frustrated patient. I was the patient who went from one doctor to the next for years with absolutely no success. As my virtually flawless management of IBD has proven many years later, I'm doing something right. There is something to this natural medicine stuff, and I am walking proof. I find that some of the better providers in natural medicine are the ones who were either sick themselves with a given condition, or they passionately treated a sick loved one. It's not until you live the tortured life of a patient that you appreciate every aspect of its significance.

My past experiences are by no means unique. What was unique was my refusal to accept the futility of incompetence and drugs as a way of life. A significant percent of IBD patients go on to have some internal body part removed at some point in time. I refused to walk around with a colostomy bag at any point in my life. I refused to take drugs for years, drugs that would tear away at my bones and immune system. As you read this chapter, you will be able to relate to my past frustrations. It is my hope that this inspires you to apply as many principles as possible discussed in this book to your own health. There is hope for you. Remember this, there is a biochemical explanation for what's going on inside your body. You don't suffer from a drug deficiency. Once you've found the underlying cause, the path is clearer for your success. There is hope.

I can remember when it began. I was 23 and stationed in Germany. I had bought a jar of what looked like a tasty pre-made sauce to have with a meal, and shortly after its consumption I was off to the bathroom with explosive diarrhea. It stuck out in my mind as odd, since that had never happened to me before. I chalked it up to something, and went on. Weeks later, on a weekend trip in East Germany, we ate lunch at a Chinese restaurant. Yes, they have lots of Chinese restaurants there too. Within about 20-30 minutes I was racing for a bathroom with explosive diarrhea again.

Those were the first two incidences that stand out clearly in my mind. My disease, or more accurately, my hypersensitivity was very slow to develop. I would have these "attacks" only occasionally in those first few years. I never really made any connection or gave it much thought. Plus, I had a mother who had been diagnosed with IBS. She would say, "You got the IBS from me." So we just chalk these things up to fate I guess.

When I started my masters degree in nutrition at Florida State, I would still have the occasional attack, but with a little more frequency. I can remember a certain Florida fast food chain ruining me whenever I ate there. I didn't do it often, but when I did, I regretted it. I went on to develop a pain in the lower right quadrant of my abdomen. Reasonably enough, I suspected some involvement of the appendix, not knowing any better. They dismissed the appendix theory, which was the right call. This may be the only right call made until years later. They had no answers, however.

I saw several doctors over the course of the next couple of years. Again, no answers. I would get the occasional spot of blood following a bowel movement, and, justifiably, would be quite concerned. At the time, I suspected colon cancer, because that's all I knew to which I could attribute something like this.

I began to make some connections between eating out and my problems, but it was still unclear. There were inconsistencies. Still, at this point in time, I was attempting to cook most of my own meals, and not drink any alcohol. I would summarize these years as having symptoms more often than in previous years, but still sporadic enough to not cause me to "cross that line of concern".

Upon graduation, I moved back to New England. We started a life in New Hampshire, and all was great, or mostly. My occasional problem became more consistent. I would be traveling for work, and have to eat many meals on the road for lunch, and sometimes dinner. This was a change over preparing my own meals, but I didn't entirely pick up on the connection due to continued inconsistencies, and the need to accommodate my career. Often times after finishing a lunch somewhere, I'd be racing down the highway at 80-90 mph to get to a bathroom for yet another round of explosive diarrhea 20-30 minutes after eating. I got to know all the spots where the accessible bathrooms were located. I have heard this same story from many others. It's embarrassing, but you are not alone.

During this time I lost a significant amount of weight, and my body odor was not appealing, I had frequent headaches, frequent foul gas, I often needed a nap after lunch, I looked like hell, I couldn't recuperate from my work-outs, and when I had an attack, I was wiped out for the day. Sounds just like the kind of guy you'd like to date, doesn't it?

I had seen a number of healthcare providers over this time as well. All of them but one were entirely useless. I heard lines like, "It's in your head", "It's stress", and "There's nothing I can do". There was one set of occurrences that will always stand out in my mind. I had lunch at a chain restaurant with my manager. While at the table talking, I had those familiar rumblings. He was talking about some damn thing, but I could only concentrate on my issue down below. I had to excuse myself, race to the bathroom, and do my thing. This time there was an added bonus. The entire bowl was red, red from my blood. Of course I was in shock, but got a hold of myself, and finished the day with him. That evening, we were over-nighting somewhere in Connecticut. I had another attack. By the way, some days I'd have 2, 3, or even 4 of them. Like earlier in the day, the toilet bowl was fully red. This time I went to the hospital, where some brave woman took a look and informed me that I had fissures in my anus. Just the thing a man wants to hear at thirty. So as a follow-up back in New Hampshire, I decided on seeing a new doctor. This one was a gastroenterologist. I mention his specialty only because it is supposed to imply some expertise in matters pertaining to the health of the GI tract. Upon performing the same look-and-see procedure, he confirmed the fissures. I explained my story to him, and here's what he told me. "There's nothing I can do for you. We'll just have to put you on Prednisone for the rest of your life." This man was obviously an idiot who didn't want to pursue the possibility of other means of care for his patients. He chose either not to immerse himself in the knowledge of his profession, or to consider anything other than a drug to treat symptoms. There are many others like him. Either I was just a dollar sign to him, or he was just fed up with his career. Either way, I question his value to his patients.

Let's be honest here. He wasn't the only one who couldn't help, or, more accurately, he didn't know enough to help. No one had any answers. I stopped seeing doctors since they were, for all intents and purposes, useless. I dragged on for another 18 months or so until I had "the breakdown". I now weighed as much as I did when I was a sophomore in high school, and was on the bathroom floor in tears. I looked at food with fear. I spent way too much of my time in the bathroom. I was a very sick man, and after progressively getting worse over several years, I had no answers. Not only was I in pain, but I was also concerned for my future. When you're sick, and you don't know why, crazy thoughts enter your mind. You appreciate life a little more. You look at your kids a little longer.

At this low point in my illness, I did an important thing. I crossed the line. Once you do cross that line, you will do anything it takes to get better. It becomes the focus of your being. You take control of something that has taken control of you. When I crossed the line, I didn't care what the cost, how much the effort, I was going to get better. I had always been very athletic, and it was gone. Even during those first several years of this problem I was still in great shape because it was a relatively rare occurrence, and I always exercised. At this point, my illness was every day, all day long. I looked like the walking dead, and I wasn't going to take this shit any more.

This book exists for many of you who too have "crossed the line," regardless of your disease. You are ready to do what it takes, you just need some honest guidance. Still many of you have yet to cross that line. Until then, you'll accept your disease as if it were your destiny.

At this critical point, I decided to go back and see one of my previous GI docs. He had performed the first colonoscopy on me years ago. In the interim, he had brought on board a couple of nurse practitioners who were dabbling in natural medicine. They began to discuss and suggest some things that no one had done before. Topics were addressed that were new to me, and to this day, are new to modern medicine to a large degree. I spent the next 8 months in and out of their office.

A stool analysis showed significant dysbiosis. With that in mind we ran a gut permeability test as well, which was a waste of money, not because it's not worthwhile, but because the results could not be interpreted. Two months later I was suffering from acute esophagitis, or GERD, which is not uncommon in these cases. So, I had an upper endoscopy done where the doc has the pleasure of checking you out from the other end for a change. The inflammation and ulcerations weren't ideal, but were treatable.

At this time, they sold me a number of products. One of them was called uva ursi. She probably should not have "prescribed" it, but it did spur on my thought process and research even more. She probably was not aware that uva ursi in the dose prescribed over the duration prescribed can be hepatotoxic, and she should have been pulling LFTs on me, but was not. In other words, she gave me an herb that over time at higher doses has the ability to wear away at the liver, and she should have tested my liver accordingly. However, with that said, this was the one indication to me in all my years of illness to date that something could work. For one month, I was able to eat anything. I thought I was cured. I was eating anything I wanted, with no explosive diarrhea. Then, unfortunately I reverted back to exactly where I was before. I had gone back to refill my "prescription" for this foul drink, but my 30-day reprieve was over. Of course I was disheartened, but I was also shown the benefit, albeit temporarily, of natural medicine, even in ill-conceived usage. Nothing else to date had helped. Another of her recommendations had good intentions, but all things considered, was a poor thought. She suggested I make my own yogurt, and the beneficial bacteria would help my GI tract. I could use honey to flavor it, and this should help, in addition to the extremely expensive probiotic I was already buying, on top of a couple other items. Well, the yogurt idea is not good for numerous reasons, as you've read in the chapter on IBD. In addition to those listed in that chapter, she should have not suggested I eat any sugars, milk and honey included, as I most assuredly, and I did, have systemic candida. She did make other good recommendations, such as including raw garlic in the diet, and some ideas on what to read.

A few months later I had some other labs done, which among other results included mild anemia, which makes a lot of sense. Also in the same month, he performed a second colonoscopy on me. I was the new beneficiary of a disease called Crohn's. I had a diagnosis, which took how many years?

This is where many providers and patients stop. "I have my diagnosis." "I can now tell people there's an official reason why I feel like hell." The provider is usually thinking, "OK, let's prescribe a drug to ameliorate the symptoms of the patient." Both continue on this unhealthy track, all the while your body is less and less vital. I refused to go down this path. Just like when I refused that GI doc who offered to me a steroid for the rest of my life, I was not going to rest with a diagnosis. I didn't want to live this way. We'd been gathering data, but I wasn't any better. I was in fear of food. I dreaded having to contemplate what to eat, because my menu selection was rapidly being diminished. In retrospect, the only thing the colonoscopy served to do was to provide me with a diagnosis. It still didn't address why I was sick. Sure, I heard the autoimmune line along the way. This is where you're told Crohn's is a disease that, for some reason, causes your own immune system to attack your GI tract, and there's nothing more you can do than feed it with steroids. Well, I wasn't biting on that line, and thank God I didn't.

With my diagnosis in hand, I put myself on some supplements, but I was a bit skeptical. I had spent good money back in the spring from my nurse practitioner on supplements with sometimes very strange ingredients, which had done me no long-term good whatsoever. I was beginning to question the competence of the nurse practitioner, so I stepped up the efforts on my research and began to take control of my condition. I can tell you in retrospect what exactly should have been done in regards to the use of the supplements, and more importantly food avoidance. Unfortunately at that time, I did not know, and neither did my provider. You may be thinking, "Guy, you had a master's in nutrition, how couldn't you?" That's true, but natural medicine at that time, at that school, was not a part of the curriculum. With that said, my new program helped me to feel mildly better over the whole month following the colonoscopy. As I modified my program, I went on to do even better where it's reported in my file that, "In greater than one month Guy has had no attacks of severe diarrhea following meals."

Later I had a food allergy panel and another stool analysis done. It showed my bifido-bacterium content had barely budged with all of those probiotics, and all of that money. It still showed no signs of parasites. My food allergy panel showed very mild allergies to just a couple of items.

My next move was to meet with the doctor, and we decided on a pharmacologic bug-killing spree. He had suspected, and I believe wisely so, that I had systemic candida, as well as pathogenic bacteria overladen in my gut. For 30 days, I was on an antifungal and antibiotic. This served to reduce the overall pathogen burden within my GI tract, and thus reduce the combined immune-inflammation combination that had been causing me so much trouble. As I look back, I know I could have likely accomplished this naturally.

At about that same time, I made the big discovery. I had a reaction to a canned food. I decided to check out the ingredients, and picked up on a preservative. I then checked the old jar of mayo in the fridge that hadn't been touched in months. Same preservative. I then went through the grocery store, looking at the ingredients of foods I had suspected, and found very similar sounding preservatives. I then did more research on preservatives, chain restaurants, and processed foods. I had at long last found the connection. I had a chemical sensitivity to preservatives. So it would seem that the initial impetus for my inflammation was due to chemical sensitivities. Once set in motion, the other downstream symptoms are bound to occur in those with certain genetic predispositions.

Chemical sensitivities usually don't just spring up on their own. Should you take antibiotics for any reason, which I had done years previously, then your good bacteria may be drastically reduced, while yeast takes over. Yeast then proliferates in the gut, bores holes through the gut, and among many other horrible things, can cause chemical sensitivities. As I had been on several rounds of antibiotics in college, then drank yeast laden beers in Germany, it only stands to reason that a slow and gradual take-over of yeast was my downfall. I remember having a terrible case of thrush as my problems got worse. Thrush is a yeast infiltration of the mouth. This is a clear symptom of systemic yeast out of control. The yeast created a chemical sensitivity. The chemical sensitivity caused inflammation, and the whole circle just fed itself as my health spiraled downward.

Over the next year or so I changed my eating habits. I prepared as much food as possible at home. I still traveled for work, but carted around a cooler containing foods I made each morning. I made it a point to analyze every label I could. Sure there were some hard learned lessons along the way, but I got better. I still had the occasional problem, but much less frequently. I could have shortened my recovery curve, but didn't have that knowledge yet. I was putting weight back on, and was very pleased with my progress.

I WAS IN CHARGE OF MY OWN HEALTH. As time passed, I would go on to test and refine things to a flawless degree. It is a condition that requires management. I am not "cured," but my IBD is managed to such a point that it seems much like a cure. I had put together a phenomenal combination of diet, supplementation, and continued monitoring and education. As I reflect back, at one point in time, I was a very sick man who was told I could not be helped, and now I am the picture of health. I went on to, and continue to help others mostly in the area of GI issues, but in other aspects of natural medicine as well.

So what happened? How did I get so sick? First, let's not rule out a genetic connection. I evidently inherited a genetic flaw or compromise of sorts from my mother, and she in turn did so from her father. For her, the issues were not as severe and didn't begin until her late twenties. Mine for the most part began at that time, but were much more severe. Now, there has to be an offender, an initial insult to the system. Some people, those who have been gifted with an iron stomach, or more precisely an iron GI tract, will never have to worry. However, there are those of us, and the list is growing, who do. In fact, gastrointestinal complaints are the number one reason for patient visits. The original offense can come from a number of sources. The challenge is to identify the offender, treat the symptoms, heal the body, and prevent it from happening again. The goal should not be to mask the problem with drugs that treat symptoms. Drugs may be fine in the short term, but you must get to the root of the problem and the resolution.

If you recall, in retrospect my first reaction was easily identified as the pre-made sauce and its fair share of preservatives. As time has gone by over these many years, more and more nasty preservatives have found their way into our food under a variety of different names, and curiously enough, GI issues are becoming wildly out of control. For whatever reason, I had sensitivity to these chemicals, and still have to this day. I have found that many others have the same issue. My problem was that I did not recognize it quickly enough to avoid a long list of health issues that snowballed over time. The science of processing food has been making great strides in the past 20 years, but our bodies have not been able to keep up. The progression of my disease and that of others seems to be correlated with the increased processing of our foods. The connection of IBD to chemicals has not been addressed to the best of my knowledge. I think a big piece of the equation is missing for many.

After having lived this illness for years, and seen this in many people and patients, I have come to identify it very quickly. In the past month, I resolved this issue for a patient in two phone calls. I accomplished in a few minutes on the phone, with one lab, and a host of supplements used over two months, what it took me many years, lots of pain and consternation, and boatloads of money to do. She had been having severe GI upset for some time. We talked about her diet. The fact that she had just had another "attack" following a meal at a Chinese restaurant (notice a pattern here) got me on the chemical trail. Not being too presumptive, I still ran a food allergy panel on her for the top culprits. She came up clean. While we were awaiting those results, I put her on a hypoallergenic diet. She "fell off the wagon" once during this time, and paid the price with the usual trip to the bathroom. How did she pay the price? She went out to dinner. Pre-made food anyone? I explained to her about inflammation, preservatives, and prepared foods. She understood, and redoubled her efforts on food made at home, you know, the stuff no one seems to eat anymore. I also put her on supplements to help with digestion, reduce inflammation, kill potential pathogens, replenish any malnutrition, and rebuild the immune system, not in that order, and not all at the same time. Within a couple of weeks, she was great, and has been since. The beauty of this story is that not only did she not suffer needlessly for years, but catching the inflammation in time prevented any food allergies from developing.

I must also add to her story that she had seen many other doctors before me. She had done what so many others do, which is after the frustration in dealing with the current model of medicine, she saw a natural medicine provider. As you recall from the chapter on natural medicine, providers come in various levels of capability. Suffice it to say, she previously saw someone who was less than competent. Upon my consultation, the problem was quickly resolved. Let this book and my experience help you. Learn from the mistakes made by others. Be the most active participant in your own healthcare. After all, what's more important than your health?

Chapter 17   Closing Thoughts

"The doctor of the future will give no medicine, but will instruct his patient in the care of the human frame, in diet, and in the cause and prevention of disease." (Thomas Edison)

We're living in Thomas Edison's future, and we're at a crossroads. We can continue to go down the path we've been on for so long, or we can adopt a new paradigm. Change for many is a scary thing. It contains the unknown. However, chapter one emphasized the many pitfalls of the known, current conventional medicine.

We now fortunately have many people converting or trying to convert to preventative and natural/integrative medicine. It can be a challenging transition, with many pitfalls. That was the purpose in writing this book. I hope you have gained an appreciation for all aspects of natural medicine. Clearly all diseases and concerns for all people cannot be properly addressed in one book. My goal was to highlight many of the strengths and concerns within natural/integrative medicine so you can make informed decisions.

There are a number of premises and unique concepts I've tried to emphasize. Some are:

- You know your body best, it is your life, and you have the most vested interest in its welfare. Be the primary advocate for your own health, and for your children.
- The current system is mostly broken. Enormous evidence of greed and corruption highlight the fact that you are simply a source of revenue.
- Natural medicine is more complex than walking into a health food store to buy a bottle off the shelf. The unique diagnostics, the philosophy, and treatment through a qualified practitioner skilled in your condition offer up great possibilities.
- Nutrition is half of natural medicine. Preventative medicine is ideal.
- Inflammatory bowel disease is the manifestation of genes, pathogens, allergies, and/or chemical sensitivities.

453

- Cutting edge gene research is highlighting the differences between us, and natural medicine offers the amazing potential to compensate for these flaws. For the first time in human history we can take preventative medicine to another level.

- There is an enormous amount of data available, which can be cut and used to prove just about any cause under the sun. It's the complete and unbiased analysis of the data that points you in the right direction.

- Use your common sense.

- As large multinational and pharmaceutical companies become bigger players in natural medicine, it implies that it is of value, contrary to what you may have heard. Its value hinges on appropriate care, a proper regimen, and patient compliance.

- There is a biochemical explanation for whatever ails you. Whether a pathogen, a toxin, or something else, it is not in your head.

I quoted and referenced many authors for a couple main reasons. I want you to gain an appreciation for the wealth of data out there, of which you are not exposed. I want you to realize that there are thousands and M.D.s, PhD.s, and other researchers who support my thoughts and statements. Those who value the aspects of natural medicine aren't "fringe conspiracy nuts" with no evidence in support of our cause, we're every day people, many transformed from the conventional medical community, with loads of supportive clinical data, only some of which you have been exposed to in this book.

Some of the concepts of this book point to an illness pyramid, much like the food guide pyramid. At the very bottom would be toxins, pathogens, nutrition, genes, lethargy, emotions, and metabolism. Above this are the now familiar inflammation, oxidation, glycosilation, hormonal decline, and metabolic inadequacies. Atop the pyramid is your disease state. You don't have cancer, heart disease, rheumatoid arthritis, or asthma. You have inflammation, oxidation, glycosilation, and/or metabolic inadequacies. You have these because of one or more factors on the first tier. Address the root cause of your chronic degenerative disease.

If you hear something enough times it becomes true. For example, the battle of Bunker Hill was actually fought on Breed's Hill. You wouldn't know it unless you've been exposed to the facts. Likewise, dairy is not necessarily good for you and your bones. This is but one of many flaws in the current food and medical system. Through marketing, habit, and repetition these things become dogmatic. People will defend something, even when they don't have all the information. It seems we're always forced to choose a side, whether it's sports, politics, or something else. Be on your own side, pick from the best of natural and conventional medicine as you see fit to establish your own healthcare model. Be your own well-informed advocate.

References

Chapter 1 - Our Current Healthcare Model

1. Lazarou J, et al. Incidence of adverse drug reactions in hospitalized patients: a meta-analysis of prospective studies. *JAMA*. 1998 Apr 15:279(15):1200-5.
2. Weinstein RA. Nosocomial infection update. *Emerg Infect Dis.* 1998 Jul-Sep;4(3):41620
3. Johnson JA, Bootman JL. Drug related morbidity and mortality and the economic impact of pharmaceutical care. *Am J Health Syst Pharm*. 1997 Mar 1;54(5):554-8
4. Zhan C, Miller M. Excess length of stay, charges, and mortality attributable to medical injuries during hospitalization. *JAMA* 2003;290;1868-74
5. Wald H, Shojania KG. Incident reporting. In: Shojania KG, Duncan BW, McDonald KM, et al, eds. *Making Health Care Safer: A Critical Analysis of Patient Safety Practices* . Rockville, MD : Agency for Healthcare Research and Quality; 2001:chap 4. Evidence Report/Technology Assessment No. 43. AHRQ publication 01-E058
6. Vincent C, Stanhope N, Crowley-Murphy M. Reasons for not reporting adverse incidents: an empirical study. *J Eval Clin Pract*. 1999 Feb;5(1):13-21
7. Null G, et al. Death by Medicine, *Life Extension Magazine*, August 206
8. Leape LL. Error in medicine. *JAMA* . 1994 Dec 21;272(23):1851-7
9. Singh G. Gastrointestinal complications of prescription and over-the-counter nonsteroidal anti-inflammatory drugs:A view from the ARAMIS database. *Am J Ther* 2000;7:115-21
10. Blot WJ, McLaughlin JK. Over the counter non-steroidal anti-inflammatory drugs and risk of gastrointestinal bleeding. *J Epidemiol Biostat* 2000;5(2);137-142
11. Nourjah P et al. *Pharmacoepidemiol Drug Saf* 15 398-405 2006
12. Tewari SN and Wilson AK. Deglycyrrhizinated licorice in duodenal ulcer. *Practitioner* 1972;210:820-5
13. Kassir ZA. Endoscopic controlled trial of four drug regimens in the treatments of chronic duodenal ulcer. *Irish Med J* 1985:78;153-6
14. Canner PL, et al. Fifteen-year mortality in coronary drug project patients:long-term benefit with niacin. *J Am Coll Cardiol* 1986,8;1245-55
15. Deodhar SD et al. Preliminary studies on anti-rheumatic activity of curcumin. Ind J Med, 1980;71:632-4
16. Murray M and Pizzorno J. *Encyclopedia of Natural Medicine*. 760
17. Murray M and Pizzorno J. *Encyclopedia of Natural Medicine* 397

Chapter 2 - Natural Medicine

1. Staehle HJ et al. *J Dent Res* 84 1066-69 2005
2. Ludtke R et al. *Complimentary Therapies in Medicine* 9 141-45 2001
3. Peterson K Journal of manipulative and physiological therapeutics 19 1996

Chapter 3 - Inflammatory Bowel Disease

1. Sawai T et al. The effect of phospholipids and fatty acids on tight-junction permeability and bacterial translocation. *Pediatr Surg Int* 2001 17 269-74
2. Haapamaki MM et al. Gene expression of group 2 phospolipase A2 in intesting in Crohn'd disease. 1999 *Am J Gastroenterol* 94 713-20

3. Pruzansky W et al. Inhibition of extracellular release of proinflammatory secretory phospolipase A2 (sPLA2) by sulphasalazine: a novel mechanism of anti-inflammatory activity. 1997 *Biochem Pharmacol* 53 1901-07

4. Gersemann M et al. Crohn's disease-defect in innate defense. *World J Gastroenterol* 2008 Sep 28 14(36) 5499-5503

5. IBID

6. Andersen AFR. Ulcerative Colitis: an allergic phenomenon. 1942 *Amer J Digest* Dis 9 91-98

7. Rowe AH. Chronic ulcerative colitis-allergy in its etiology. 1942 *Ann Intern Med* 17 83-100

8. Truelove SC. Ulcerative colitis provoked by milk. *BMJ* 154-160 Jan 21 1961

9. Nanda R et al. Food intolerance and the irritable bowel syndrome. *Gut* 1989 Aug 30(8) 1099-104

10. Workman EM et al. Diet in the management of Crohn's disease. *Hum Nutr Appl Nutr* 1984 Dec 38(6) 469-73

11. Behr M and Kapur V. The evidence for mycobacterium paratuberculosis in Crohn's disease. *Curr Opin Gastroenterol* 2008 24(1)17-21

12. Bibiloni R et al. The bacteriology of biopsies differs between newly diagnosed, untreated, Crohn's disease, and ulcerative colitis patients. *Journal of Medical Microbiology* 2006 55 1141-49

13. Darfeuille-Michaud A et al. Presence of adherent Escherichia coli strains in ileal mucosa of patients with Crohn's disease. *Gastroenterology* 1998 Dec 115(6) 1405-13

14. Frank D et al. Molecular-phylogenetic characterization of microbial community imbalances in human inflammatory bowel diseases. *PNAS* Aug 21 2007 vol 104 no 34

15. Hulin SJ et al. Sulphide-induced energy deficiency in colonic cells is prevented by glucose but not by butyrate. *Aliment Pharmacol Ther* 16 325-31 2002

16. IBID

17. IBID

18. Gaudier E et al. Butyrate specifically modulates MUC gene expression in intestinal epithelial goblet cells deprived of glucose. Am J Physiol Gastrointest Liver Physiol 287 G1168-74 2004.

19. IBID

20. Toy L et al. Defective expression of GP180, a novel CD8 ligand on intestinal epithelial cells, in inflammatory bowel disease. *J Clin Invest* 1997 100:2062-2071

21. Sanchez-Munoz F et al. Role of cytokines in inflammatory bowel disease. *World J Gastroenterol* 2008 Jul 21 14(27) 4280-88

22. Kozuch P and Hanauer S. Treatment of inflammatory bowel disease: a review of medical therapy. *World J Gastroenterol* 2008 Jan 21 14(3) 354-77

23. IBID

24. Olmsted County MN

25. Kozuch P and Hanauer S. Treatment of inflammatory bowel disease: a review of medical therapy. *World J Gastroenterol* 2008 Jan 21 14(3) 354-77

26. National Cooperative Crohn's Disease Study *NCCDS*

27. Sanchez-Munoz F et al, Role of cytokines in inflammatory bowel disease. *World J Gastroenterol* 2008 Jul 21 14(27) 4280-88

28. IBID

29. Murray M and Pizzorno J. *Encyclopedia of Natural Medicine* 2nd ed. p 609

30. Jones VA et al. Food intolerance: a major factor in the pathogenesis of irritable bowel syndrome. *Lancet* 1982 2(8308) 1115-7

31. MacDermott R, Treatment of irritable bowel syndrome in outpatients with inflammatory bowel disease using a food and beverage intolerance, food and beverage avoidance diet. *Inflamm Bowel Dis* 2007 13 91-96

32. Petitpierre M et al. Irritable bowel syndrome and hypersensitivity to food. *Ann Allergy* 1985 54(6)538-40

33. Boero M et al. Candida overgrowth in gastric juice of peptic ulcer subjects on short and long-term treatment with H2-receptor antagonists. *Digestion* 28 1983 158-63

34. Gupta I et al, Effects of Boswellia serrata gum resin in patients with ulcerative colitis. *Eur J Med Res* 1997 Jan 2(1) 37-43

35. Gupta I et al. Effects of gum resin of Boswellia serrate in patients with chronic colitis. *Planta Med* 2001 Jul 67(5) 391-5

36. Gerhardt H et al. Therapy of active Crohn's disease with boswellia serrate extract H 15. *Z Gastroenterol* 2001 Jan 39(1) 11-17

37. Almallah YZ et al. Distal procto-colitis, natural cytotoxicity, and essential fatty acids. *Am J Gastroenterol* 1998 May 93(5) 804-9

38. Belluzzi A et al. Effect of an enteric-coated fish-oil preparation on relapses in Crohn's disease. *N Engl J Med* 1996 334 1557-60

39. Lorenz R et al. Supplementation with n-3 fatty acids from fish oil in chronic inflammatory bowel disease-a randomized, placebo-controlled, double-blind cross-over trial. *J Intern Med Suppl* 1989 731 225-32

40. Stenson WF et al. Dietary supplementation with fish oil in ulceratice colitis. *Ann Intern Med* 1992 116(8) 609-14

41. MacLean C et al. Systemic review of the effects of n-3 fatty acids in inflammatory bowel disease. *Am J Clin Nutr* 2005 82 611-9

42. Bibiloni R et al. The bacteriology of biopsies differs between newly diagnosed, untreated, Crohn's disease, and ulcerative colitis patients. *Journal of Medical Microbiology* 2006 55 1141-49

43. Takaishi H et al. Circulation autoantibodies against purified colonic mucin in ulcerative colitis. *J Gastroenterol* 2000 35(1) 20-7

44. Treede I et al. Anti-inflammatory effects of phosphatidylcholine. *J of Biological Chem* vol 282 no 37 27155-164 2007

45. Gibson PR and Muir JG. Reinforcing the mucus: a new therapeutic approach for ulcerative colitis. *Gut* 54 900-03 2005

46. Stremmel W et al. Phosphatidylcholine for steroid-refractory ulcerative colitis. *Ann Intern med* 2007 147 603-10

47. Stremmel et al. Retarded release phosphatidylcholine benefits with chronic active ulcerative colitis. *Gut* 2005 54 966-71

48. Treede I et al. Anti-inflammatory effects of phosphatidylcholine. *J of Biological Chem* vol 282 no 37 27155-164 2007

49. Aggarwal B and Shishodia S. Suppression of nuclear factor-kappa B activation pathway by spice-derived phytochemicals: reasoning for seasoning. *Anderson cancer center University of Texas Invited review for Annals of the New York Academy of Sciences*

50. Shakibaei M et al. Suppression of NF-KB activation by curcumin leads to inhibition of expression of cyclo-oxygenase-2 and matrix metalloproteinase-9 in human articular chondrocytes: implications for the treatment of osteoarthritis. *Biochemical Pharmacology* 2007 73 1343-1445

51. Aggarwal B and Shishodia S. Suppression of nuclear factor-kappa B activation pathway by spice-derived phytochemicals: reasoning for seasoning. *Anderson cancer center University of Texas Invited review for Annals of the New York Academy of Sciences*

52. IBID

53. Clarke J and Mullin G. A review of complementary and alternative approaches to immunomodulation. *Nutr in Clin Pract* 2008 23 49-62
54. IBID
55. IBID
56. Hanai H et al. Curcumin maintenance therapy for ulcerative colitis: randomized, multicenter, double-blind, placebo-controlled trial. *Clin Gastroenterol Hepatol* 2006 4(12) 1502-6
57. Gonzales A and Orlando R. Curcumin and resveratrol inhibit nuclear factor-kappa-B-mediated cytokine expression in adipocytes. *Nutrition And Metabolism* 2008 5 17
58. May B et al. Efficacy of a fixed peppermint oil/caraway oil combination in non-ulcer dyspepsia. *Arzneimittelforschung* 1996 46(12) 1149-53
59. Alternative Medicine Review Monographs vol 1 p 33
60. Clarke J and Mullin G. A review of complementary and alternative approaches to immunomodulation. *Nutr in Clin Pract* 2008 23 49-62
61. Schleithoff S et al. Vitamin D supplementation improves cytokine profiles in patients with congestive heart failure: a double-blind, randomized, placebo-controlled trial. *Am J Clin Nutr* 2006 83 754-9
62. Stio M et al. The vitamin D analogue TX 527 NF-Kappa B activation in peripheral blood mononuclear cells of patients with Crohn's disease. *J Steroid Biochem Mol Biol* 2007 103(1) 51-60
63. Bartels LE et al 1,25 dihydroxyvitamin D3 and dexamethasone increase interleukin-10 production in CD4+ T cells from patients with Crohn's disease. *Int Immunopharmacol* 2007 7(13) 1755-64
64. Dubinsky M etal Immunogenetic phenotypes in inflammatory bowel disease. *World J Gastroenterol* 2006 Jun 21 12(23)3645-50

Chapter 4 - Bone Health

1. Feskanich D et al. Milk, dietary calcium, and bone fractures in women: a 12 year prospective study. *Am J Public Health* 87 992-97 1997
2. Bolland M et al. Vascular events in healthy older women receiving calcium supplementation: randomized controlled trial. *BMJ* 336 262-66 2008
3. Winzenberg T et al. Effects of calcium supplementation on bone density in healthy children: meta-analysis of randomized controlled trials. *BMJ* doi:10.1136/bmj.38950.561400.55
4. Weinsier RL Krumdieck CL. Dairy foods and bone health: examination of the evidence. *Am J Clin Nutr* 72 681-9 2000.
5. Lanou A et al. Calcium, dairy products, and bone health in children and young adults: a reevaluation of the evidence. *Pediatrics* 115 736-43 2005
6. Reid I et al. Effect of calcium supplementation on bone loss in postmenopausal women. *N Engl J Med* 328 460-4 1993
7. Reid I et al. Long-term effects of calcium supplementation on bone loss and fractures in postmenopausal women: a randomized controlled trial. *Am J Med* 98 329-30 1995
8. Reid I et al, Randomized controlled trial of calcium supplementation in healthy, non-osteoporotic, older men. *Arch Intern Med* 168 2276-82 2008
9. Cadogan J et al. Milk intake and bone mineral acquisition in adolescent girls: randomized, controlled, intervention trial. *BMJ* 315 1255-60 1997
10. Nowson C et al. A co-twin study of the effect of calcium supplementation on bone density during adolescence. *Osteoporosis Int* 7 219-25. 1997
11. Hegsted M. Fractures, calcium, and the modern diet. *Am J Clin Nutr* 74 571-3 2001

12. Weaver C et al. Choices for achieving adequate dietary calcium with a vegetarian diet. *Am J Clin Nutr* 70 543s-8s 1999

13. Lanou A et al. Calcium, dairy products, and bone health in children and young adults: a reevaluation of the evidence. *Pediatrics* 115 736-43 2005

14. Breslau N et al. Relationship of animal protein-rich diet to kidney stone formation and calcium metabolism. *J Clin Endocrinol Metab* 66 140-146 1988

15. IBID

16. Tschope W Ritz E. Sulfur-containing amino acids are a major determinant of urinary calcium. *Mineral Electrolyte Metab* 11:137 1985.

17. Dawson-Hughes B et al. Treatment with potassium bicarbonate lowers calcium excretion and bone resorption in older men and women. *J Clin Endocrinol Metab* 94 96-102 2009

18. Maurer M et al. Neutralization of western diet inhibits bone resorption independently of K intake and reduces cortisol secretion in humans. *Am J Physiol Renal Physiol* 284 f32-40 2003

19. Dawson-Hughes B et al. Treatment with potassium bicarbonate lowers calcium excretion and bone resorption in older men and women. *J Clin Endocrinol Metab* 94 96-102 2009

20. Frassetto L, Sebastian A. Age and systemic acid-base equilibrium: analysis of published data. *J Gerontol A Biol Sci Med Sci* 51 B91-99

21. Matkovic V et al. Urinary calcium, sodium, and bone mass of young females. *Am J Clin Nutr* 62 417-25 1995.

22. Zakardas M et al. Sodium chloride supplementation and urinary calcium excretion in postmenopausal women. *Am J Clin Nutr* 50 1088-94 1989

23. Curhan G et al. A Prospective Study of Dietary Calcium and Other Nutrients and the Risk of Syptomatic Kidney Stones. *NEJM* Vol 328 P 833-38 1993

24. Barilla DE et al. Renal Oxalate Excretion Following Oral Oxalate loads in patients with ileal disease and with renal and absorptive hypercalciurias: effect of calcium and magnesium. *Am J Med* 1978 64 579-85

25. Hall P. Nephrolithiasis: Treatment, causes, and prevention. *Cleveland Clinic Journal of Medicine* 76 583-591 2009

26. Borghi L et al. Comparison of two diets for the prevention of recurrent stones in idiopathic hypercalciuria. *NEJM* 346 77-84 2002

27. Borghi L et al. Urinary volume, water, and recurrences in idiopathic calcium nephrolithiasis: a 5 year randomized prospective study. *J Urol* 155 839-43 1996

28. Parmar, M. Kidney Stones. *BMJ* 328 1420-1425 2004

29. Danpure C. Molecular Etiology of Primary Hyperoxaluria type 1: new directions for treatment. *Am J Nephrol* 25 303-310 2005

30. Hall P. Nephrolithiasis: Treatment, causes, and prevention. *Cleveland Clinic Journal of Medicine* 76 583-591 2009

31. Williams EL et al. Primary hyperoxaluria type 1: update and additional mutation analysis of the AGXT gene. *Hum Mutat* 30 910-17 2009

32. Danpure C. Molecular Etiology of Primary Hyperoxaluria type 1: new directions for treatment. *Am J Nephrol* 25 303-310 2005

33. Shaw W. The role of oxalates in autism and chronic disorders. *Wise Traditions* 11 40-47 2010

34. Uotila L. The metabolic functions and mechanisms of vitamin K. *Scand J Clin Lab Invest Suppl* 201, 109-17, 1990

35. Pizzorno L and Pizzorno J. Vitamin K, beyond coagulation to uses in bones, vascular, and anti-cancer metabolism. *Integrative Medicine* 7 24-30 2008

36. Shearer M et al. Chemistry, nutritional sources, tissue distribution, and metabolism of vitamin K with special reference to bone health. *J Nutr* 126 1181S-86S 1996
37. Shearer M et al. Chemistry, nutritional sources, tissue distribution, and metabolism of vitamin K with special reference to bone health. *J Nutr* 126 1181S-86S 1996
38. Ikeda Y et al. Intake of fermented soybeans, natto, is associated with reduced bone loss in postmenopausal women:Japanese population-based osteoporosis (JPOS) study. *J Nutr* 136 1323-28 2006
39. Knapen MH et al. Vitamin K2 supplementation improves hip bone geometry and bone strength indices in postmenopausal women. *Osteoporosis Int* 18 963-72 2007
40. Bugel S. Vitamin K and bone health. *Proceeding of the Nutrition Society* 62 839-43 2003
41. Kamao M et al. Vitamin K content of foods and dietary vitamin K intake in Japanese young women. *J Nutr Sci Vitaminol* 53 464-470 2007
42. Knapen MH et al. Vitamin K2 supplementation improves hip bone geometry and bone strength indices in postmenopausal women. *Osteoporosis Int* 18 963-72 2007
43. Adams J and Pepping J. Vitamin K in the treatment and prevention of osteoporosis and arterial calcification. *Am J Health-syst Pharm* 62 1574-81 2005
44. Vergnaud P et al. Undercarboxylated osteocalcin measured with a specific immunoassay predicts hip fracture in elderly women: the EPIDOS study. *J Clin Endocrinol Metab* 82 719-24 1997
45. Adams J and Pepping J. Vitamin K in the treatment and prevention of osteoporosis and arterial calcification. *Am J Health-syst Pharm* 62 1574-81 2005
46. Schurgers L et al. Vitamin K-containing dietary supplements: comparison of synthetic vitamin K1 and natto-derived menaquinone-7. *Blood* 109 3279-83 2007
47. Schurgers L et al. Vitamin K-containing dietary supplements: comparison of synthetic vitamin K1 and natto-derived menaquinone-7. *Blood* 109 3279-83 2007
48. Knapen MH, et al. Vitamin K2 supplementation improves hip bone geometry and bone strength indices in postmenopausal women. *Osteoporosis Int* 18 963-72 2007
49. Shiraki M et al. Vitamin K (menatetronone) effectively prevents fractures and sustains lumbar bone mineral density in osteoporosis. *J Bone Miner Res* 15 515-21 2000
50. Pizzorno L and Pizzorno J. Vitamin K, beyond coagulation to uses in bones, vascular, and anti-cancer metabolism. *Integrative Medicine* 7 24-30 2008
51. Knapen MH, et al. Vitamin K2 supplementation improves hip bone geometry and bone strength indices in postmenopausal women. *Osteoporosis Int* 18 963-72 2007
52. Adams J and Pepping J. Vitamin K in the treatment and prevention of osteoporosis and arterial calcification. *Am J Health-syst Pharm* 62 1574-81 2005
53. Feskanich D, et al. Vitamin K intake and hip fractures in women: a prospective study. *Am J Clin Nutr* 69 74-79 1999
54. Cockayne S et al. Vitamin K and the prevention of fractures. *Arch Intern Med* 166 1256-61 2006
55. Iwamoto J et al. Effect of combined administration of vitamin D3 and vitamin K2 on bone mineral density of the lumbar spine in postmenopausal women with osteoporosis. *J Orthop Sci* 5 546-51 2000
56. Ushiroyama T et al. Effect of continuous combined therapy with vitamin K2 and vitamin D3 on bone mineral density and coagulofibrinolysis function in postmenopausal women. *Maturitas* 41 211-21 2002

Chapter 5 - Methylation

1. Benevenga N. Consideration of betaine and one-carbon sources of N5-methyl-tetrahydrofolate for use in homocystinuria and neural tube defects. *Am J Clin Nutr* 2007 85 946-9.
2. Sanz A et al. Methionine restriction decreases mitochondrial oxygen radical generation and leak as well as oxidative damage to mitochondrial DNA and proteins. *FASEB J* 2006 Jun;20(8):1064-73.
3. Sanz A et al. Methionine restriction decreases mitochondrial oxygen radical generation and leak as well as oxidative damage to mitochondrial DNA and proteins. *FASEB J* 2006 Jun;20(8):1064-73.
4. Sanz A et al. Methionine restriction decreases mitochondrial oxygen radical generation and leak as well as oxidative damage to mitochondrial DNA and proteins *FASEB J* 2006 Jun;20(8):1064-73.
5. Shcherbatykh I and Carpernter D. The Role of Metals in the Etiology of Alzheimer's Disease. *Journal of Alzheimer's Disease* 11 2007 191-205.
6. Shcherbatykh I and Carpernter D. The Role of Metals in the Etiology of Alzheimer's Disease. *Journal of Alzheimer's Disease* 11 2007 191-205.
7. Shcherbatykh I and Carpernter D. The Role of Metals in the Etiology of Alzheimer's Disease. *Journal of Alzheimer's Disease* 11 2007 191-205.
8. Domingo Jose. Aluminum and other metals in Alzheimer's disease. *Journal of AD* 10 2006 331-341.
9. Miller A. The methionine-homocysteine cycle and its effects on cognitive diseases. *AMR* 8 1 2003.
10. Miller A. The methionine-homocysteine cycle and its effects on cognitive diseases. *AMR* 8 1 2003.
11. Clarke R et al. Folate, Vitamin B12, and serum total homocysteine levels in confirmed alzheimers disease. *Arch Neurol* 1998 55 1449-55.
12. Boldyrev A and Johnson P. Homocysteine and its derivatives as possible modulators of neuronal and non-neuronal cell glutamate receptors in Alzheimer's disease. *J of Alz Dis* 11 2007 219-28.
13. Seshadri S et al. Plasma homocysteine as a risk factor for dementia and Alzheimer's disease. *NEJM* 2002 346 476-83.
14. Selley ML et al. The effect of increased concentrations of homocysteine on the concentration of (E)-4-hydroxy-2-nonenal in the plasma and cerebrospinal fluid of patients with Alzheimer's disease. *Neurobiol Aging* 2002 23 3 383-8.
15. Finkelstein JD. Metabolic Regulatory Properties of S-adenosylmethionine and S-Adenosylhomocysteine. *Clin Chem Lab Med* 2007 45 (12) 1694-9.
16. Lindenbaum J et al. Neuropsychiatric disorders caused by cobalamin deficiency in the absence of anemia or macrocytosis. *NEJM* 1988 318 1720-28.
17. Ikeda T et al. Treatment of Alzheimer-type dementia with intravenous mecobalamin. *Clin Ther* 1992 14(3) 426-37.
18. Kuszczyk M et al. Homocysteine-induced acute excitotoxicity in cerebellar granule cells in vitro is accompanied by PP2A-mediated dephosphorylation of tau. *Neurochem Int* 2009 Jul-Aug;55(1-3):174-80. Epub 2009 Feb 24.
19. Zieminska E and Lazarewicz JW. Excitotoxic neuronal injury in chronic homocysteine neurotoxicity studied in vitro: the role of NMDA and group I metabotropic glutamate receptors. *Acta Neurobiol Exp* 2006;66(4):301-9.
20. Ho P et al. Multiple aspects of homocysteine neurotoxicity: glutamate excitotoxicity, kinase hyperactivation and DNA damage. *J Neurosci Res* 2002 Dec 1;70(5):694-702.

21. Montgomery SA et al. Meta-analysis of double blind randomized controlled clinical trials of acetyl-L-carnitine versus placebo in the treatment of mild cognitive impairment and mild Alzheimer's Disease. *Int Clin Phsychopharmacol* 2003 Mar;18(2):61-71.
22. Shults CW et al. Effects of coenzyme Q10 in early Parkinson disease: evidence of slowing of the functional decline. *Arch Neurol* 2002 Oct;59(10):1541-50.)
23. Akaike A et al. Protective effects of a vitamin B12 analog, methylcobalamin, against glutamate cytotoxicity in cultured cortical neurons. *Eur J Pharmacol* 1993 Sep 7;241(1):1-6.
24. Savage DG et al. Sensitivity of serum methylmalonic acid and total homocysteine determinations for diagnosing cobalamin and folate deficiencies. *AM J Med* 1994 Mar;96(3):239-46.
25. Steenge GR et al. Betaine supplementation lowers plasma homocysteine in healthy men and women. *J Nutr* 2003 133 1291-95.
26. Schwab U et al. Betaine supplementation decreases plasma homocysteine concentrations but does not affect body weight, body composition, or resting energy expenditure in human subjects. *Am J Clin Nutr* 2002 76 961-7.
27. Olthof MR et al. Low dose betaine supplementation leads to immediate and long-term lowering of plasma homocysteine in healthy men and women. *J Nutr* 2003 Dec;133(12):4135-8.
28. Afthan G et al. The effect of low doses of betaine on plasma homocysteine in healthy volunteers. *Br J Nutr* 2004 Oct;92(4):665-9.
29. Ueland PM et al. Betaine: a key modulator of one-carbon metabolism and homocysteine status. *Clin Chem Lab Med* 2005 43 (10) 1069-75.
30. Schwab U et al. Betaine supplementation decreases plasma homocysteine concentrations but does not affect body weight, body composition, or resting energy expenditure in human subjects. *Am J Clin Nutr* 2002 76 961-7.
31. Schwab U et al. Orally administered betaine has an acute and dose dependent effect on dserum betaine and plasma homocysteine concentrations in healthy humans. *J Nutr* 2006 136 34-38.
32. Schwab U et al. Orally administered betaine has an acute and dose dependent effect on dserum betaine and plasma homocysteine concentrations in healthy humans. *J Nutr* 2006 136 34-38.
33. Craig S. Betaine in Human Nutrition. *Am J Clin Nutr* 2004 80 539-49.
34. Olthof MR and Verhoef P. Effects of betaine intake on plasma homocysteine concentrations and consequences for health. *Curr Drug Metab* 2005 6 15-22.
35. Zeisel SH. Betaine supplementation and blood lipids: fact or artifact. *Nutr Rev* 2006 64 77-79.
36. Barak A et al. Betaine, Ethanol, and the liver: a review. *Alcohol* 13 1996 395-98.
37. Kharbanda KK. Role of transmethylation reactions in alcoholic liver disease. *World J Gastroenterol* 2007 13 4947-54.
38. Kharbanda KK. Role of transmethylation reactions in alcoholic liver disease. *World J Gastroenterol* 2007 13 4947-54.
39. Detich N et al. The Methyl donor SAMe Inhibits active demethylation of DNA. *J Biol Chem* 2003 278 20812-820.
40. Soeken KL et al. Safety and efficacy of S-adenosylmethionine (SAMe) for osteoarthritis. *J Fam Pract* 2002 May;51(5):425-30.
41. Derflinger T et al. *Better Breast Health for Life* p9 2005.
42. Ravel C et al. Lack of association between genetic polymorphisms in enzymes associated with folate metabolism and unexplained reduced sperm counts. *PLoS One* 2009 Aug 6;4(8):e6540.

43. Yang QH et al. Prevalence and effects of gene-gene and gene-nutrient interactions on serum folate and serum total homocysteine concentrations in the United States: findings from the third National Health and Nutrition Examination Survey DNA Bank. *AM J Clin Nutr* 2008 Jul;88(1):232-46.

44. Siva A et al. The heritability of plasma homocysteine, and the influence of genetic variation in the homocysteine methylation pathway. *QJM* 2007 Aug;100(8):495-9. Epub 2007 Jul 17.

45. Yang QH et al. Prevalence and effects of gene-gene and gene-nutrient interactions on serum folate and serum total homocysteine concentrations in the United States: findings from the third National Health and Nutrition Examination Survey DNA Bank. *AM J Clin Nutr* 2008 Jul;88(1):232-46.

46. Sharp L and Little J. Polymorphisms in genes involved in folate metabolism and colorectal neoplasia" A HuGE review. *Am J of Epidemiology* 159 2004 423-443.

47. Sharp L and Little J. Polymorphisms in genes involved in folate metabolism and colorectal neoplasia" A HuGE review. *Am J of Epidemiology* 159 2004 423-443.

48. Scazzone C et al. Methionine Synthase Reductase (MTRR) A66G polymorphism is not related with plasma homocysteine concentration and risk for vascular disease. *Exp Mol Pathol* 2009 Feb 4. [Epub ahead of print].

49. Botto N et al. Genetic polymorphisms in folate and homocysteine metabolism as risk factors for DNA damage. *Eur J Hum Genet* 2003 Sep;11(9):671-8.

50. Botto N et al. Genetic polymorphisms in folate and homocysteine metabolism as risk factors for DNA damage. *Eur J Hum Genet* 2003 Sep;11(9):671-8.

51. Botto N et al. Genetic polymorphisms in folate and homocysteine metabolism as risk factors for DNA damage. *Eur J Hum Genet* 2003 Sep;11(9):671-8.

52. Sharp L and Little J. Polymorphisms in genes involved in folate metabolism and colorectal neoplasia" A HuGE review. *Am J of Epidemiology* 159 2004 423-443.

Chapter 6 - Vascular Health

1. Bradley R and Oberg E. Integrative treatments to reduce risk for cardiovascular disease. **IMCJ** 8 26-32 2009

2. Abramson J. Overdosed America the Broken Promise of American Medicine. *Harper Perinnial*

3. Abramson J. Overdosed America the Broken Promise of American Medicine. *Harper Perennial*

4. Choudhry N et al. Relationships between authors of clinical practice guidelines and the pharmaceutical industry. *JAMA* 287 612-17 2002

5. Abramson J. Overdosed America the Broken Promise of American Medicine. Harper Perennial

6. IBID

7. IBID

8. Carey J. Do cholesterol drugs do any good? *Business Week* January 17 2008

9. IBID

10. Carey J. Do cholesterol drugs do any good? *Business Week* January 17 2008 (with my own commentary added)

11. Vos E and Rose C. Questioning the benefits of statins. *CMAJ* 173 2005 doi:10.1503/cmaj.1050120

12. Pedersen T et al. High-dose atorvastatin vs usual-dose simvastatin for secondary prevention after myocardial infarction. The IDEAL study: A randomized controlled trial. *JAMA* 294 2437-2445 2005

13. Ravnskov U et al. Should we lower cholesterol as much as possible? *BMJ* 332 1330-32 2006
14. LaRosa JC et al. Intensive lipid lowering with Atorvastatin in patients with stable coronary disease. *NEJM* 352 1425-35
15. Brugts JJ et al. The benefits of statins in people without established cardiovascular disease but with cardiovascular risk factors: meta-analysis of randomized controlled trials. *BMJ* 2009;338:b2376
16. Moride Y et al. Clinical and public health assessment of benefits and risks of statins in primary prevention of coronary events: resolved and unresolved issues. *Can J Cardiol* 24 293-300 2008
17. CHOUDRY
18. Thavendiranathan P et al. Primary prevention of cardiovascular diseases with statin therapy. *Arch Intern Med* 166 2307-13 2006
19. Carey J. Do cholesterol drugs do any good? *BusinessWeek* January 17 2008
20. IBID
21. IBID
22. Nissen S. The Jupiter trial: key findings, controversies, and implications. *Current Cardiology Reports* 11 81-82 2009
23. Mora S and Ridker PM. Justification for the use of statins in primary prevention: an intervention trials evaluating rosuvastatin (JUPITER)—can C-reactive protein be used to target statin therapy in primary prevention? *Am J Cardiol* 97 33a-41a 2006
24. Liao JK. Does it matter whether or not a lipid-lowering agent inhibits Rho kinase? *Curr Atheroscler Rep* 9 384-88 2007
25. IBID
26. Kronmal RA et al. Total serum cholesterol levels and mortality risk as a function of age. A report based on the Framingham data. *Arch Intern Med* 153 1065-73 1993
27. IBID
28. Rogers S. *The Cholesterol Hoax*. Sand Key Company Inc 2008 ISBN: 978-1-887202-06-0
29. Rogers S. *The Cholesterol Hoax*. Sand Key Company Inc 2008 ISBN: 978-1-887202-06-0 p185
30. Pauling L. *How to Live Longer and Feel Better*. Oregon State University Press 2006 p 43-44
31. Witztum J and Steinberg D. Role of oxidized low density lipoprotein in atherogenesis. *J Clin Invest* 88 1785-1792 1991
32. Rogers S. *The Cholesterol Hoax*. Sand Key Company Inc 2008 ISBN: 978-1-887202-06-0 p 56, 92-93, 115
33. Witztum J and Steinberg D. Role of oxidized low density lipoprotein in atherogenesis. *J Clin Invest* 88 1785-1792 1991
34. Toborek M et al. Unsaturated fatty acids selectively induce an inflammatory environment in human endothelial cells. *Am J Clin Nutr* 75 119-25 2002
35. Wallin R et al. Arterial calcification: a review of mechanisms, animal models, and the prospects for therapy. *Med Res Rev* 21 274-301 2001
36. Packard RRS et al. Innate and adaptive immunity in atherosclerosis. *Semin Immunopathol* 31 2009 doi: 10.1007/s00281-009-0153-8
37. Libby P. Inflammation and cardiovascular disease mechanisms. *Am J Clin Nutr* 83 s456-60 2006
38. Berliner JA et al. Atherosclerosis: basic mechanisms. *Circulation* 91 2488-2496 1995
39. Staprans I et al. Oxidized cholesterol in the diet accelerates the development of atherosclerosis in LDL receptor – and apolipoprotein E-deficient mice. *Arterioscler Thromb Vasc Biol* 20 7-8-14 2000
40. Toborek M et al. Unsaturated fatty acids selectively induce an inflammatory environment in human endothelial cells. *Am J Clin Nutr* 75 119-25 2002

41. Wallin R et al. Arterial calcification: a review of mechanisms, animal models, and the prospects for therapy. *Med Res Rev* 21 274-301 2001
42. Berliner JA et al. Atherosclerosis: basic mechanisms. *Circulation* 91 2488-2496 1995
43. Libby P. Inflammation and cardiovascular disease mechanisms. *Am J Clin Nutr* 83 s456-60 2006
44. Packard RRS et al. Innate and adaptive immunity in atherosclerosis. *Semin Immunopathol* 31 2009 doi: 10.1007/s00281-009-0153-8
45. Staprans I et al. Oxidized cholesterol in the diet accelerates the development of atherosclerosis in LDL receptor – and apolipoprotein E-deficient mice. *Arterioscler Thromb Vasc Biol* 20 7-8-14 2000
46. Boger RH. Asymmetric Dimethylarginine (ADMA) and cardiovascular disease: insights from prospective clinical trials. *Vasc Med* 10 S19-25 2005
47. Zoccali C. The endothelium as a target in renal disease. *J Nephrol* 20 s39-44 2007
48. Szuba A and Podgorski M. Asymmetric Dimethylarginine (ADMA) a novel cardiovascular risk factor – evidence from epidemiological and prospective clinical trials. *Pharmacological Reports* 58 s16-20 2006
49. Schnabel R et al. Asymmetrical dimethyarginine and the risk of cardiovascular events and deaths in patients with coronary artery disease: results from the AtheroGene study. *Circ Res* 97 e53-59 2005
50. Valkonen VP et al. Risk of acute coronary events and serum concentration of asymmetrical dimethylarginine. *Lancet* 358 2127-28 2001
51. Lu TM et al. Plasma levels of asymmetrical dimethylarginine and adverse cardiovascular events after percutaneous coronary intervention. *Eur Heart J* 24 1912-19 2003
52. Nijveldt RJ et al. Asymmetrical dimethylarginine (ADMA) in critically ill patients: high plasma ADMA concentration is an independent risk factor for ICU mortality. *Clin Nutr* 22 23-30 2003
53. Palm F et al. Dimethylarginine dimethyaminohydrolase (DDAH): expression, regulation, and function in the cardiovascular and renal systems. *Am J Physiol Heart Circ Physiol* 293 H3227-45 2007
54. Valkonen PV et al. DDAH gene and cardiovascular risk. *Vasc Med* 10 s45-48 2005
55. Palm F et al. Dimethylarginine dimethyaminohydrolase (DDAH): expression, regulation, and function in the cardiovascular and renal systems. *Am J Physiol Heart Circ Physiol* 293 H3227-45 2007
56. Zakrzewicz D and Eickelberg O. From arginine methylation to ADMA: A novel mechanism with therapeutic potential in chronic lung diseases. *BMC Pulmonary Med* 9 2009 doi:10.1186/1471-2466-9-5
57. Landim MBP et al. Asymmetric Dimethylarginine (ADMA) and endothelial dysfunction: implications for atherogenesis. *Clinics* 64 471-78 2009
58. Palm F et al. Dimethylarginine Dimethyaminohydrolase (DDAH): expression, regulation, and function in the cardiovascular and renal systems. *Am J Physiol Heart Circ Physiol* 293 H3227-45 2007
59. Landim MBP et al. Asymmetric Dimethylarginine (ADMA) and endothelial dysfunction: implications for atherogenesis. *Clinics* 64 471-78 2009
60. Boger RH. Asymmetric Dimethylarginine (ADMA) and cardiovascular disease: insights from prospective clinical trials. *Vasc Med* 10 S19-25 2005
61. Nygard O et al. Plasma homocysteine levels and mortality in patients with coronary artery disease. *N Engl J Med* 337 230-6 1997
62. IBID
63. Robinson K et al. Hyperhomocysteinemia and low pyridoxal phosphate. Common and independent reversible risk factors for coronary artery disease. *Circulation* 92 2825-30 1995

64. Nygard O et al. Plasma homocysteine levels and mortality in patients with coronary artery disease. *N Engl J Med* 337 230-6 1997

65. Albert CM et al. Effect of folic acid and B vitamins on risk of cardiovascular events and total mortality among women at high risk for cardiovascular disease. *JAMA* 299 2027-36 2008

66. Lonn E et al. Homocysteine lowering with folic acid and B vitamins in vascular disease. *N Engl J Med* 354 1567-77 2006

67. Imura N et al. Chemical methylation of inorganic mercury with methylcobalamin, a vitamin B12 analog. *Science* 172 1248-49 1971

68. Salonen JT et al. Intake of mercury from fish, lipid peroxidation, and the risk of myocardial infarction and coronary, cardiovascular, and any death in eastern Finnish men. *Circulation* 91 645-55 1995

69. Virtanen J et al. Mercury, fish oils, and risk of acute coronary events and cardiovascular disease, coronary heart disease, and all-cause mortality in men in eastern Finland. *Arterioscler Thromb Vasc Biol* 25 228-33 2005

70. Choi A et al. Methylmercury exposure and adverse cardiovascular effects in Faroese Whaling men. *Environ Health Perspect* 117 367-72 2009

71. Guallar E et al. Mercury, fish oil and the risk of myocardial infarction. *NEJM* 347 1747-54 2002

72. No Author. A randomized, controlled trial of aspirin in persons recovered from myocardial infarction. *JAMA* 243 661-69 1980

73. Fowkes FG et al. Aspirin for prevention of cardiovascular events in a general population screened for a low ankle brachial index: a randomized controlled trial. *JAMA* 303 841-48 2010

74. He J et al. Aspirin and risk of hemorrhagic stroke. *JAMA* 280 1930-35 1998

75. Rogers S. The High Blood Pressure Hoax. Sand Key Company Inc. 2005 ISBN: 1-887202-05-6

76. Beulens JWJ et al. High dietary menaquinone intake is associated with reduced coronary calcification. *Atherosclerosis* 2008 doi: 10.1016/j.atherosclerosis.2008.07.010

77. Schurgers LJ et al. Regression of warfarin-induced medial elastocalcinosis by high intake of vitamin K in rats. *Blood* 109 2823-31 2007

78. Adams J and Pepping J. Vitamin K in the treatment and prevention of osteoporosis and arterial calcification. *Am J health-Syst Pharm* 62 1574-81 2005

79. Schurgers regression of, Wallin R et al. Effects of the blood coagulation vitamin K as inhibitor of arterial calcification. *Thromb Res* 122 411-417 2008

80. Wallin R et al. Arterial calcification: a review of mechanisms, animal models, and the prospects for therapy. *Med Res Rev* 21 274-301 2001

81. Danziger J. Vitamin K-dependent proteins, warfarin, and vascular calcification. *Clin J Am Soc Nephrol* 3 1504-10 2008

82. IBID

83. Beulens JWJ et al. High dietary menaquinone intake is associated with reduced coronary calcification. *Atherosclerosis* 2008 doi: 10.1016/j.atherosclerosis.2008.07.010

84. Koos R et al. Relation of oral anticoagulation to cardiac valvular and coronary calcium assessed by multislice spiral computed tomography. *Am J Cardiol* 96 747-9 2005

85. Spronk HMH et al. Tissue-specific utilization of menaquinone-4 results in the prevention of arterial calcification in warfarin-treated rats. *J Vasc Res* 40 531-37 2003

86. Luo G et al. Spontaneous calcification of arteries and cartilage in mice lacking matrix Gla protein. *Nature* 386 78-81 1997

87. Danziger J. Vitamin K-dependent proteins, warfarin, and vascular calcification. *Clin J Am Soc Nephrol* 3 1504-10 2008

88. Herrmann Sm et al. Polymorphisms of the human matrix Gla protein MGP gene, vascular calcification, and myocardial infarction. *Arterioscler Thromb Vasc Biol* 20 2386-93 2000

89. Jono S et al. 1,25-dihydroxyvitamin D3 increases in-vitro vascular calcification by modulating secretion of endogenous parathyroid hormone-related peptide. *Circulation* 98 1302-06 1998

90. IBID

91. Bolland M et al. Vascular events in healthy older women receiving calcium supplementation: randomized controlled trial. *BML* doi:10.1136/bmj.39440.525752.BE

92. IBID

93. Pohle K et al. Coronary calcifications in young patients with first, unheralded myocardial infarction: a risk factor matched analysis by electron beam tomography. *Heart* 89 625-28 2003

94. Taylor A et al. Coronary calcium independently predicts incident premature coronary heart disease over measured cardiovascular risk factors. *J Am Coll Cardiol* 46 807-14 2005

95. Witteman JC et al. Aortic calcified plaques and cardiovascular disease (the Framingham study) *Am J Cardiol* 66 1060-64 1990

96. Shaw LJ et al. Coronary artery calcium as a measure of biologic age. *Atherosclerosis* 188 112-19 2006

97. Jie KS et al. Vitamin K intake and osteocalcin levels in women with and without aortic atherosclerosis: a population-based study. *Atherosclerosis* 116 117-23 1995

98. Jie KG et al. Vitamin K status and bone mass in women with and without aortic atherosclerosis: a population-based study. *Calcif Tissue Int* 59 352-56 1996

99. Budoff M and Gul K Expert. Review on coronary calcium.

100. Danziger J. Vitamin K-dependent proteins, warfarin, and vascular calcification. *Clin J Am Soc Nephrol* 3 1504-10 2008

101. Adams J and Pepping J. Vitamin K in the treatment and prevention of osteoporosis and arterial calcification. *Am J Health-Syst Pharm* 62 1574-81 2005

102. Pizzorno L and Pizzorno J. Vitamin K beyond coagulation to uses in bone, vascular, and anti-cancer metabolism. *Integrative Medicine* 7 24-30 2008

103. Ornish D et al. Intensive lifestyle changes for reversal of coronary heart disease. *JAMA* 280 2001-07 1998

104. de Lorgeril M et al. Mediterranean diet, traditional risk factors, and the rate of cardiovascular complications after myocardial infarction. *Circulation* 99 779-85 1999

105. Gey FK et al. Inverse correlation between plasma vitamin E and mortality from ischemic heart disease in cross-cultural epidemiology. *Am J Clin Nutr* 53 326s-34s 1991

106. Riemersma RA et al. Low plasma vitamins E and C. Increased risk of angina in Scottish men. *Ann NY Acad Sci* 570 291-5 1989

107. Reaven P et al. Effects of oleate-rich and linoleate-rich diets on the susceptibility of low density lipoprotein to oxidative modification in mildly hypercholesterolemic subjects. *J Clin Invest* 91 668-76 1993

108. Toborek M et al. Unsaturated fatty acids selectively induce an inflammatory environment in human endothelial cells. *Am J Clin Nutr* 75 119-25 2002

109. Reaven P et al. Effects of oleate-rich and linoleate-rich diets on the susceptibility of low-density lipoprotein to oxidative modification in mildly hypercholesterolemic subjects. *J Clin Invest* 91 668-76 1993

Chapter 7 - Dietary choices

1. Chopra D et al. *Alternative Medicine is Mainstream* 2009
2. IBID
3. IBID
4. Nathan C. Epidemic inflammation: pondering obesity. *Mol Med* 14 485-92 2008
5. IBID
6. Thalman S and Meier C. Local adipose tissue depots as cardiovascular risk factors. *Cardiovascular Res* 75 690-701 2007
7. Montecucco F et al. Insulin resistance: a proinflammatory state mediated by lipid-induced signaling dysfunction and involved in atherosclerotic plaque instability. *Mediators Inflamm* 2008 2008 767623
8. IBID
9. IBID
10. Nathan C. *Mol Med* 2008 Jul-Aug;14(7-8):485-92
11. Wellen K and Hotamisligil G. Obesity-induced inflammatory changes in adipose tissue. *J Clin Invest* 112 1785-88 2003
12. Rudin E and Barzilai N. Inflammatory peptides derived from adipose tissue. *Immun Ageing* 2 1-3 2005
13. White M. IRS proteins and the common path to diabetes. *Am J Physiol Endocrinol Metab* 283 E413-22 2002
14. Montecucco F et al. Insulin resistance: a proinflammatory state mediated by lipid-induced signaling dysfunction and involved in atherosclerotic plaque instability. *Mediators Inflamm* 2008 2008 767623
15. Rudin E and Barzilai N. Inflammatory peptides derived from adipose tissue. *Immun Ageing* 2 1-3 2005
16. Rabe K. Adipokines and insulin resistance. *Mol Med* 14 741-51 2008
17. IBID
18. Rudin E and Barzilai N. Inflammatory peptides derived from adipose tissue. *Immun Ageing* 2 1-3 2005
19. Ye J. Role of insulin in the pathogenesis of free fatty acid-induced insulin resistance in skeletal muscle. *Endocrine, Metabolic & Immune Disorders – Drug Targets* 7 65-74 2007
20. IBID
21. IBID
22. Montecucco F et al. Insulin resistance: a proinflammatory state mediated by lipid-induced signaling dysfunction and involved in atherosclerotic plaque instability. *Mediators Inflamm* 2008 2008 767623
23. IBID
24. Boden G and Laakso M. Lipids and glucose in type 2 diabetes: what about the B-cell and the mitochondria? *Diabetes Care* 28 986-87 2005
25. Stefan MN. Elevated plasma nonesterified fatty acids are associated with deterioration of acute insulin response in IGT but not NGT. *Am J Physiol Endocrinol Metab* 284 E1156-61 2003
26. Poitout V et al. Regulation of the insulin gene by glucose and fatty acids. *J Nutr* 136 873-76 2006
27. Maedler K. Distinct effects of saturated and monounsaturated fatty acids on B-cell turnover and function. *Diabetes* 50 69-76 2001
28. El-Assaad W. *Endocrinology* 144;9: 4154-4163
29. Maedler K. Distinct effects of saturated and monounsaturated fatty acids on B-cell turnover and function. *Diabetes* 50 69-76 2001
30. IBID

31. El-Assaad JW. Saturated fatty acids synergize with elevated glucose to cause pancreatic beta-cell death. *Endocrinology* 144 4154-63 2003
32. Maassen JA. Fatty acid-induced mitochondrial uncoupling in adipocytes as a key protective factor against insulin resistance and beta cell dysfunction: a new concept in the pathogenesis of obesity-associated type 2 diabetes mellitus. *Diabetologia* 50 2036-2041 2007
33. IBID
34. Montecucco F et al. Insulin resistance: a proinflammatory state mediated by lipid-induced signaling dysfunction and involved in atherosclerotic plaque instability. *Mediators Inflamm* 2008 2008 767623
35. Thalman S and Meier C. Local adipose tissue depots as cardiovascular risk factors. *Cardiovascular Res* 75 690-701 2007

Chapter 8 - Dairy

1. Bischoff S and Crowe S. Gastrointestinal food allergy: new insights into pathophysiology and clinical perspectives. *Gastroenterology* 128 1089-1113 2005
2. Ahmed T and Fuchs G. Gastrointestinal allergy to food: A review. *J Diarrhoeal Dis Res* 15 211-23 1997
3. Carroccio A and Iacono G. Review article: chronic constipation and food hypersensitivity – an intriguing relationship. *Aliment Pharmacol Ther* 24 1295-1304 2006
4. Ahmed T and Fuchs G. Gastrointestinal allergy to food: A review. *J Diarrhoeal Dis Res* 15 211-23 1997
5. Ibid
6. Salvatore S and Vandenplas Y. Gastroesophageal reflux and cow milk allergy: is there a link? *Pediatrics* 110 972-84 2002
7. Ahmed T and Fuchs G. Gastrointestinal allergy to food: A review. *J Diarrhoeal Dis Res* 15 211-23 1997
8. Host A. Cow's milk allergy. *J R Soc Med* 90 S34-39 1997
9. Ibid
10. Ahmed T and Fuchs G. Gastrointestinal allergy to food: A review. *J Diarrhoeal Dis Res* 15 211-23 1997
11. Ibid
12. Host A. Cow's milk allergy. *J R Soc Med* 90 S34-39 1997
13. Firer MA et al. Humoral immune response to cow's milk in children with cow's milk allergy. Relationship to the time of clinical response to cow's milk challenge. *Int Arch Allergy Appl Immunnol* 84 173-77 1987
14. Bischoff S and Crowe S. Gastrointestinal food allergy: new insights into pathophysiology and clinical perspectives. *Gastroenterology* 128 1089-1113 2005
15. Iacono G et al. Chronic constipation as a symptom of cow milk allergy. *J Pediatr* 126 34-39 1995
16. Nsouli TM et al. Role of food allergy in serious otitis media. *Ann Allergy* 73 215-19 1994
17. Carroccio A et al. Chronic constipation and food intolerance: a model of proctitis causing constipation. *Scand J Gastroenterol* 40 33-42 2005
18. Salo OP et al. Milk causes a rapid urticarial reaction on the skin of children with atopic dermatitis and milk allergy. *Acta Derm Venereol* 66 438-42 1986
19. Hill Dj et al. Cow milk allergy within the spectrum of atopic disorders. *Clin Exp Allergy* 24 1137-43 1994
20. Pelto L et al. Milk hypersensitivity – key to poorly defined gastrointestinal symptoms in adults. *Allergy* 53 307-10 1998

21. Iacono G. Chronic constipation as a symptom of cow milk allergy. *J Pediatr* 126 34-39 1995

22. Iacono G et al. Intolerance of cow's milk and chronic constipation in children. *N Engl J Med* 338 1100-4 1998

23. Host A. Cow's milk allergy. *J R Soc Med* 90 S34-39 1997

24. Salvatore S and Vandenplas Y. Gastroesophageal reflux and cow milk allergy: is there a link? *Pediatrics* 110 972-84 2002

25. Host A. Cow's milk allergy. *J R Soc Med* 90 S34-39 1997

26. Salvatore S and Vandenplas Y. Gastroesophageal reflux and cow milk allergy: is there a link? *Pediatrics* 110 972-84 2002

27. Kelly KJ et al. Eosinophilic esophagitis attributed to gastroesophageal reflux: improvement with an amino-acid based formula. *Gastroenterology* 109 1503-12 1995

28. Hill DJ et al. Challenge confirmation of late-onset reactions to extensively hydrolyzed formulas in infants with multiple food protein intolerance. *J Allergy Clin Immunol* 96 386-94 1995

29. Karjalainen J et al. A bovine albumin peptide as a possible trigger of insulin-dependent diabetes mellitus. *N Engl J Med* 327 302-7 1992

30. Savilahti E et al. Children with newly diagnosed insulin-dependent diabetes mellitus have increased levels of cow's milk antibodies. *Diabetes Res* 7 137-40 88

31. Saukkonen T et al. significance of cow's milk protein antibodies as risk factor for childhood IDDM: interactions with dietary cow's milk intake and HLA-DQB1 genotype. *Diabetologia* 41 72-8 1998

32. Birgisdottir BE et al. Lower consumption of cow's milk protein A1 beta-casein at 2 years of age, rather than consumption among 11-14 year old adolescents, may explain the lower incidence of type 1 diabetes in Iceland than in Scandinavia. *Ann Nutr Metab* 50 177-83 2006

33. Cavallo MG et al. Cell-mediated immune response to beta casein in recent-onset insulin-dependent diabetes: implications for disease pathogenesis. 348 926-28 1996

34. Knip M et al. Environmental triggers and determinants of type 1 diabetes. *Diabetes* 54 S125-36 2005

35. Ibid

36. Ibid

37. Hypponen E et al. Intake of vitamin D and risk of type 1 diabetes: a birth-cohort study. *Lancet* 358 1500-3 2001

38. Pedersen LB et al. 1,25-dihydroxyvitamin D3 reverses experimental autoimmune encephalomyelitis by inhibiting chemokine synthesis and monocyte trafficking. *J Neurosci Res* 85 2480-90 2007

39. Harrison LC and Honeyman MC. Cow's milk and type 1 diabetes: the real debate is about mucosal immune function. *Diabetes* 48 1501-07 1999

40. Gerstein HC. Cow's milk exposure and type 1 diabetes mellitus. A critical overview of the clinical literature. *Diabetes Care* 17 13-9 1994

41. Harrison LC and Honeyman MC. Cow's milk and type 1 diabetes: the real debate is about mucosal immune function. *Diabetes* 48 1501-07 1999

42. Ibid

43. Knip M et al. Environmental triggers and determinants of type 1 diabetes. *Diabetes* 54 S125-36 2005

44. Ibid

45. Ibid

46. Ibid

47. Ibid

48. Ibid

49. Ibid
50. Feskanich D et al. Milk, dietary calcium, and bone fractures in women: a 12-year prospective study. *Am J Publ Health* 87 992-7 1997
51. Cumming RG and Klineberg RJ. Case-control study of risk factors for hip fractures in the elderly. *Am J Epidemiol* 139 493-503 1994
52. Walker AR et al. The influence of numerous pregnancies and lactations on bone dimensions in South African Bantu and Caucasian mothers. *Clin Sci* 42 189-96 1972
53. Reidhead P. 'Richard Burroughs, DVM: On FDA and Posalic(R).' *The Milkweed,* January 2006
54. 'Report of the Canadian Veterinary Medical Association Expert Panel on rBST,' *Prepared for Health Canada,* November 1998.
55. Cohen, R. Milk – *The Deadly Poison.* 1997 p 60
56. Campbell MJ. IGF status is altered by tamoxifen in patients with breast cancer. *Mol Pathol* 54 307-10 2001
57. Grimberg A. Mechanisms by which IGF-1 may promote cancer. *Cancer Boil Ther* 2 630-5 2003
58. LeRoith D and Roberts CT. The insulin-like growth factor system and cancer. *Cancer Lett* 195 127-37 2003
59. Karasik A et al. Insulin-like growth factor-1 (IGF-1) and IGF-binding protein-2 are increased in cyst fluids of epithelial ovarian cancer. *J Clin Endocrinol Metab* 78 271-6 1994
60. Fuchs CS et al. Plasma insulin-like growth factors, insulin-like binding protein-3, and outcome in metastatic colorectal cancer: results from intergroup trial N9741. *Clin Cancer Res* 14 8263-9 2008
61. Garner MJ et al. Dietary risk factors for testicular carcinoma. *Int J Cancer* 106 934-41 2003
62. Giovannucci E. Nutritional factors in human cancers. *Adv Exp Med Biol* 472 29-42 1999
63. Van Schaik G et al. Trends in somatic cell counts, bacterial counts, and antibiotic residue violations in New York State during 1999-2000. *J Dairy Sci* 85 782-9 2002
64. Wong S et al. Recalls of foods and cosmetics due to microbial contamination reported to the U.S. Food and Drug Administration. *Food Prot* 63 113-6 2000
65. Grosvenor C et al. Hormones and growth factors in milk. Endocr Rev 14 710-28 1992
66. Franscini N et al Prion protein in milk. *PloS ONE.* 1 e71 2006
67. Buehring GC et al. Humans have antibodies reactive with bovine leukemia virus. *AIDS Res Hum Retroviruses* 19 1105-13 2003
68. Grant IR et al. Incidence of mycobacterium paratuberculosis in bulk raw and commercially pasteurized cow's milk from approved dairy processing establishments in the United Kingdom. 68 2428-35 2002
69. Abubakar I et al. Detection of mycobacterium avium subspecies paratuberculosis from patients with crohn's disease using nucleic acid-based techniques: a systematic review and meta-analysis. *Inflamm Bowel Dis* 14 401-10 2008
70. Feller M et al. Mycobacterium avium subspecies paratuberculosis and Crohn's disease: a systematic review and meta-analysis. *Lancet Infect Dis* 7 607-13 2007

Chapter 9 - Iron

1. Murray M and Pizzorno J. Encyclopedia of Natural Medicine, revised 2nd edition p236
2. Murray M and Pizzorno .J Encyclopedia of Natural Medicine, revised 2nd edition p236
3. Pizarro F et al. Iron status with different feeding regimens; relevance to screening and prevention of iron deficiency. *J Pediatr* 118 687-92 1991
4. Pisacane A et al. Iron status in breast-fed infants. *J Pediatr* 127 429-31 1995

5. McMillan JA et al. Iron sufficiency in breast-fed infants and the availability of iron from human milk. *Pediatrics* 58 686 1976
6. Sardi B. *The Iron Time Bomb* 1999
7. McCord J. Effects of positive iron status at a cellular level. *Nutr Revs* 54 85-88 1996
8. Hulthen L et al. Effect of a mild infection on serum ferritin concentration – clinical and epidemiological implications. *Eur J Clin Nutr* 52 376-9 1998
9. Carrier J et al. Exacerbation of dextran sulfate sodium-induced colitis by dietary iron supplementation: role of NF-KappaB. *Int J Colorectal Dis* 21 381-7 2006
10. McCord JM Iron, free radicals, and oxidative injury. *Sem in Hem* 35 5-12 1998
11. Sardi B. The Iron Time Bomb. 1999 p. 80
12. Kiechl S et al. Body iron stores and the risk of carotid artherosclerosis: prospective results from the Bruneck study. *Circulation* 96 3300-07 1997
13. Tuomainen TK et al. Association between body iron stores and the risk of acute myocardial infarction in men. *Circulation* 97 1461-66 1998
14. Robinson RW et al. Increased incidence of coronary heart disease in women castrated prior to the menopause. *Arch Intern Med* 104 908 1959
15. Ritterband Ab et al. Gonadal function and the development of coronary heart disease. *Circulation* 27 237 1963
16. Gordon T et al. Menopause and coronary heart disease: the Framingham study. *Ann Intern Med* 89 157 1978
17. Roest M et al. Heterozygosity for a hereditary hemochromatosis gene is associated with cardiovascular death in women. *Circulation* 100 1268-73 1999
18. IBID
19. Tuomainen TP et al. Increased risk of acute myocardial infarction in carriers of the hemochromatosis gene Cys282Tyr mutation: a prospective cohort study in men in eastern Finland. Circ 100 1274-79 1999
20. Bulaj ZJ et al. Clinical and biochemical abnormalities in people heterozygous for hemochromatosis. *NEJM* 335 1799-1805 1996
21. Zacharski L et al. Decreased cancer risk after iron reduction in patients with peripheral artery disease: results from a randomized trial. J Natl Canceer Inst 100 996-1002 2008
22. Nelson R et al Body iron stores and risk of colonic neoplasia. *J of Natl Cancer Inst* 86 455-60 1994.
23. Selby JV and Friedman GD. Epidemiologic evidence of an association between body iron stores and risk of cancer. *Int J Cancer* 41 677-82 1988
24. Milman N et al. Iron status markers in patients with small cell carcinoma of the lung. Relation to survival. *Br J cancer* 64 895-8 1991
25. Stevens RG et al. Body iron stores and the risk of cancer. *NEJM* 319 1047-52 1988
26. Reizenstein P. Iron, free radicals and cancer. *Med Oncol Tumor Pharmacother* 8 229-33 1991
27. Hjalgrim H et al. Cancer incidence in blood transfusion recipients. *J Natl Cancer Inst* 99 1864-74 2007
28. Yeh JJ et al. Effect of blood transfusion on outcome after pancreaticoduodenectomy for exocrine tumour of the pancreas. *Br J Surg* 94 466-72 2007
29. Meyers DG et al. A historical cohort study of the effect of lowering body iron through blood donation on incident cardiac events. *Transfusion* 42 1135-39 2002
30. Meyers DG et al. Possible association of a reduction in cardiovascular events with blood donation. *Heart* 78 188-93 1997
31. Tuomainen TP et al. Cohort study of relation between donating blood and risk of myocardial infarction in 2682 men in eastern Finland. *BMJ* 314 793-4 1997
32. Edgren G et al. Improving health profile of blood donors as a consequence of transfusion safety efforts. *Transfusion* 47 2017-24 2007

33. Kato J et al. Long-term phlebotomy with low-iron diet therapy lowers risk of development of hepatocellular carcinoma from chronic hepatitis C. *J Gastroenterol* 42 830-6 2007

34. Rockey DC and Cello JP. Evaluation of the gastrointestinal tract in patients with iron-deficiency anemia. *NEJM* 329 1691-5 1993

35. Sardi B. *The Iron Time Bomb* 1999 p. 35

Chapter 10 - Our Ideal Diet

1. Cohen MN and Armelagos CJ. Editors Summation. In: Cohen MN, Armelagos CJ, editors. Paleopathology at the origins of agriculture. New York: *Academic Press*, 1984:585-601

2. Larsen CS. Dietary reconstruction and nutritional assessment of past peoples: the bioanthropologic record. In: Kiple KF Ornelas KC, eds The Cambridge World History of Food, vol 1. Cambridge: *Cambridge Univ Press*, 2000:13-34.

3. Eaton SB et al. Paleolithic nutrition revisited: A twelve year retrospective on its nature and implications. *Eur J Clin Nutr* 51 207-16 1997

4. Eaton SB et al. Evolutionary health promotion: A consideration of common counterarguments. *Prev Med* 34 119-123 2002

5. Eaton SB et al. Evolutionary health promotion: A consideration of common counterarguments. *Prev Med* 34 119-123 2002

6. Mazess R and Mather W. Bone mineral content of north Alaskan Eskimos. *Am J Clin Nutr* 27 916-25 1974

7. Krajcovicova-Kudlackova M et al. Homocysteine levels in vegetarians versus omnivores. *Ann Nutr Metab* 44 135-8 2000

8. Remer T et al. Increased risk of iodine deficiency with vegetarian nutrition. *Br J Nutr* 81 45-9 1999

9. Willett W. Lessons from dietary studies in Adventists and questions for the future. *Am J Clin Nutr* 78 539S-43S 2003

10. Daniel K, *The Whole Soy Story, the dark side of America's favorite health food*. 2005

11. Daniel K, *The Whole Soy Story, the dark side of America's favorite health food*. 2005

12. Daniel K, *The Whole Soy Story, the dark side of America's favorite health food*. 2005

13. Setchell KD et al. Exposure of infants to phyto-oestrogens from soy-based infant formula. *Lancet* 3530 815-6 1997

14. Franke A and Custer L. Diadzein and genistein concentrations in human milk after soy consumption. *Clinical Chemistry* 42 955-64 1996

(Chapter 11 - Supplement Quality)

Chapter 12 - Vitamin D

1. MCKenna MJ. Differences in vitamin D status between countries in young adults and the elderly. *Am J Med* 93 69-77 1992

2. Bhattoa HP et al. Prevalence and seasonal variation of hypovitaminosis D and its relationship to bone metabolism in community dwelling postmenopausal Hungarian women. *Osteoporos Int* 15 447-51 2004

3. Cheng S et al. Association of low 25-hydroxyvitamin D concentrations with elevated parathyroid hormone concentrations and low cortical bone density in early pubertal and prepubertal Finnish girls. *Am J Clin Nutr* 78 485-92 2003

4. Tangpricha V et al. Vitamin D insufficiency among free-living healthy young adults. *Am J Med* 2002 112 659-62

5. Mathieu C and Badenhoop K. Vitamin D and type 1 diabetes mellitus: state of the art. *Trends Endocrinol Metab* 16 261-66 2005

6. Ibid

7. Hypponen E et al. Intake of vitamin D and risk of type 1 diabetes: a birth-cohort study. *Lancet* 358(9292) 1500-3 2001

8. Palomer X et al. Role of vitamin D in the pathogenesis of type 2 diabetes mellitus. *Diabetes Obes Metab* 10 185-97 2008

9. Garland CF et al. The role of vitamin D in cancer prevention. *Am J Public Health* 96 252-61 2006

10. Chen TC et al. Prostatic 25-hydroxyvitamin D-1-alpha hydroxylase and its implication in prostate cancer. *J Cell Biochem* 88 315-22 2003

11. Garland CF et al. The role of vitamin D in cancer prevention. *Am J Public Health* 96 252-61 2006

12. Grant WB et al. An estimate of cancer mortality rate reductions in Europe and the U.S. with 1,000 IU of oral vitamin D per day. *Recent Results Cancer Res* 174 225-34 2007

13. Gorham ED et al. Optimal vitamin D status for colorectal cancer prevention: a quantitative meta-analysis. *Am J Prev Med* 32 210-6 2007

14. Lappe JM et al. Vitamin D and calcium supplementation reduces cancer risk: results of a randomized trial. *Am J Clin Nutr* 85 1586-91 2007

15. Garland C et al. What is the dose-response relationship between vitamin D and cancer risk. *Nutr Revs* 65 S91-S95 2007

16. Gorham ED et al. Optimal vitamin D status for colorectal cancer prevention: a quantitative meta-analysis. *Am J Prev Med* 32 210-6 2007

17. Vestergaard P and Mosekilde L. Cohort study on effects of parathyroid surgery on multiple outcomes in primary hyperparathyroidism. *BMJ* 327 530-4 2003

18. Dobnig H et al. Independent association of low serum 25-hydroxyvitamin D and 1,25-hydroxyvitamin D levels with all-cause and cardiovascular mortality. *Arch Intern Med* 168 1340-9 2008

19. Giovannucci E et al. 25-hydroxyvitamin D and risk of myocardial infarction in men: a prospective study. *Arch Intern Med* 168 1174-80 2008

20. Pfeifer M et al. Effects of a short-term vitamin D-3 and calcium supplementation on blood pressure and parathyroid hormone levels in elderly women. *J Clin Endocrinol Metab* 86 1633-1637 2001

21. Forman JP et al. Plasma 25-hydroxyvitamin D levels and risk of incident hypertension. Hypertension 49 1063-1069 2007

22. Melamed ML et al. Serum 25-hydroxyvitamin D levels and the presence of peripheral arterial disease: results from NHANES 2001-2004. *Arterioscler Thromb Vasc Biol* 28 1179-85 2008

23. Watson KE et al. Active serum vitamin D levels are inversely correlated with coronary calcification. *Circulation* 96 1755-60 1997

24. Wang TJ et al. Vitamin D deficiency and risk of cardiovascular disease. *Circulation* 117 503-11 2008

25. Hampton T. Experts urge early investment in bone health. *JAMA* 291 811-12 2004

26. Burge R et al. Incidence and economic burden of osteoporosis-related fractures in the U.S., 2005-2025. *J Bone Miner Res* 22 465-75 2007

27. Trivedi DP et al. Effect of four monthly oral vitamin D3 (cholecalciferol) supplementation on fractures and mortality in men and women living in the community: randomized double blind controlled trial. *BMJ* 326 469-72 2003

28. Chapuy MC et al. Vitamin D3 and calcium to prevent hip fractures in the elderly women. *N Engl J Med* 327 1637-42 1992

29. O'brien KO. Combined calcium and vitamin D supplementation reduces bone loss and fracture incidence in older men and women. *Nutr Revs* 56 148-58 1998
30. Plotnikoff GA and Quigley JM. Prevalence of severe hypovitaminosis D in patients with persistent, nonspecific musculoskeletal pain. *Mayo Clin Proc* 78 1463-70 2003
31. Prabhala A et al. Severe myopathy associated with vitamin D deficiency in western New York. *Arch Intern Med* 160 1199-203 2000
32. Plotnikoff GA and Quigley JM. Prevalence of severe hypovitaminosis D in patients with persistent, nonspecific musculoskeletal pain. *Mayo Clin Proc* 78 1463-70 2003Al Faraj S and Al Mutairi K Spine 2003 28 177-79
33. Nesby-O'Dell S et al. Hypovitaminosis D prevalence and determinants among African American and white women of reproductive age: third national health and nutrition examination survey, 1988-1994. *Am J Clin Nutr* 76 187-92 2002
34. Talwar SA et al. Dose response to vitamin D supplementation among postmenopausal African America women. *Am J Clin Nutr* 86 1657-62 2007

Chapter 13 - Vitamin A

1. Rothman KJ, et al. Teratogenicity of high vitamin A intake. *N Engl J Med* 333 1369-73 1995
2. Melhus H et al. Excessive dietary intake of vitamin A is associated with reduced bone mineral density and increased risk for hip fracture. *Ann Intern Med* 129 770-78 1998
3. Feskanich D et al. Vitamin A intake and risk fractures among postmenopausal women. *JAMA* 287 47-54 2002
4. Strobel M et al. The importance of beta-carotene as a source of vitamin A with special regard to pregnant and breastfeeding women. *Eur J Nutr* 46 1/1-1/20 (suppl 1) 2007
5. Berger SG et al. Malnutrition and morbidity are higher in children who are missed by periodic vitamin A capsule distribution for child survival in rural Indonesia. *J Nutr* 137 1328-33 2007
6. Berger SG et al. Malnutrition and morbidity are higher in children who are missed by periodic vitamin A capsule distribution for child survival in rural Indonesia. *J Nutr* 137 1328-33 2007
7. Fallon S and Enig M. Vitamin A Saga. *Wise Traditions* March 2002
8. Strobel M et al. The importance of beta-carotene as a source of vitamin A with special regard to pregnant and breastfeeding women. *Eur J Nutr* 46 1/1-1/20 (suppl 1) 2007
9. Tang G et al. Spinach or carrots can supply significant amounts of vitamin A as assessed by feeding with intrinsically deuterated vegetables. *Am J Clin Nutr* 82 821-28 2005
10. Strobel M et al. The importance of beta-carotene as a source of vitamin A with special regard to pregnant and breastfeeding women. *Eur J Nutr* 46 1/1-1/20 (suppl 1) 2007
11. Tang G. Bioconversion of dietary provitamin A carotenoids to vitamin A in humans. *Am J Clin Nutr* 91 1468S-73S 2010
12. Semba R. Vitamin A as "anti-infective" theapy, 1920-1940. *J Nutr* 129 783-91 1999
13. IBID
14. IBID
15. IBID
16. IBID
17. IBID
18. Werler MM et al. Maternal vitamin A supplementation in relation to selected birth defects. *Teratology* 42 497-503 1990
19. Martinez-Frias ML and Salvador J. Epidemiological aspects of prenatal exposure to high dose vitamin A in Spain. *Eur J Epidemiol* 6 118-23 1990

20. Hartmann S et al. Exposure to retinyl esters, retinol, and retinoic acids in non-pregnant women following increasing single and repeated oral doses of vitamin A. *Ann Nutr Metab* 49 155-64 2005
21. IBID
22. IBID
23. Mastroiacovo P et al. High vitamin A intake in early pregnancy and major malformations: a multicenter prospective controlled study. *Teratology* 59 7-11 1999
24. Hartmann S et al. Exposure to retinyl esters, retinol, and retinoic acids in non-pregnant women following increasing single and repeated oral doses of vitamin A. *Ann Nutr Metab* 49 155-64 2005
25. Weigand UW et al. Safety of vitamin A: recent results. *Int J Vitam Nutr Res* 68 411-16 1998
26. Strobel M et al. The importance of beta-carotene as a source of vitamin A with special regard to pregnant and breastfeeding women. *Eur J Nutr* 46 1/1-1/20 (suppl 1) 2007
27. IBID
28. IBID
29. Feskanich D et al. Vitamin A intake and risk fractures among postmenopausal women. *JAMA* 287 47-54 2002
30. Melhus H et al. Excessive dietary intake of vitamin A is associated with reduced bone mineral density and increased risk for hip fracture. *Ann Intern Med* 129 770-78 1998
31. Michaelson K et al. Serum retinol levels and the risk of fracture. *N Engl J Med* 348 287-94 2003
32. Barker ME et al. Serum retinoids and beta-carotene as predictors of hip and other fractures in elderly women. *J Bone Miner Res* 20 913-20
33. Kawahara TN et al. Short-term vitamin A supplementation does not affect bone turnover in men. *J Nutr* 132 1169-72 2002
34. McDonald HM et al. Nutritional associations with bone loss during the menopausal transition: evidence of a beneficial effect of calcium, alcohol, and fruit and vegetable nutrients and of a detrimental effect of fatty acids. *AM J Clin Nutr* 79 155-65 2004
35. Caire-Juvera G et al. Vitamin A and retinol intakes and the risk of fractures among participants of the Women's Health Initiative Observational Study. *Am J Clin Nutr* 89 323-30 2009
36. Sanchez-Martinez R et al. The retinoid X receptor ligand restores defective signaling by the vitamin D receptor. *EMBO Reports* 7 1030-34 2006
37. Bettuon D et al. Retinoid X receptor is a nonsilent major contributor to vitamin D receptor-mediated transcriptional activation. *Molecular Endocrinology* 17 2320-28 2003
38. Aburto A et al. The influence of vitamin A on the utilization and amelioration of toxicity of cholecalciferol, 25-hydroxycholecalciferol, and 1,15 dihydroxycholecalciferol in young broiler chickens. *Poultry Science* 77 585-593 1998
39. Oliva A et al. Effect of retinoic acid on osteocalcin gene expression in human osteoblasts. *Biochem Biophys Res Commun* 191 908-14 1993
40. Linden V. Vitamin D and myocardial infarction. *Br Med J* 3 647-58 1974
41. Rajasree S et al. Serum 25-hydroxyvitamin D3 levels are elevated in South Indian patients with ischemic heart disease. *Eur J Epidemiol* 17 567-571 2001
42. Moon J et al. Hypothesis: etiology of atherosclerosis and osteoporosis: are imbalances in the calciferol endocrine system implicated? *J Am Coll Nutr* 11 567-83 1992
43. Cannell J et al. Cod liver oil, vitamin A toxicity, frequent respiratory infections, and the vitamin D deficiency epidemic. *Annals of Otology, Rhinology, and Laryngology* 117 864-70 2008
44. IBID

45. Price P et al. Warfarin-induced artery calcification is accelerated by growth and vitamin D. *Arterioscler Thromb Vasc Biol* 20 317-27 2000

46. Schurgers L et al. Oral Anticoagulant treatment: friend or foe in cardiovascular disease. *Blood* 104 3231-3232 2004

47. Spronk HM et al. Tissue-specific utilization of menaquinone-4 results in the prevention of arterial calcification in warfarin-treated rats. *J Vasc Res* 40 531-7 2003

48. Vermeer C et al. Vitamin K and the urogenital tract. *Haemostasis* 246-57 1986

49. Arora P et al. Vitamin A status in children with asthma. *Pediatr Allergy Immunol* 13 223-226 2002

50. IBID

51. Mizuno Y et al. Serum vitamin A concentrations in asthmatic children in Japan. *Pediatrics international* 48 261-64 2006

52. Main ANH et al. Vitamin A deficiency in crohn's disease. *Gut* 24 1169-75 1983

53. Zaiger G et al. Vitamin A exerts its activity at the transcriptional level in the small intestine. *Eur J Nutr* 43 259-66 2004

54. Fernandez-Banares F et al. Vitamin status in patients with inflammatory bowel disease. *Am J Gastroenterol* 84 744-78 1989

55. Kuroki F et al. Multiple vitamin status in Crohn's disease. Correlation with disease activity. *Dig Dis Sci* 38 1614-18 1993

56. Bousvaros A et al. Vitamins A and E serum levels in children and young adults with inflammatory bowel disease: effect of disease activity. *JPGN* 26 129-35 1998

57. Wright JP et al. Vitamin A therapy in patients with Crohn's disease. *Gastroenterology* 88 512-14 1985

58. Stephensen C et al. Vitamin A is excreted in the urine during acute infection. *Am J Clin Nutr* 60 388-92 1994

59. Dong P et al. Expression of retinoic acid receptors in the intestinal mucosa and the effect of vitamin A on mucosal immunity. *Nutrition* 2009 doi:10.1016/jj.nut.2009.08.011

60. Zaiger G et al. Vitamin A exerts its activity at the transcriptional level in the small intestine. *Eur J Nutr* 43 259-66 2004

61. Kang S et al. High and low vitamin A therapies induce distinct FoxP3+ T-cell subsets and effectively control intestinal inflammation. *Gastroenterology* 137 1391-1402 2009

62. Biesalski H and Nohr D. New aspects in vitamin A metabolism: the role of retinyl esters as systemic and local sources for retinol in mucous epithelia. *J Nutr* 134 3453S-57S 2004

63. Mucida D et al. From the diet to the nucleus: vitamin A and tgf-beta join efforts at the mucosal interface of the intestine. *Semin Immunol* 21 14-21 2009

64. Reifen R et al. Vitamin A deficiency exacerbates inflammation in a rat model of colitis through activation of nuclear factor-KB and collagen formation. *J Nutr* 132 2743-47 2002

65. Lee H et al. Cutting edge: inhibition of NF-KB mediated TSLP expression by retinoid X receptor. *The Journal of Immunology* 181 5189-93 2008

66. Kang S et al. Vitamin A metabolites induce gut-homing Fox-P3+ regulatory T-cells. *The Journal of Immunology* 179 3724-33 2007

67. Mora JR and von Andrian UH. Role of retinoic acid in the imprinting of gut-homing IgA-secreting cells. *Semin Immunol* 21 28-35 2009

68. Fagarasan S and Honjo T. Intestinal IgA synthesis: regulation of front-line body defenses. *Nat Rev Immunology* 3 63-72 2003

69. Suri-Payer E and Fritzsching B. Regulatory T cells in experimental autoimmune disease. *Springer Semin Immunopathol* 28 3-16 2006

70. Reifen R et al. Vitamin A deficiency exacerbates inflammation in a rat model of colitis through activation of nuclear factor-KB and collagen formation. *J Nutr* 132 2743-47 2002

71. Mucida D et al. From the diet to the nucleus: vitamin A and tgf-beta join efforts at the mucosal interface of the intestine. *Semin Immunol* 21 14-21 2009

72. Mora JR and von Andrian UH. Role of retinoic acid in the imprinting of gut-homing IgA-secreting cells. *Semin Immunol* 21 28-35 2009

73. Lee H et al. Cutting edge: inhibition of NF-KB mediated TSLP expression by retinoid X receptor. *The Journal of Immunology* 181 5189-93 2008

74. Dong P et al. Expression of retinoic acid receptors in the intestinal mucosa and the effect of vitamin A on mucosal immunity. *Nutrition* 2009 doi:10.1016/jj.nut.2009.08.011

75. Kang S et al. Vitamin A metabolites induce gut-homing Fox-P3+ regulatory T-cells. *The Journal of Immunology* 179 3724-33 2007

76. Biesalski H and Nohr D. New aspects in vitamin A metabolism: the role of retinyl esters as systemic and local sources for retinol in mucous epithelia. *J Nutr* 134 3453S-57S 2004

Chapter 14 - Probiotics

1. Ng SC et al. Mechanisms of action of probiotics: recent advances. *Inflamm Bowel Dis* 15 300-10 2009

2. Yoshioka H et al. Development and differences of intestinal flora in the neonatal period in breast-fed and bottle-fed infants. *Pediatrics* 72 317-21 1983

3. Kailasapathy K and Chin J. Survival and therapeutic potential of probiotic organisms with reference to lactobacillus acidophilus and bifidobacterium spp. *Immunology and Cell Biology* 78 80-88 2000

4. Shah NP. Probiotic bacteria: selective enumeration and survival in dairy foods. Symposium: Probiotic bacteria accepted Oct 7 1999 School of life sciences and technology, Victoria University of Technology

5. Coudeyras S et al. Adhesion of human probiotic lactobacillus rhamnosus to cervical and vaginal cells and interaction with vaginosis-associated pathogens. *Infectious Disease in Obstetrics and Gynecology* volume 2008 Article ID 549640 doi 10.1155/2008/549640

6. Anukam K et al. Augmentation of antimicrobial metronidazole therapy of bacterial vaginosis with oral probiotic lactobacillus rhamnosus GR-1 and lactobacillus reuteri RC-14: randomized, double-blind, placebo controlled trial. *Microbes Infect* 8 1450-54 2006

7. Reid G et al. Oral probiotics can resolve urogenital infections. *FEMS Immunol Med Microbiol* 30 49-52 2001

8. Martinez RC et al. Improved treatment of vulvovaginal candidiasis with fluconazole plus probiotic lactobacillus rhamnosus GR-1 and lactobacillus reuteri RC-14. *Lett Appl Microbiol* 48 269-74 2009

9. Singh J et al. Bifidobacterium longum, a lactic acid-producing intestinal bacterium inhibits colon cancer and modulates the intermediate biomarkers of colon carcinogenesis. *Carcinogenesis* 18 833-41 1997

10. Le MG et al. Consumption of dairy produce and alcohol in case-control study of breast cancer. *J Natl Cancer Inst* 77 633-66 1986

11. Veer P et al. Consumption of fermented milk products and breast cancer: a case-control study in the Netherlands. *Cancer Research* 49 4020-23 1989

12. Leyer GJ et al. Probiotic effects on cold and influenza-like symptom incidence and duration in children. *Pediatrics* 124 e172-79 2009

13. Weizman Z et al. Effect of probiotic infant formula on infections in child care centers: comparison of two probiotic agents. *Pediatrics* 115 5-9 2005

14. Tubelius P et al. Increasing work-place healthiness with the probiotic lactobacillus reuteri: a randomized, double-blind placebo-controlled study. Environmental Health: A Global Access Science Source. *Environmental Health* 4:25 2005

15. Rosenfeldt V et al. Effect of probiotics on gastrointestinal symptoms and small intestinal permeability in children with atopic dermatitis. *J Pediatr* 145 612-16 2004
16. Wickens K et al. A differential effect of 2 probiotics in the prevention of eczema and atopy: a double-blind, randomized, placebo-controlled trial. *J Allergy Clin Immunol* 122 788-94 2008
17. Rautava S et al. Probiotics during pregnancy and breast-feeding might confer immunomodulatory protection against atopic disease in the infant. *J allergy Clin Immunol* 109 119-21 2002
18. Gruber C et al. Randomized, placebo-controlled trial of lactobacillus rhamnosus GG as treatment of atopic dermatitis in infancy. *Allergy* 62 1270-76 2007
19. Betsi GI et al. Probiotics for the treatment of prevention of atopic dermatitis: a review of the evidence from randomized controlled trials. *Am J Clin Dermatol* 9 93-103 2008
20. Johnston BC et al. Probiotics for pediatric antibiotic-associated diarrhea: a meta-analysis of randomized placebo-controlled trials. *CMAJ* 175 377-83 2006
21. Hickson M et al. Use of probiotic lactobacillus preparation to prevent diarrhea associated with antibiotics: randomized double-blind placebo controlled trial. *BMJ* doi:10.1136/bmj.39231.599815.55)
22. Hookman P and Barkin J. Clostridium diificile associated infection, diarrhea and colitis. *World J Gastroenterol* 15 1554-80 2009
23. IBID
24. Johnston BC et al. Probiotics for pediatric antibiotic-associated diarrhea: a meta-analysis of randomized placebo-controlled trials. *CMAJ* 175 377-83 2006
25. Basu S et al. Efficacy of lactobacillus rhamnosus GG in acute watery diarrhea of Indian children: a randomized controlled trial. *J Pediatr Child Health* 43 837-42 2007
26. Basu S et al. Effect of lactobacillus GG in persistent diarrhea in Indian children: a randomized controlled trial. *J Clin Gastroenterol* 41 756-60 2007
27. Szymanski H et al. Treatment of acute infectious diarrhea in infants and children with a mixture of three lactobacillus rhamnosus strains – a randomized, double-blind, placebo-controlled trial. *Aliment Pharmacol Ther* 23 247-53 2005
28. Johnston BC et al. Probiotics for pediatric antibiotic-associated diarrhea: a meta-analysis of randomized placebo-controlled trials. *CMAJ* 175 377-83 2006
29. Hickson M et al. Use of probiotic lactobacillus preparation to prevent diarrhea associated with antibiotics: randomized double-blind placebo controlled trial. *BMJ* doi:10.1136/bmj.39231.599815.55)
30. Lin H. Small intestinal bacterial overgrowth: a framework for understanding irritable bowel syndrome. *JAMA* 292 852-58 2004
31. McFarland LV and Dublin S. Meta-analysis of probiotics for the treatment of irritable bowel syndrome. *World J Gastroenterol* 14 2650-61 2008
32. Jimenez MB. Treatment of irritable bowel syndrome with probiotics. An etiopathogenic approach at last? *Rev Esp Enferm Dig* 101 553-64 2009
33. IBID
34. Pimentel M et al. Eradication of small intestinal bacterial overgrowth reduces symptoms of irritable bowel syndrome. *Am J Gastroenterol* 95 3503-06 2000
35. Jimenez MB. Treatment of irritable bowel syndrome with probiotics. An etiopathogenic approach at last? *Rev Esp Enferm Dig* 101 553-64 2009
36. IBID
37. McFarland LV and Dublin S. Meta-analysis of probiotics for the treatment of irritable bowel syndrome. *World J Gastroenterol* 14 2650-61 2008
38. Lin H. Small intestinal bacterial overgrowth: a framework for understanding irritable bowel syndrome. *JAMA* 292 852-58 2004
39. IBID

40. IBID
41. Jimenez MB. Treatment of irritable bowel syndrome with probiotics. An etiopathogenic approach at last? *Rev Esp Enferm Dig* 101 553-64 2009
42. McFarland LV and Dublin S. Meta-analysis of probiotics for the treatment of irritable bowel syndrome. *World J Gastroenterol* 14 2650-61 2008
43. Saggioro A. Probiotics in the treatment of irritable bowek syndrome. *J Clin Gastroenterol* 38 S104-6 2004
44. Amenta M et al. Diet and chronic constipation. Benefits of oral supplementation with symbiotic zir fos (bifidobacterium longum W11 + FOS Actilight) *Acta Biomed* 77 157-62 2006
45. Bu LN et al. Lactobacillus casei rhamnosus Lcr35 in children with chronic constipation. *Pediatr Int* 49 485-90 2007
46. Gawronska A et al. A randomized double-blind placebo-controlled trial of lactobacillus GG for abdominal pain and disorder in children. *Aliment Pharmacol Ther* 25 177-84 2007
47. Zocco MA et al. Efficacy of lactobacillus GG in maintaining remission of ulcerative colitis. *Aliment Pharmacol Ther* 23 1567-74 2006
48. Fujimori S et al. High dose probiotic and prebiotic cotherapy for remission induction of active Crohn's disease. *J Gastroenterol Hepatol* 22 1199-204 2007
49. Miele E et al. Effect of a probiotic preparation (VSL#3) on induction and maintenance of remission of children with ulcerative colitis. *Am J Gastroenterol* 104 437-43 2009
50. Packey CD and Sartor RB. Commensal bacteria, traditional and opportunistic pathogens, dysbiosis and bacterial killing in inflammatory bowel disease. *Curr Opin Infect Dis* 22 292-301 2009
51. Ott SJ et al. Reduction in diversity of the colonic mucosa associated bacterial microflora in patients with active inflammatory bowel disease. *Gut* 53 685-93 2004
52. Packey CD and Sartor RB. Commensal bacteria, traditional and opportunistic pathogens, dysbiosis and bacterial killing in inflammatory bowel disease. *Curr Opin Infect Dis* 22 292-301 2009
53. Isolauri E et al. Probiotics: a role in the treatment of intestinal infection and inflammation? *Gut* 50 Siii54-iii59 2002
54. Sartor RB. Microbial influences in inflammatory bowel diseases. *Gastroenterology* 134 577-94 2008
55. Frank DN et al. Molecular-phylogenetic characterization of microbial community imbalances in human inflammatory bowel diseases. The National Academy of Sciences of the USA supporting evidence at http://www.pnas.org/content/suppl/2007/08/06/0706625104.DC1.
56. Packey CD and Sartor RB. Commensal bacteria, traditional and opportunistic pathogens, dysbiosis and bacterial killing in inflammatory bowel disease. *Curr Opin Infect Dis* 22 292-301 2009
57. Ott SJ et al Reduction in diversity of the colonic mucosa associated bacterial microflora in patients with active inflammatory bowel disease. Gut 53 685-93 2004
58. Frank DN et al. Molecular-phylogenetic characterization of microbial community imbalances in human inflammatory bowel diseases. The National Academy of Sciences of the USA supporting evidence at http://www.pnas.org/content/suppl/2007/08/06/0706625104.DC1.
59. Packey CD and Sartor RB. Commensal bacteria, traditional and opportunistic pathogens, dysbiosis and bacterial killing in inflammatory bowel disease. *Curr Opin Infect Dis* 22 292-301 2009
60. Baumgart M et al. Culture independent analysis of ileal mucosa reveals a selective increase in invasive Escherichia coli of novel phylogeny relative to depletion of Clostridiales in Crohn's disease involving the ileum. *ISME J* 1 403-18 2007

Chapter 15 - Fish Oil

1. Vrablik M et al. Omega-3 fatty acids and cardiovascular disease risk: do we understand the relationship? *Physiol Res* S19-26 2009
2. Manger MS et al. Dietary intake of n-3 long-chain polyunsaturated fatty acids and coronary events in Norwegian patients with coronary artery disease. *Am J Clin Nutr* (May 19, 2010) doi: 10.3945/ajcn.2010.29175
3. Albert Cm et al. Fish consumption and risk of sudden cardiac death. *JAMA* 279 23-28 1998
4. Albert Cm et al. Blood levels of long chain n-3 fatty acids and the risk of sudden death. *N Engl J Med* 346 1113-18 2002
5. Burr ML et al. Effects of changes in fat, fish, and fibre intakes on death and myocardial reinfarction: diet and reinfarction trial (DART). *Lancet* 2 757-61 1989
6. Vrablik M et al. Omega-3 fatty acids and cardiovascular disease risk: do we understand the relationship? *Physiol Res* S19-26 2009
7. Yokoyama M et al. Effects of eicosapentaenoic acid on major coronary events in hypercholesterolaemic patients (JELIS): a randomized open-label, blinded endpoint analysis. *Lancet* 369 1090-98 2007
8. Saito Y et al. Effects of EPA on coronary artery disease in hypercholesterolemic patients with multiple risk factors: subanalysis of primary prevention cases from the Japan EPA lipid intervention study (JELIS). *Atherosclerosis* 200 135-40 2008
9. Hotline Editorial. The results of the GISSI-Prevenzione trial in the general framework of secondary prevention. *European Heart Journal* 21 949-52 2000
10. Siscovick DS et al. Dietary intake and cell membrane levels of long-chain n-3 polyunsaturated fatty acids and the risk of primary cardiac arrest. *JAMA* 274 1363-67 1995
11. Hotline Editorial. The results of the GISSI-Prevenzione trial in the general framework of secondary prevention. *European Heart Journal* 21 949-52 2000
12. Vrablik M et al. Omega-3 fatty acids and cardiovascular disease risk: do we understand the relationship? *Physiol Res* S19-26 2009
13. Murray M and Pizzorno J. *Encyclopedia of Natural Medicine.* revised second edition p771
14. Murray M and Pizzorno J. *Encyclopedia of Natural Medicine.* revised second edition p775-76
15. Murray M and Pizzorno J. *Encyclopedia of Natural Medicine.* revised second edition p775
16. IBID
17. Murray M and Pizzorno J. *Encyclopedia of Natural Medicine.* revised second edition p779-80
18. Navarro E et al. Abnormal fatty acid pattern in rheumatoid arthritis. A rationale for treatment with marine and botanical lipids. *J of Rheumatology* 27 298-303 2000
19. Cleland LG et al. Clinical and biochemical effects of dietary fish oil supplements in rheumatoid arthritis. *J Rheumatol* 15 1471-5 1988
20. Fortin P et al. Validation of meta-analysis: the effects of fish oil in rheumatoid arthritis. *J of Clinical Epidemiology* 48 1379-90 1995
21. Van der Tempel H et al. Effects of fish oil supplementation in rheumatoid arthritis. *Annals of the Rheumatic Diseases* 49 76-80 1990
22. Cleland LG et al. Reduction of cardiovascular risk factors with long-term fish oil treatment in early rheumatoid arthritis. *J of Rheumatology* 33 1973-79 2006
23. Murray M and Pizzorno J. *Encyclopedia of Natural Medicine.* revised second edition p 776-77
24. Murray M and Pizzorno J. *Encyclopedia of Natural Medicine.* revised second edition p 777
25. Murray M and Pizzorno J. *Encyclopedia of Natural Medicine.* revised second edition p 771
26. Saldeen T. All About Omega-3 The Vitamin from the Ocean p68 2006

27. Al MDM et al. Maternal essential fatty acid patterns during normal pregnancy and their relationships with the neonatal essential fatty acid status. *Br J Nutr* 74 55-68 1995

28. Al MDM et al. Long-chain polyunsaturated fatty acids, pregnancy, and pregnancy outcome. *Am J Clin Nutr* 71 285s-91s 2000

29. Challis JR et al. Prostaglandins and mechanisms of preterm birth. *Reproduction* 124 1-17 2002

30. Wathes D et al. Polyunsaturated fatty acids in male and female reproduction. *Biol Reprod* 77 190-201 2007

31. Reece MS et al. Maternal and perinatal long-chain fatty acids: possible roles in preterm birth. *Am J Obstet Gynecol* 176 907-14 1997

32. Olsen SF et al. Gestational age in relation to marine n-3 fatty acids in maternal erythrocytes: a study of women in the Faroe Islands and Denmark. *Am J Obstet Gynecol* 164 1203-9 1991

33. Olsen SF et al. Randomized controlled trial of effect of fish-oil supplementation on pregnancy duration. *Lancet* 339 1003-7 1992

34. Olsen SF et al. Randomized clinical trials of fish oil supplementation in high risk pregnancies. Fish oil trials in pregnancy (FOTIP) team. *BJOG* 107 382-95 2000

35. Smuts CM et al. A randomized trial of docosahexaenoic acid supplementation during the third trimester of pregnancy. *Obstet Gynecol* 101 469-79 2003

36. Olsen SF and Secher NJ. Low consumption of seafood in early pregnancy as a risk factor for preterm delivery: prospective cohort study. *BMJ* 324 447-50 2002

37. Makrides M and Gibson R. Long-chain polyunsaturated fatty acid requirements during pregnancy and lactation. *Am J Clin Nutr* 71 307s-11s 2000

38. Uauy R et al. Role of essential fatty acids in the function of the developing nervous system. *Lipids* 31 s167-s176 1996

39. Uauy R et al. Role of essential fatty acids in the function of the developing nervous system. *Lipids* 31 s167-s176 1996

40. Makrides M and Gibson R. Long-chain polyunsaturated fatty acid requirements during pregnancy and lactation. *Am J Clin Nutr* 71 307s-11s 2000

41. Uauy R et al. Role of essential fatty acids in the function of the developing nervous system. *Lipids* 31 s167-s176 1996

42. Uauy R et al. Role of essential fatty acids in the function of the developing nervous system. *Lipids* 31 s167-s176 1996

43. Uauy R et al. Role of essential fatty acids in the function of the developing nervous system. *Lipids* 31 s167-s176 1996

44. Helland I et al. Maternal supplementation with very-long-chain n-3 fatty acids during pregnancy and lactation augments children's IQ at four years of age. *Pediatrics* 111 e39-e44 2003

45. Helland I et al. Effect of supplementing pregnant and lactating mothers with n-3 very-long-chain fatty acids on children's IQ and body mass index at 7 years of age. *Pediatrics* 122 e472-9 2008

46. Al MDM et al. Long-chain polyunsaturated fatty acids, pregnancy, and pregnancy outcome. *Am J Clin Nutr* 71 285s-91s 2000

47. Murray M and Pizzorno J. *Encyclopedia of Natural Medicine.* revised second edition p 388

48. Lin PY and Kuan-Pin S. A meta-analytic review of double-blind, placebo-controlled trials of antidepressant efficacy of omega-3 fatty acids. *J Clin Psychiatry* 68 1056-61 2007

49. Freeman MP et al. Randomized dose-ranging pilot trial of omega-3 fatty acids for postpartum depression. *Acta Psychiatr Scand* 113 31-5 2006

50. Murray M and Pizzorno J. *Encyclopedia of Natural Medicine.* revised second edition p 412

51. Saldeen T. All About Omega-3 The Vitamin from the Ocean p45 2006

52. De Caterina R et al. n-3 fatty acids in the treatment of diabetic patients. *Diabetes Care* 30 1012-26 2007

53. Delarue J et. al Effects of fish oil on metabolic responses to oral fructose and glucose loads in healthy humans. *Am J Physiol* 270 E353-62 1996

54. Borkman M et al. Effects of fish oil supplementation on glucose and lipid metabolism in NIDDM. *Diabetes* 38 1314-19 1989

55. Axelrod L et al. Effects of a small quantity of omega-3 fatty acids on cardiovascular risk factors in NIDDM. *Diabetes Care* 17 37-45 1994

56. Glauber H et al. Adverse metabolic effect of omega-3 fatty acids in non-insulin-dependent diabetes mellitus. *Annals of Internal Medicine* 108 663-668 1988

57. Vessby B et al. Polyunsaturated fatty acids may impair blood glucose control in type 2 diabetic patients. *Diabetic Medicine* 9 126-33 1992

58. Popp-Snijders C et al. Dietary supplementation of omega-3 polyunsaturated fatty acids improves insulin sensitivity in non-insulin-dependent diabetics. *Diabetes Research* 4 141-147 1987

59. De Caterina R et al n-3 fatty acids in the treatment of diabetic patients. Diabetes Care 30 1012-26 2007

60. Carpentier Y et al. n-3 fatty acids and the metabolic syndrome. *Am J Clin Nutr* 83 1499S-504S 2006

61. Galgani J et al. Effect of the dietary fat quality on insulin sensitivity. *British Journal of Nutr* 100 471-79 2008

62. Grundt H et al. Increased lipid peroxidation during long-term intervention with high doses of n-3 fatty acids (PUFAs) following an acute myocardial infarction. *Eur J Clin Nutr* 57 793-800 2003

63. Gonzalez M et al. Lipid peroxidation products are elevated in fish oil diets even in the presence of added antioxidants. *J Nutr* 122 2190-95 1992

64. Kinsella JE. Dietary n-3 polyunsaturated fatty acids of fish oils, autooxidation ex vivo and peroxidation in vivo implications. *Nutritional and toxicological consequences of food processing.* Edited by M Friedman, Plenum Press, New York 1991

65. IBID

66. Altomare E et al. Increased lipid peroxidation in type 2 poorly controlled diabetic patients. *Diabete Metab* 18 264-71 1992

67. Luostarinen R et al. Vitamin E supplementation counteracts the fish oil-induced increase of blood glucose in humans. *Nutr Res* 15 953-68 1995